Where Women Have No Doctor:
A health guide for women

A. August Burns

Ronnie Lovich

Jane Maxwell

Katharine Shapiro

Editor: Sandy Niemann
Assistant editor: Elena Metcalf

The Hesperian Foundation
Berkeley, California, USA

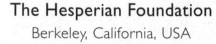

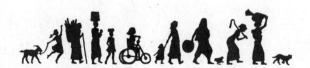

The Hesperian Foundation and the contributors to *Where Women Have No Doctor* do not assume liability for the use of information contained in this book. This book should not replace properly supervised, hands-on training. If you are not sure what to do in an emergency situation, you should try to get advice and help from people with more experience or from local medical and health authorities.

This health guide can be improved with your help. We would like to hear about your experiences, traditions and practices. If you are a midwife, traditional birth attendant, village health worker, doctor, nurse, mother, or anyone with suggestions for ways to make this book better meet the needs of your community, please write to us. Thank you for your help.

Copyright © 1997 by The Hesperian Foundation. All rights reserved.

The Hesperian Foundation encourages others to copy, reproduce or adapt to meet local needs any or all parts of this book, including the illustrations, provided that the parts reproduced are distributed free or at cost—not for profit.

Any organization or person who wishes to copy, reproduce or adapt any or all parts of this book for commercial purposes must obtain permission from the Hesperian Foundation.

Before beginning any translation or adaptation of this book or its contents, please contact the Hesperian Foundation for suggestions about adapting the information in the book, updates on the information provided, and to avoid the duplication of efforts. Please send the Hesperian Foundation a copy of any materials in which text or illustrations from this book have been used.

First edition: June 1997.
Printed in the USA by George Lithograph.
ISBN: 0-942364-25-2 paper

Library of Congress Cataloging-in-Publication Data

Where women have no doctor : a health guide for women / by A. August
        Burns ... [et al.] ; edited by Sandy Niemann, assistant editor, Elena
        Metcalf.
                        p.   cm.
                Includes bibliographical references and index.
                ISBN 0-942364-25-2 (pbk. : alk. paper)
                1. Women--Health and hygiene. 2. Women's health services.
        3. Community health aides. 4. Medicine, Popular.   I. Burns, A.
        August (Arlene August), 1952-   . II. Niemann, Sandy.
        RA564.85.W46   1997   97-19421
        613'.04244--dc21   CIP

The Hesperian Foundation
PO Box 11577
Berkeley, California 94712-2577 USA

Credits:

Project coordinator: Jane Maxwell

Art coordination:
Deborah Wolf and August Burns

Design and production:
Elena Metcalf and Jane Maxwell

Book format: Laughing Bear Associates, Montpelier, Vermont

Cover design: Sara Boore

Cover scans and layout:
Paul Marcus and Shareen Harris

Field testing coordination:
Katharine Shapiro, Deborah Wolf, August Burns, and Elsa Aegerter

Additional writing:
Susan McCallister, Elena Metcalf, Sandy Niemann and Sarah Shannon

Medical editor: Melissa Smith

Additional research: Ronnie Lovich

Additional medicines research:
Todd Jailer and Brian Linde

Copy editor: John Kadyk

Proof readers: Marc Polonsky, Lorraine Mann, and Rose Hauer

Index: Ty Koontz

Production manager:
Susan McCallister

Illustrations

The artists deserve special mention. The skill and sensitivity with which they have so gracefully illustrated this book gives it a quality that we hope will allow women all over the world to feel connected with each other. The artists are:

Namrata Bali (India)
Silvia Barandier (Brazil)
Jennifer Barrios (USA)
Sara Boore (USA)
Mariah Boyd-Boffa (USA)
Heidi Broner (USA)
May Florence Cadiente (Philippines)
Barbara Carter (USA)
Yuni Cho (Korea)
Elizabeth Cox (Papua New Guinea)
Christine Eber (USA)
Regina Faul-Doyle (USA)
Victoria Francis (Switzerland)
Sandy Frank (USA)
Lianne Friesen (Canada)
Jane Wambui Gikera (Kenya)
Susie Gunn (Guatemala)
May Haddad (Lebanon)
Anna Kallis (Cyprus)
Ceylan Karasapan-Crow (USA)
Delphine Kenze (Central African Republic)
Susan Klein (USA)
Joyce Knezevich (USA)
Gina Lee (USA)
Bekah Mandell (USA)
June Mehra (UK)

Naoko Miyamoto (Japan)
Gabriela Núñez (Peru)
Sarah Odingo (Kenya)
Rose Okong'o Olendi (Kenya)
Rosa Oviedo (Nicaragua)
Kate Peatman (USA)
Sara Reilly-Baldeschwieler (UK)
Petra Röhr-Rouendaal (Germany)
Leilani Roosman (UK)
Lucy Sargeant (USA)
Felicity Savage King (UK)
Carolyn Shapiro (USA)
Akiko Aoyagi Shurtleff (Japan)
Pat Siddiq (Afghanistan)
Nisa Smiley (USA)
Fatima Jubran Stengel (Palestine)
Suma (India)
Dovile Tomkute-Veleckiene (Lithuania)
Andrea Triguba (USA)
Anila Vadgama (India)
Lihua Wang (China)
Liliana Wilson (USA)
Fawzi Yaqub (Turkey)

Cover Photographs:

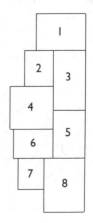

1. *Mauritania* by Lauren Goodsmith

2. *India* by Renée Burgard

3. *China* by Guo Hui Fen

4. *Uzbekistan* by Gilberte Vansintejan

5. *Papua New Guinea* by Elizabeth Cox

6. *Morocco* by Lauren Goodsmith

7. *Democratic Republic of Congo* by Gilberte Vansintejan

8. *Mexico* by Suzanne C. Levine

Thanks:

It is impossible to adequately thank all the people who made *Where Women Have No Doctor* a reality. This book started as a good idea shared by a small group of women and ended up as a remarkable international collaboration spanning 5 continents. Now we find ourselves wanting to thank everyone who helped, but simply listing their names does not do justice to the tremendous and generous contributions so many have made: from the groups of women who met early on to discuss topics related to women's health care, and who later reviewed chapters we wrote based on what they told us; to others who sent us original materials or reviewed (often several times) different sections of the book; to others who wrote drafts of chapters; to the specialists in women's health care who reviewed parts of or the entire manuscript; and to the artists—women from 23 countries—whose illustrations reflect just how diverse a project this was. We thank you all, for through your combined efforts, this book now rightfully belongs to any woman who reads or uses it.

Wholehearted thanks to the following friends of Hesperian for their work on writing specific chapters, or for contributing the time or ideas that helped complete them:

Abortion: Judith Winkler of IPAS, and Judith Tyson

Breastfeeding: Felicity Savage King, Helen Armstrong, Judy Canahuati, and Nikki Lee

Female Circumcision: Jane Kiragu, Leah Muuya, Joyce Ikiara, the women of Mandaeleo Ya Wanawake, Nahid Toubia and Zeinab Eyega of Rainbo, Grace Ebun Delano, Abdel Hadi El-Tahir, Inman Abubakr Osman, and Dehab Belay

Mental Health: Carlos Beristain

Pregnancy: Suellen Miller

Rape and **Violence:** Elizabeth Shrader Cox

Sex Workers: Eka Esu-Williams

Women with Disabilities: Judith Rogers, Pramila Balasundaram, and Msindo Mwinyipembe

In addition, we are deeply indebted to Sara Boore, Heidi Broner, Regina Faul-Doyle, Susan Fawcus, Blanca Figueroa, Sadja Greenwood, May Haddad, Richard Laing, Lonny Shavelson, Richard Steen, and Deborah Wachtel, for their constant availability and selfless efforts in ways too diverse and numerous to mention. It's hard to imagine what we would have done without them.

Thanks also to the following groups of women in different countries who contributed so much of their time, hearts and minds to review these materials and enrich the book: in Bangladesh: The Asia Foundation; in Botswana: Thuso Rehabilitation Centre, Maun; in Brazil: the Association of Community Health Workers of Canal do Anil, and the health educators of Itaguai; in Cyprus, Egypt, Jordan, Lebanon, Palestine, Syria and Yemen: the many groups of women who are members of the Arab Resource Collective; in El Salvador: the women of Morazán and Chalatenango; in Ethiopia: the groups of women who met in Addis Ababa; in Ghana: The Association of Disabled Women, Dorma Ahenkro, the school girls of Wa, and the women of Korle Bu; in Honduras: the women of Urraco Pueblo; in India: CHETNA, SEWA, Streehitikarini, the women of Bilaspur, Madhya Pradech, and the exiled women of Tibet; in Kenya: Mandaeleo Ya Wanawake—from the districts of Machakos, Kitui, Kerugoya and Murang'a—the Dagoretti Clinic Community Health Workers, the Mwakimai Self Help Group of Kisi, Crescent Medical Aid, the women of Population and Health Services (PHS) of Nairobi, and the women of VOWRI, Nairobi; in Mexico: the women of Ajoya, and the community health promotors of Oaxaca; in Nigeria: the Nigeria Youth AIDS Programme; in Papua New Guinea: the East Sepik Women and Children's Health Project; in the Philippines: GABRIELA, HASIK, LIKKHAN, REACHOUT, and the People's Organizations for Social Transformation; in Sierra Leone: the women of Matatie Village; in the Solomon Islands: the women of Gizo; in Uganda: the Kyakabadiima Women's Group, and WARAIDS; and in Zimbabwe: the Women's Action Group.

And heartfelt gratitude to the countless others who gave so freely of their time and talents, especially:

Hilary Abell	Kathy Attawell	Amie Bishop	Sandra Tebben	Karen Cooke
Jane Adair	Elizabeth de Avila	Edith Mukisa	Buffington	Kristin Cooney
Niki Adams	Enoch Kafi Awity	Bitwayiki	Elizabeth Bukusi	Chris Costa
Christine Adebajo	Marie Christine N.	Michael Blake	Elliot Burg	Elizabeth Cox
Vida Affum	Bantug	Paulina Abrefa	May Florence Cadiente	Clark Craig
Stella Yaa Agyeiwaa	David Barabe	Boateng	Indu Capoor	Betty Crase
Baldreldeen Ahmed	Naomi Baumslag	Simone Bodemo	Ward Cates	Mitchell Creinin
Felicia Aldrich	Barbara Bayardo	Nancy Bolan	Mary Catlin	Bonnie Cummings
Bhim Kumari Ale	Carola Beck	Peter Boland	Denise Caudill	George Curlin
Jennifer Alfaro	Rayhana Begum	Bill Bower	Barbara Chang	Philip Darney
Thomas Allen	Medea Benjamin	Christine Bradley	Amal Charles	Sarah Davis
Nancy Aunapu	Marge Berer	Paula Brentlinger	Andrew Chetley	John Day
Adrianne Aron	Denise Bergez	Verna Brooks	Casmir Chipere	Grace Ebun Delano
Fred Arradondo	Stephen Bezruchka	Mary Ann Buckley	Lynne Coen	David de Leeuw
Rosita Arvigo	Pushpa Bhatt	Sharon Burnstien	Louise Cohen	Junice L. Demeterio-
Leonida Atieno	Deborah Bickel	Mary Ann Burris	Mark Connolly	Melgar

Lorraine Dennerstein
Kathy DeReimer
Maggie Diaz
Gerri Dickson
Becky Dolhinow
Efua Dorkenoo
Brendon Doyle
Sunun Duangchan
Deborah Eade
Beth Easton
Christine Eber
Tammy Edet
Abdel Hadi El-Tahir
Erika Elvander
Li Enlin
John Ensign
Nike Esiet
Steven A. Esrey
Clive Evian
Zeinib Eyega
Melissa Farley
Betty Farrell
Anibal Faundes
Sharon Fonn
Claudia Ford
Diane Jinto Forte
Daphne Fresle
Anita Gaind
Loren Galvão
Monica Gandhi
Sabry Khaill Ghobrial
Gayle Gibbons
Marta Ginebreda
Lynn Gordon
Nora Groce
Gretchen Gross
Dora Gutierrez
Ane Haaland
Kathleen Haley
Shirley Hamber
Janie Hampton
Joanne Handfield
Barbara Harrington
Richard Harvey

Fauzia Muthoni Hassan
Elizabeth Hayes
Lori Heise
N.S. Hema
Shobha Menon-Hiatt
Hans Hogerzeil
Jane Holdsworth
Nap Hosang
Douglas Huber
Ellen Israel
Genevieve Jackson
Jodi Jacobson
Carol Jenkins
Signy Judd
Margaret Kaita
Mustapha Kamara
Tom Kelly
Mary Kenny
Joyce Kiragu
Susan Klein
Ahoua Koné
Zoe Kopp
Anna Kretsinger
Diana Kuderna
Anuradha Kumar
Dyanne Ladine
Martín Lamarque
Joellen Lambiotte
Kathleen Lankasky
Lin Lap-Chew
Hannah Larbie
BA Laris
Laura Laski
Carolyn Lee
Jessica Lee
Pam Tau Lee
Susan Lee
Felicia Lester
Abby Levine
Cindy Lewis
Sun Li
Peter Linde
Betsy Liotus
Stephanie Lotane

Susan Lovich
Nellie Luchemo
NP Luo
Esther Galima Mabry
Martha Macintyre
Margaret Mackenzie
Rebecca Magalhães
Monica Maher
Fardos Mohamed Mahmoud
Lisa Maldonado
J. Regi Manimagala
Karin Manzone
Alan Margolis
Kathy Martinez
Rani Marx
Sitra Maunaguru
Danielle Mazza
Pat Mbetu
Dorothy Mbori-Ngacha
Gary Mcdonald
Sandy McGunegill
Katherine McLaughlin
Molly Melching
Tewabetch Mengistu
Tasibete Meone
Sharon Metcalf
Ann Miley
Jan Miller
Kathy Miller
Donald Minkler
Eric Mintz
Barbara Mintzes
Linda Mirabele
Nanette Miranda
David Modersbach
Rahmat Mohammad
Gail Montano
Maristela G. Monteiro
Mona Moore
David Morley
Sam Muziki
Arthur Naiman
Nancy Newton

Elizabeth Ngugi
Eunice Njovana
Folashade B. Okeshola
Peaches O'Reilly
Emma Ottolenghi
Mary Ellen Padorski
Lauri Paolinetti
Jung Eun Park
Sarah Parsons
Laddawan Passar
Palavi Patel
Jamel Patterson
Andrew Pearson
María Picos
Gita Pillai
Linda J. Poole
Malcolm Potts
Alice Purdy
Robert Quick
Zahida Qureshi
Lisa Raffel
Rita Raj-Hashim
Narmada Ranaweera
Rebecca Ratcliff
Augusta Rengill
Dawn Roberts
Kama Rogo
Nancy Russel
Carolyn Ryan
Mira Sadgopal
Valdete Sala
Estelle Schneider
Kimberly Schultz
Violet Senna
Shalini Shah
Nicolas Sheon
Mira Shiva
Kathy Simpson
Mohindra Singh
Elise Smith
Cathy Solter
Barbara de Souza
Judith Standly
Fatima Jubran Stengel

Kay Stone
Marianne Stone-Jimenez
Eleanor Sullivan
Susan Sykes
Michael Tan
Linda Teitjen
Judith Timyan
Susan Toft
Rikka Transgrud
Nhumey Tropp
Barbara Trott
Sandy Truex
Ilana Trumbull
Janis Tunder
Nanette Tver
Aruna Uprety
Gilberte Vansintejan
Sarah Verbiest
Carol Vlassoff
Bea Vuylsteke
Bela Wabi
Martha Wambui
Judith Wasserheit
Ruth Waswa
Barbara Waxman
Jane Weaver
Vivienne Wee
Ellen Weis
Rachel West
Eve Whang
Kate White
Wil Whittington
Laura Wick
Pawana Wienrawee
Christine van Wijk
Everjoyce Win
Kathryn Wirogura
Erin Harr Yee
Irene Yen
Rokeya Zaman
Marcie Zellner
Kaining Zhang
Lisa Ziebel
Margot Zimmerman

The following persons and groups kindly gave us permission to use their artwork: Family Care International for numerous drawings by Regina Faul-Doyle from their book *Healthy Women, Healthy Mothers: An Information Guide*; Macmillan Press Ltd., for Janie Hampton's drawing on page 60 from *Healthy Living, Healthy Loving*; the Environmental and Development Agency, New Town, South Africa for the drawing on page 395 from their magazine, *New Ground*; Honto Press for Akiko Aoyagi Shurtleff's drawing on page 411 from *Culinary Treasures of Japan*; the Movimento de Mulheres Trabalhadoras Rurais do Nordeste for the drawing on page 17 from *O Que É Gênero?*; and the Colectivo de Mujeres de Matagalpa and the Centro de Mujeres de Masaya for the drawing on page 338 from their manual *¡Más allá de las lágrimas!*.

We also thank the following foundations and individuals for their generosity in financially supporting the project: Catalyst Foundation; Conservation, Food and Health Foundation; C.S. Fund; Domatila Barrios de Chungara Fund; Ford Foundation; Greenville Foundation; John D. and Catherine T. MacArthur Foundation; Norwegian Agency for Development Cooperation; David and Lucile Packard Foundation; San Carlos Foundation; Swedish International Development Cooperation Agency; Kathryn and Robert Schauer; and Margaret Schink. Thanks also to the many individuals who made contributions to match a Catalyst Foundation grant. Finally, a special thanks to Luella and Keith McFarland for their early support and encouragement, and to Davida Coady for believing in this project and pushing it forward during a difficult time.

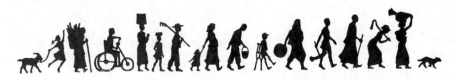

About this Book:

This book was written to help women care for their own health, and to help community health workers or others meet women's health needs. We have tried to include information that will be useful for those with no formal training in health care skills, and for those who do have some training.

Although this book covers a wide range of women's health problems, it does not cover many problems that commonly affect both women and men, such as malaria, parasites, intestinal problems, and other diseases. For information on these kinds of problems, see *Where There Is No Doctor* or another general medical book.

Sometimes the information in this book will not be enough to enable you to solve a health problem. When this happens, get more help. Depending on the problem, we may suggest that you:

- *see a health worker*. This means that a trained health worker should be able to help you solve the problem.
- *get medical help*. This means you need to go to a clinic that has trained medical people or a doctor, or a laboratory where basic tests are done.
- *go to a hospital*. This means you need to see a doctor at a hospital that is equipped for emergencies, for surgery, or for special tests.

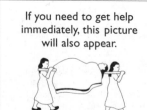

If you need to get help immediately, this picture will also appear.

TRANSPORT!

How to Use this Book:

Finding information in the book

To find a topic you want to know about, you can use either the list of Contents or the Index.

The **Contents**, at the front of the book, lists the chapters in the order in which they appear. There is also a list of contents at the beginning of every chapter. Each topic on this list appears on the numbered page listed as a large heading (words in big, dark letters).

The **Index**, or Yellow Pages at the back of the book, lists all the important topics covered in the book, in the order of the alphabet (a, b, c, d...).

To find information about the medicines used in this book, look in the **Green Pages** toward the back of the book. Page 485 gives more information about using medicines and the Green Pages.

If you do not understand the meanings of some of the words used in this book, you may find them in the **List of Difficult Words** that starts on page 544. The first time these words appear in a chapter, they are *printed in slanted letters, like this*. You can also look up the word in the index to see if it is explained in another part of the book.

Many chapters end with a section called 'Working for Change'. These sections give suggestions for working to improve women's health in your community.

Finding information on a page

To find information on a page, first look over the whole page. You will see that the page is divided into 2 parts: a large, main column and a small column on the outside of the page. The main column gives most of the information about a topic. The small column has additional information that can help you better understand the topic.

Whenever you see a picture of a book in the small column, this means more information about a topic can be found in another part of the book. The words under the book say what the topic is. The page number on the book says where that topic can be found. If there are several topics, the book is shown once and the topics and their page numbers are listed below.

166
foods rich in protein

What the different things on a page mean:

Most pages have several **headings**. The headings in the small column give the general topic that is being discussed on that page. The headings in the main column give more specific topics.

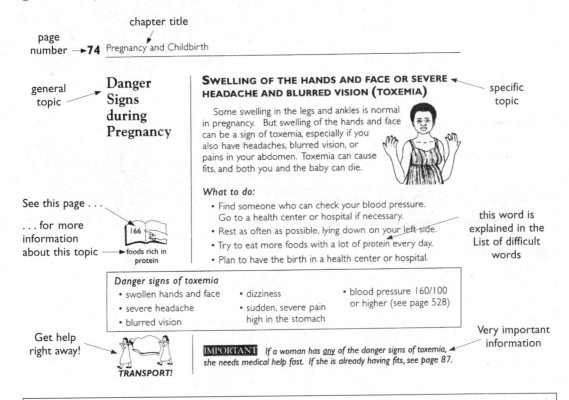

chapter title

page number → **74** Pregnancy and Childbirth

general topic →

Danger Signs during Pregnancy

SWELLING OF THE HANDS AND FACE OR SEVERE HEADACHE AND BLURRED VISION (TOXEMIA) ← specific topic

Some swelling in the legs and ankles is normal in pregnancy. But swelling of the hands and face can be a sign of toxemia, especially if you also have headaches, blurred vision, or pains in your abdomen. Toxemia can cause fits, and both you and the baby can die.

What to do:
• Find someone who can check your blood pressure. Go to a health center or hospital if necessary.
• Rest as often as possible, lying down on your left side.
• Try to eat more foods with a lot of *protein* every day.
• Plan to have the birth in a health center or hospital.

See this page . . .
. . . for more information about this topic →

166
foods rich in protein

this word is explained in the List of difficult words

Danger signs of toxemia
• swollen hands and face
• severe headache
• blurred vision
• dizziness
• sudden, severe pain high in the stomach
• blood pressure 160/100 or higher (see page 528)

Get help right away! →

TRANSPORT!

IMPORTANT *If a woman has any of the danger signs of toxemia, she needs medical help fast. If she is already having fits, see page 87.*

Very important information

Some pages also contain **medicine boxes**, which look like this:

These boxes tell you the amount of medicine to give, how often to give it, and for how long. Sometimes we recommend medicines without putting them in a box. In either case, **look up each medicine in the Green Pages before using it.**

Medicine for Breast Infection		
Medicine	**How much to take**	**When and how to take**
dicloxicillin . . . . 250 mg	. . . .	4 times a day for 10 days. Take at least 30 minutes before eating food.
If you cannot find this or are allergic to penicillin, take:		
erythromycin . . . . 500 mg	. . . .	4 times a day for 10 days.

Important: If a breast infection is not treated early, it will get worse. The hot and painful swelling will feel as if it is filled with liquid (abscess). If this happens, follow the treatment described here, AND see a health worker who has been trained to drain an abscess using sterile equipment.

Contents:

Chapter 1

Women's Health Is a Community Issue

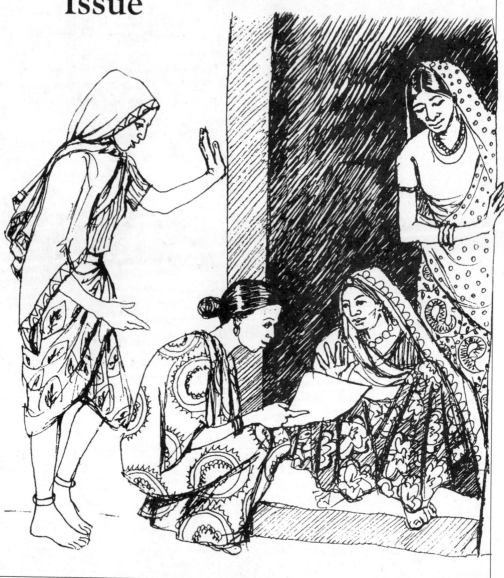

When a woman is healthy, she has the energy and strength to do her daily work, to fulfill the many roles she has in her family and community, and to build satisfying relationships with others. In other words, a woman's health affects every area of her life. Yet for many years, 'women's health care' has meant little more than maternal health services such as care during pregnancy and birth. These services are necessary, but they only address women's needs as mothers. Except for the ability to produce babies, a woman's health needs have been treated as no different from a man's.

➤ *Good health is more than the absence of disease. Good health means the well-being of a woman's body, mind, and spirit.*

In this book we offer a different view of women's health. First, we believe that every woman has a right to complete health care, throughout her life. A woman's health care should help her in all areas of life—not just in her role as a wife and mother. Second, we believe that a woman's health is affected not just by the way her body is made, but by the social, cultural, and economic conditions in which she lives.

While men's health is also affected by these factors, women as a group are treated differently from men. They usually have less power and fewer resources, and lower status in the family and community. This basic inequality means that:

- more women than men suffer from poverty.
- more women than men are denied the education and skills to support themselves.
- more women than men lack *access* to important health information and services.
- more women than men lack control over their basic health care decisions.

This larger view helps us understand the underlying (root) causes of women's poor health. Improving women's health includes treating their health problems, but it also requires changing the conditions of their lives so they can gain more power over their own health.

When this happens, everyone—the woman, her family and community—benefits. A healthy woman has a chance to fulfill all of her potential. Plus, she will have healthier babies, be better able to care for her family, and can contribute more to her community. This kind of view also helps us see that a woman's health problem is almost never her problem alone. Women's health is a community issue.

Women Are More at Risk for Disease and Poor Health

➤ *Not getting enough good food can keep a girl from growing properly, and can lead to serious health problems.*

eating to stay healthy

Because a woman's body is different from a man's, and because of the basic inequalities between men and women, women face a greater risk of disease and poor health. Here are some of the health problems that affect women most:

Poor nutrition

Poor *nutrition* is the most common and disabling health problem among women in poor countries. Starting in childhood, a girl is often given less food to eat than a boy. As a result, she may grow more slowly and her bones may not develop properly (which may later cause difficulty during childbirth). The problem worsens as she becomes a young woman, because her need for good food increases as her workload increases, and as she starts her *monthly bleeding*, becomes pregnant, and breastfeeds.

Without enough good food, she may begin to suffer from general poor health, including *exhaustion*, weakness, and *anemia*. If a woman who is already *malnourished* becomes pregnant, she is more likely to have serious complications with childbirth, such as heavy bleeding, *infection*, or a baby that is born too small.

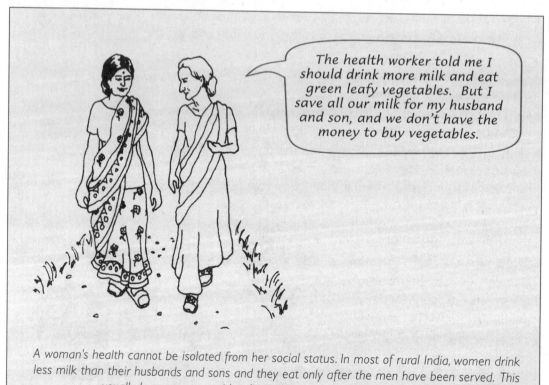

The health worker told me I should drink more milk and eat green leafy vegetables. But I save all our milk for my husband and son, and we don't have the money to buy vegetables.

A woman's health cannot be isolated from her social status. In most of rural India, women drink less milk than their husbands and sons and they eat only after the men have been served. This usually leaves women with a limited diet, and it also tells about how she is valued.
—CHETNA, Ahmedabad, India

Reproductive health problems

Sexually transmitted diseases (STDs), including *HIV/AIDS*. A woman is physically more at risk for getting STDs and AIDS than a man. That is because a man's *semen* stays inside her and the *germs* it carries can pass through the lining of the *vagina* into her blood. And, since a woman often has no signs of infection, she may not get treatment.

But the problem is really a social one. Women often have little control over decisions about sex and often cannot refuse *unsafe sex*. As a result, 165 million women get an STD every year, and 1.65 million became infected with HIV in 1995 alone. Without treatment, STDs can cause disabling pain, severe *pelvic inflammatory disease (PID), infertility,* problems during pregnancy, and an increased risk of cervical *cancer.* HIV/AIDS causes death.

Frequent pregnancies. In many parts of the world, 1/3 to 1/2 of young women become mothers before they are 20 years old. Without *family planning,* many of these women will not have time to get strong again between births. This puts a woman at risk for poor health and complications of pregnancy and childbirth. Frequent childbirth also means she is less able to control her own life, to get an education, and to learn skills to support herself.

Complications from pregnancy and birth. In the last 30 years, the number of infant deaths has been greatly reduced. Yet the number of women who die from pregnancy and birth has not. Every minute, one woman dies from a problem related to pregnancy. Every minute, 30 women develop a lasting health problem related to pregnancy. This means that over time, about a quarter of all women living in poor countries will be seriously affected by *complications* from pregnancy and birth.

Unsafe abortion. When a woman tries to end a pregnancy by having an unsafe *abortion,* she risks her life. But every day about 50,000 women and girls try to end their pregnancies in unsafe ways because they have no way to get a safe abortion. Many are left unable to have children or with lasting pain, infection, and other health problems.

Female circumcision. Female *circumcision,* in which part or all of a girl's outer *genitals* are cut off, can cause serious health problems. These include *pelvic* and *urine* system infections, sexual and emotional problems, and difficulties during childbirth. Yet despite these problems, it continues to be widely practiced. Every year about 2 million girls are circumcised, mostly in Africa, but also in the Middle East and Asia.

261

STDs and other infections of the genitals

➤ *Because women must often have unsafe sex against their will, STDs are a social issue.*

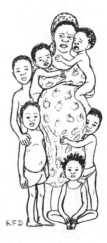

➤ *Every minute, one woman dies from a problem related to pregnancy.*

➤ *Every year 75,000 women die from unsafe abortions.*

➤ *Men and women get many of the same diseases, but women can be affected differently.*

TB, 387
alcohol and other drugs, 435

393
work

➤ *A woman faces health risks from her work inside and outside of the home. Working long hours, the 'double work day', can make her body too tired to fight disease.*

➤ *Problems with mental health can be as serious as other health problems.*

413
mental health

General medical problems

Women are more likely than men to suffer from certain health problems because of the work they do, because of poor nutrition, or from being too tired. A disease can also cause a different kind of harm to a woman than a man. For example, a woman who suffers from a disease which weakens or disfigures her may be rejected by her husband.

Once they are sick, women are less likely to seek and receive treatment until they are seriously ill. For example, *tuberculosis (TB)* is spreading among both men and women, but fewer women than men get treatment. Almost 3000 women die every day from TB—at least 1/3 of whom did not receive proper treatment or never even knew they had the disease. Other health problems that in the past affected mostly men are now risks for women, too. For example, more women are suffering from problems related to smoking cigarettes or drinking too much alcohol.

Work hazards

Women face health risks every day from the work they do. At home, lung diseases from smoke or burns from cooking fires are so common that they are considered the main work-related health problem for women. Diseases spread through water are also common, because of the amount of time women spend washing clothes, hauling water, or standing in water while farming.

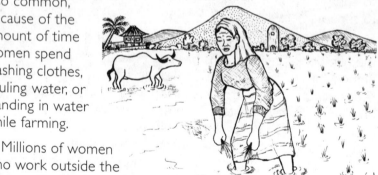

Millions of women who work outside the home suffer health problems due to unsafe conditions in the workplace. And when they come home from their jobs, they usually continue to work at home, so they end up with twice as much work. This leads to exhaustion and an increased risk of illness.

Mental health problems

Women and men have about the same risk of developing a mental health problem. Severe depression, however, affects many more women than men. It often affects women who are poor, who have experienced loss or violence, or whose communities have been destroyed or undergone great change. But women who suffer any kind of mental health problem are much less likely than men to get help.

Violence

Violence is often overlooked as a health problem. But violence can lead to serious injuries, mental health problems, physical *disabilities,* and even death. Many girls are sexually abused by family members or friends. Many women are forced to have sex or are physically abused by their partners. *Rape* and *sexual harassment* are a constant threat to all women. These kinds of violence happen in almost all parts of the world, and under all social conditions.

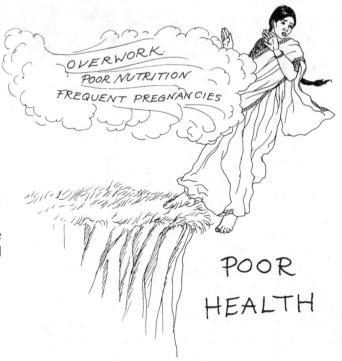

Still, most violence against women is not reported, because the police and others often blame women rather than men for the problem. The men causing the violence are rarely punished.

➤ *Women usually suffer violence from men they know. But most violence is not reported, and the men are not punished.*

violence, 313

rape and sexual assault, 327

How women are forced into a life of poor health

Although not all women suffer from the health problems described above, most will suffer from 3 of them: poor nutrition, pregnancies that are too close together, and overwork. Each of these problems affects a woman's general health and wears her body out, making her more likely to get sick. Pregnancy also makes certain medical problems—like malaria, hepatitis, diabetes, and anemia—worse, just as they make pregnancy more difficult. All these things make a woman much more likely to suffer from general poor health than a man.

OVERWORK
POOR NUTRITION
FREQUENT PREGNANCIES

POOR HEALTH

Causes of Poor Health in Women

It is easy to name the direct causes of most of women's health problems. For example, we can say that STDs are caused by different germs, poor nutrition comes from not eating enough good food, and problems during pregnancy are often caused by a lack of prenatal (before birth) care. But beneath these direct causes are 2 root causes—poverty and the low status of women—that contribute to many of women's health problems.

POVERTY

Two out of three women around the world are poor. Women are not only much more likely than men to be poor, but are most often among the poorest of the poor.

Millions of women are caught in a cycle of poverty that begins even before they are born. Babies born to women who did not get enough to eat during pregnancy are likely to be small at birth and to develop slowly. In poor families, girls are less likely than their brothers to get enough to eat, causing their growth to be further stunted. Girls are often given little or no education, so as women they must work at unskilled jobs and receive less wages than men (even if they do the same kind of work). At home, their daily work is unpaid. Exhaustion, poor nutrition, and lack of good care during pregnancy place the woman and her children at risk for poor health.

Poverty forces her to live under conditions that can cause many physical and mental health problems. For example, poor women often:

- live in bad housing, with little or no sanitation or clean water.

- do not have enough good food, and must spend precious time and energy looking for food they can afford.

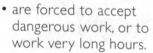

- are forced to accept dangerous work, or to work very long hours.

- cannot use medical care, even if it is free, because they cannot afford time off work or away from their families.

- are so busy struggling to survive that they have little time or energy to take care of their own needs, to plan for a better future, or to learn new skills.

- are blamed for their poverty and made to feel less important than those with more money.

Poverty often forces women into relationships in which they must depend on men for survival. If a woman depends on a man for her—or her children's—support, she may have to do things to keep him happy that are dangerous to her health. For example, she may allow him to be violent or to have unsafe sex because she fears losing his economic support.

LOW STATUS OF WOMEN

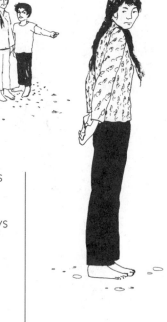

Status is the importance that a person has in the family and community. Status affects how a woman is treated, how she values herself, the kinds of activities she is allowed to do, and the kinds of decisions she is allowed to make. In most communities in the world, women have lower status than men. Women's lower status leads to discrimination—that is, being treated poorly or denied something simply because they are women. Discrimination may take different forms in different communities, but it always affects a woman's health.

Wanting sons rather than daughters. Many families value boys more than girls because boys can contribute more to the family's wealth, support their parents in old age, perform ceremonies after their parents die, and carry on the family name. As a result, girls are often breastfed for a shorter time, are given less food and medical care, and receive little or no education.

Lack of legal rights or power to make decisions. In many communities, a woman cannot own or inherit property, earn money, or get credit. If she gets divorced, she may not be allowed to keep her children or her belongings. Even if a woman has legal rights, her community's traditions may allow her little control over her life. Often a woman cannot decide how the family's money is spent or when to get health care. She cannot travel or participate in community decisions without her husband's permission.

> ➤ *Because so much of the work that women do is not recognized, they often lack legal protection in the workplace.*

When women are denied power in these ways, they must depend on men to survive. As a result, they cannot easily demand things that contribute to good health, like family planning, safer sex, enough food, health care, and freedom from violence.

Having too many children, or having children too close together. Discrimination against women can also lead them to get pregnant more often, because bearing children may be the only way that women can gain status for themselves or their partners.

> ➤ *Women make up half of the world's population, but work 2 out of every 3 hours worked in the world, receive only a tenth of the world's income, and own only a hundredth of the world's property.*

Under all these conditions, women live less healthy lives and get less health care. They also often accept their low status, because they have been raised to value themselves less than men. They may accept poor health as their lot in life and seek help only when health problems are severe or life-threatening.

> ➤ *The medical system does not provide all the services women need.*

The medical system does not meet women's needs

Poverty and discrimination in the family and community not only lead to more health problems for women, they also make the medical system less likely to provide the services women need. Government policies and the global economy may add to this problem.

In poor countries, many people do not have access to health services of any kind. (The box below explains one reason why this problem has become worse in recent years.) And because of discrimination against women, the little money that does exist will probably not be spent on women's health needs. So a woman may not be able to get good care even if she can afford to pay for it. Some reproductive health services may be provided, but to meet all of her health needs, she will probably have to travel to the capital city or perhaps even leave her country.

In many countries, the skills needed to care for women are considered 'special' and are provided only by doctors. Yet many of these services could be provided at lower cost by trained community health workers.

Debt and structural adjustment: keeping the poor poor

During the 1970s, many poor countries were pressured to borrow money from banks in rich countries. Some poor countries used this money to try to improve the lives of their people. Many new schools, hospitals, clinics, and other projects were started.

But as the banks demand that their money be paid back, the poor countries have been forced to change or "adjust" their economies. They are forced to pay these banks much of the wealth the people produce, and to make it easy for foreign companies to make money by using the poor countries' resources and labor.

As a result, poor countries can no longer spend as much money on programs that help the poor—such as schools, health centers, hospitals, and programs that help people get food and fuel at a fair price. Governments now are left with less money to pay doctors, nurses, and other health workers, or to provide medical supplies or equipment. The health of all poor people suffers from these changes, but the health of poor women and children suffers most of all.

Mira's Story

When Mira was a little girl, she dreamed of living in a big house, with electricity and a tile floor. Her husband would be handsome and kind, and she would be able to do whatever she wished. But Mira's family was poor, and she was the youngest of four daughters. Sometimes, when her father was drinking, he would beat her mother, and weep at his misfortune of having so many girls.

When Mira was 14, and old enough to be married, she cried when she learned her dreams would never come true. It was already arranged: Mira would marry a man whom her father had chosen. He had some land, and Mira's father thought the family would benefit from their marriage. Mira had no choice in the matter.

With the birth of Mira's second child—a son—her husband stopped insisting on sex so often. Mira was very glad for that. Although he did not hurt her, he had warts all over his penis that disgusted her. Over the next 20 years, she had 6 more children, including a little girl who died at age 3, and a boy who died at birth.

One day, Mira was using the latrine and she noticed a bloody discharge coming from her vagina when it wasn't time for her monthly bleeding. She had never had a health exam, but now Mira asked her husband if she might see a health worker. He replied that he didn't trust doctors, and besides, he didn't have the money to spend every time she felt worried about something.

Mira was 40 when she began to suffer constant pain low in her belly. The pain worried her, but she didn't know who to talk to about it. Some months later, Mira finally decided she had to go against her husband's wishes and get medical help. She was frightened for her life, and borrowed some money from a friend.

At the health center, Mira got some medicine for the vaginal discharge, although the health worker did not examine her first. Mira returned home that night, exhausted and upset that she had defied her husband and spent her friend's savings. As weeks passed, Mira's health continued to worsen, and she became discouraged, realizing that something was still wrong.

Finally, Mira became so weak that her husband believed she really was ill, and they begged a ride to a hospital in the big city far away. After waiting several days, Mira was seen at the hospital. Finally, she was told that she had advanced cancer of the cervix. The doctor said they could remove her womb, but that the cancer had already spread. The one treatment that might save her life was available only in another part of the country, and was very expensive. The doctor asked, "Why didn't you get regular Pap tests? If we had found this earlier, we could have treated it easily." But it was too late for that. Mira went home, and in less than two months, she died.

WHY DID MIRA DIE?

Here are some common answers to this question:

A doctor may say...

> Mira died of advanced cervical cancer because she did not get treatment earlier.

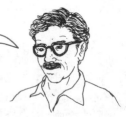

> ➤ There are many reasons why poor women get—and die from—diseases that can be prevented or cured.

Or a teacher...

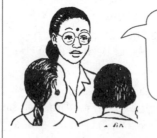

> Mira died because she didn't know she should have a Pap test done.

Or a health worker...

> Mira died because her husband exposed her to genital warts and other STDs. These put her at high risk for developing cancer of the cervix.

> ➤ For more information about cancer of the cervix, see page 377.

All these answers are correct. Women who start having sex at a young age and are exposed to genital warts **are** at a greater risk for cancer of the cervix. And if the cancer is found early (usually by having a *Pap test*), it can almost always be cured.

Yet these answers show a very limited understanding of the problem. Each of them blames one person—either Mira or her husband—and goes no further. Mira was at greater risk of dying of cervical cancer because she was a poor woman, living in a poor country.

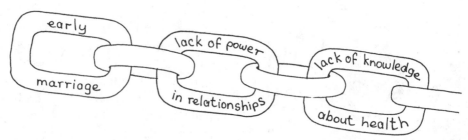

early marriage / lack of power in relationships / lack of knowledge about health

How poverty and the low status of women worked together to cause Mira's death

Mira and her family were poor, so she was forced to marry and start having sex when she was very young. As a woman, she lacked power in her relationship with her husband. She had no control over when and how many children to have, or over her husband's relationships with other women. Her family's poverty meant that she suffered from poor nutrition her whole life, which weakened her body and left her more at risk for disease.

➤ *You can explore the root causes of Mira's death or other health problems by using the excercise called "But Why?" on page 26.*

Although **Mira's community** lacked health services, the nearest health center did have some women's health services, like family planning and information about preventing HIV/AIDS. But the health workers had no information or training about other women's health problems, even such serious ones as cancer of the *cervix*. They did not know how to do a pelvic *exam* (to look at the vagina, cervix and other reproductive parts) or a Pap test. So even if Mira had gone for medical care sooner, the health worker would not have been able to help her.

As a result, Mira had to travel a long distance at great cost to see a doctor who could tell her what was wrong. By that time it was too late.

Finally, **Mira's country** was poor, with little money to spend on health care. Like the governments of many poor countries, her government chose to focus on other important health services, but not on women's health. What money her government did spend on women's health went to expensive hospitals in the big city instead of community health programs that women like Mira can get to. This meant that the services to find and treat cervical cancer—and many other women's health problems—early were not available.

Poverty and the low status of women worked against Mira at all 3 levels—in her family, in her community, and in her country—to create the health problem that caused her death.

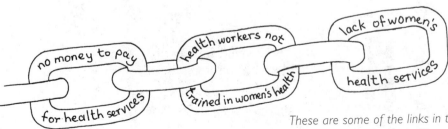

These are some of the links in the chain of causes that led to Mira's death. They are the same links that cause many of women's health problems.

Working for Change

IT DOES NOT HAVE TO BE THIS WAY

The way societies are organized forces most women into lives of poverty and poor health. But societies could be organized in a way that favors health instead of disease.

Since the causes of poor health exist at the family, community, and national levels, changes to improve women's health must happen at each of these different levels.

Working for change in your family

You can improve your health by learning about women's health problems and by making changes in your own life and in your family. Talk with your partner about what you each need to have better health, including practicing safer sex and sharing the workload fairly. You can also work to improve the health and future of your children. Here are some ideas:

➤ For other ideas of how your partner can help, see page 14.

Raising our children for a better world

How we raise our children, from the moment they are born, will determine much of what they believe and how they act as adults.

As mothers, we teach our children every day of their lives:

- When we feed our husbands and sons first, we teach our children that girls' and women's hunger is less important.
- When we send only our sons to school, we teach our children that girls do not deserve the opportunities that come from an education.
- When we teach our sons that it is manly to be violent, we raise violent men.
- When we do not speak out against violence in our neighbor's house, we teach our sons that it is acceptable for a man to beat his wife and children.

As mothers, we have the power to change who our children will become:

- We can teach our sons to be kind and compassionate, so they will grow up to be kind and compassionate husbands, fathers, and brothers.
- We can teach our daughters to value themselves, so they will expect the same from others.

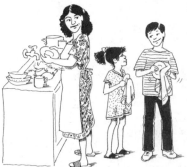

- We can teach our sons to share and take pride in household work, so their sisters, wives and daughters do not suffer the burden of overwork.
- We can teach our daughters to be more independent by finishing school or learning a skill.
- We can teach our sons to respect all women and to be responsible sexual partners.

We can raise our children for a better world.

Working for change in your community

You can improve your health and the health of other women in your community by sharing this book and by talking with them about women's health problems.

Talking with others can be hard. Women often feel shame (for example, when talking about parts of the body) or fear about what others will think. Yet talking with others is the only way to learn more about health problems and to discover their causes. Often you will find that other women are worried about the same things, and want to discuss them.

Get a small group of women together to talk about health problems in your community. Try inviting women who are friends of your friends, neighbors, or women you work with. Once you have identified a health problem that many women share, it is often helpful to meet again and invite others to discuss it and learn more. When you meet, think about the root causes of the health problem, and plan the changes you can make in your families and community. For ways to work with a group to plan and carry out actions for change, see pages 26 to 31.

➤ *Because social conditions affect them differently, women and men may need to find different solutions for the same health problems.*

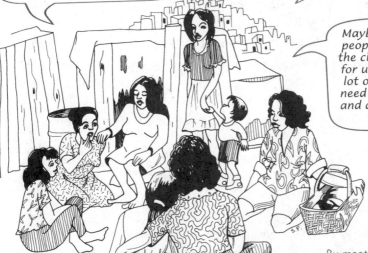

My back hurts so much these days from having to carry water all the way up the hill to my house. The health worker says I shouldn't carry heavy loads when I'm pregnant—that's how Mari lost her pregnancy. But how else would my family get water?

It isn't a problem just for women who are pregnant! My back is always hurting too. I finally got my husband to start helping me carry water every day.

I was visiting my sister the other day, and where she lives they got the city to put in some water taps close to the houses. It's great, she doesn't have to carry water very far at all. All the women love it.

Maybe we could get enough people together to convince the city to do the same thing for us. But we would need a lot of people. And we would need to know who to talk to, and decide where we wanted the water taps.

Well, we could talk with José. He's a teacher and everyone respects him. He could probably help.

By meeting with a small group of women, you can learn more about a health problem and what can be done to solve it.

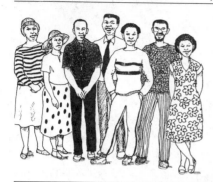

Think about involving men as well as women in discussions about women's health. It may seem difficult to talk about women's health problems with men, because this kind of talk is considered taboo, or 'women's secrets'. But since men are often in positions of power, their help can be very important. Look for men who are supportive of women, are good role models for boys, or who treat women as their equals.

HOW MEN CAN HELP

Any man can help improve women's health by:

- raising his children to respect women, and treating boys and girls as equals.
- asking women what they think, and listening to them. A man can listen to his partner's and daughters' concerns and needs, and see if together they can find a way to meet the needs of everyone in the family.
- talking with his partner about how many children they each want to have, and then taking equal responsibility for family planning.
- encouraging his partner to go for regular health exams, and helping find the money and time for her to go.
- taking turns caring for the children and doing house work.
- being faithful to his partner or, if he cannot, being honest with her and practicing safer sex when he is not with her. If a man ever gets an STD, he should tell all of his sexual partners right away, so everyone can get treatment.
- encouraging his partner to take a fair share of the food that there is to eat— even if nobody is getting very much.
- encouraging all of his children to stay in school as long as they can. The longer they can stay in school, the more choices they will have as adults, and the better their health will be.

A man can also set a good example in his community by:

- encouraging women in his community to come to meetings, and making sure that they have a chance to speak. Or by encouraging women to hold their own, separate meetings, where men will not speak.
- encouraging women to become involved in planning and running community projects.
- encouraging others to limit their use of alcohol and drugs—these contribute nothing to the community and waste money and energy. Try to plan celebrations that do not involve alcohol.
- not tolerating **any** kind of violence against women.
- teaching children how to care for their physical, mental, and sexual health and how to prevent common illnesses.
- working to change the image that a strong man is one who has sex with many women. **A strong man is a strong partner.**

Here are some other activities that can help improve health in a community:

- **Share information**. Find ways to spread information about the common health problems in your community, so that everyone will know about them.

- **Form support groups.** Women who share common problems—such as women who have survived rape or abuse, breastfeeding mothers, women with disabilities, or *sex workers*—can form groups to support each other and work together to overcome their problems.

starting a support group

In Zimbabwe, the Musasa Project was created to help women who suffered from violence, particularly violence in the home and sexual assault. Musasa found that women who were beaten by their partners were not protected by the law. Many people said that men should have power over women because that was the way it had always been. Or because it was part of their community's beliefs. These people also said that regular beatings reminded women of their 'place'.

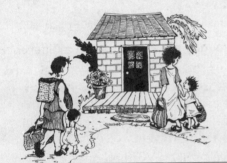

Musasa's goal is to change this attitude through public education and by counseling those who have survived violence. In this way, women, men, teachers, students, police, and health workers are learning that violence is an abuse of power. Musasa plans to set up a house where women and children can stay when they are in danger.

- **Work toward more independence.** Projects that help women earn money and improve their working conditions also help women start to make their own decisions and gain self-esteem.

In a tiny Mayan village in Guatemala, a group of women formed a weaving group. They sold their weavings through a cooperative store for women's crafts in the capital city. The women now earn more income than most of the men in their area. As a result, women have gained new status in their families and communities and have more opportunities in their lives.

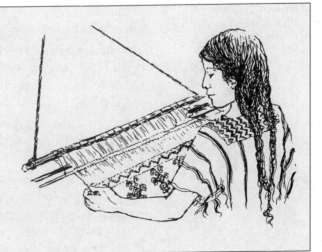

community sanitation

• **Develop community projects**. For example, try to find ways for every family in the community to get enough to eat, or to improve community *sanitation* and access to clean water.

The Green Belt movement in Kenya has involved many women in planting and protecting trees, which prevent soil erosion and provide fuel. The women's success at protecting the environment and providing fuel for their families has built their confidence and helped them earn a living.

As one Green Belt member said, "Our forests were running out because of our constant need for firewood. We meet weekly to collect seeds, to do potting and fencing, and tend the trees in our nursery. We also talk to groups and schools about the environment. In this way, we are both helping ourselves and bettering the environment."

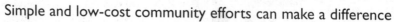

Simple and low-cost community efforts can make a difference

When you first look at a problem, it often seems very hard to make changes. But, in fact, communities can make many improvements that do not cost too much. For example, here are some of the suggestions this book contains for preventing or helping solve women's health problems:

Many women's health problems could be prevented or treated early if more health workers were trained to care for women's health.

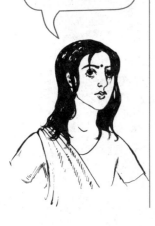

• Start a community stove project. Women often suffer from lung infections, burns, and back problems. Low-cost cook stoves that are safer, use less fuel, and produce less smoke can prevent many of these problems (see page 394).

• Establish an emergency transportation system. Many women die from complications of pregnancy, childbirth, and unsafe abortion. These deaths could often be prevented by reaching medical care quickly (see page 101).

• Low-cost cancer screening can prevent many women from dying from cervical and breast cancer. Cancers are much easier to treat if they are found early (see page 375).

• Make family planning services and good *prenatal* care accessible to all women. Doing so can prevent many deaths due to complications of pregnancy, childbirth and unsafe abortion.

• Train health workers to care for women's health. They should be trained in pelvic exams, Pap tests and visual inspection, manual vacuum aspiration (MVA), breast exams, and *counseling*. They should also learn how to use medicines for women's health.

Working for change in your country

You can improve your health, and the health of many other women in your country, by working together with other groups in different parts of the country. By working together, you can make important changes in the way your government treats women and women's health. For example, community groups can pressure the government to punish men who rape or abuse women, or to make safe abortion available. Or you can get laws passed to allow women to own or inherit property—so that women are not forced to depend on men.

Many women and men are struggling to get their governments to:

- equip rural clinics and train health workers to treat common women's health problems. This way, rural women will not be forced to go to urban hospitals for care.
- pay for people from rural and poor urban areas—especially women—to get health training. That way there will not be such a shortage of trained health workers.
- keep companies from damaging the environment and advertising products that harm people's health.

- force companies to provide fair working conditions and decent wages for women and men.
- make it easier for people to grow food for their communities, not for export.
- distribute unused land to those who have been forced from their land.

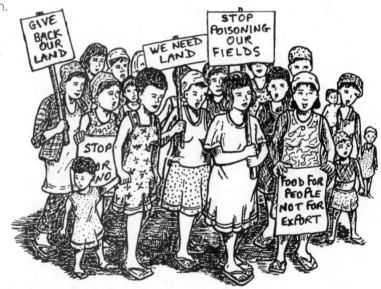

GAINING POWER OVER OUR OWN HEALTH

Just as 'women's health' means more than maternal health, it also means more than access to health care. To be truly healthy, women need the chance to make the decisions necessary for good health. And they need access to a fair share of the resources in their communities and in the world.

By joining other women and men in the struggle for health, we can demand the chance to live healthy, full, and joyful lives—free of disease, pain, and fear.

Chapter 2

In this chapter:

Solving Health Problems

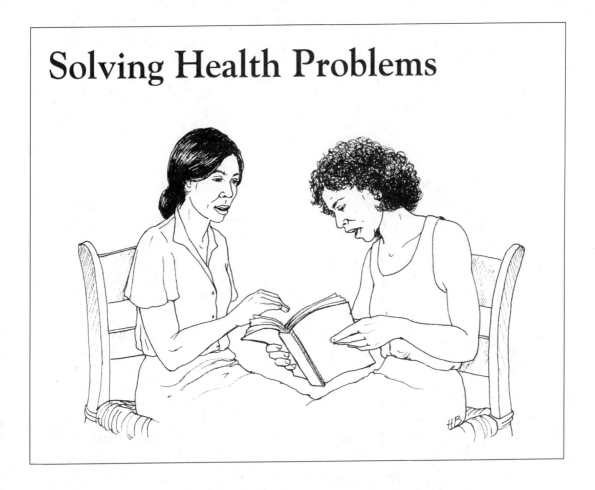

Whenever a woman has signs of a health problem, she needs information in order to solve it. She needs to know what the problem is, its cause, what can be done to treat it, and how to prevent it from happening again.

In this chapter we tell the story of one woman, Juanita, and how she solved her health problem. Although the details apply only to Juanita, the way she thinks about her problem and works to solve it can apply to all health problems. You can use this method to solve a health problem yourself or to make decisions about getting good medical care.

Juanita discovered that a lasting solution to her health problem involved looking beyond her own situation. She also had to identify the root causes of the problem in her community and country, and work to change them. Like Juanita, you and your community can use this method to identify all the causes of women's poor health—and to plan ways to make your community a healthier place for women.

➤ *Some problems must be treated with skilled medical care. But most health problems can be treated at home or can be prevented by healthy living.*

Juanita's Story

Juanita lives in a small village in the mountains of western Honduras where she and her husband grow corn on a small plot of land. Their land does not produce enough to feed their 3 children, so several times each year Juanita's husband, Raul, goes off to the coast with other men from the village to work on the banana plantations.

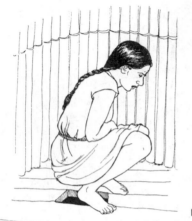

About 3 weeks after the last time her husband returned home from the coast, Juanita began to notice more *discharge* than usual from her vagina. Then she started having pain when passing *urine*. Juanita knew that something was wrong, but she had no idea what it was.

Juanita decided to ask her friend Suyapa for help. Suyapa suggested drinking teas made from corn silk, because this had helped her when she had had pain passing urine. So Juanita tried the teas—but the pain and discharge did not go away. Suyapa then recommended the remedy her friend María del Carmen had used for pains after childbirth. The local midwife had given María a cotton cloth filled with *plant medicines* to wrap around her belly. When Juanita tried the remedy and it didn't work, she thought putting the medicines inside her vagina might be better. But nothing helped, and her signs kept on bothering her.

Finally Juanita decided to go see the health worker, Don Pedro. She felt shy about having a man examine her, but by this time she was scared that something serious was wrong.

WHAT IS THE PROBLEM?

Don Pedro told Juanita that in order to help her, he needed to learn as much about the illness as possible. So he asked Juanita these questions:

Step 1: Start with doubt. This means admitting you do not know the answer yet.

Step 2: Find out as much as possible about the problem. Ask questions like these:

- *When did you first notice the problem?*
- *What signs made you suspect that something was wrong?*
- *How often do you have these signs? What are they like?*
- *Have you ever had these signs before, or has anyone in your family or community had them before?*
- *Does anything make the signs better or worse?*

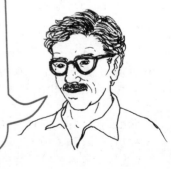

SOME ILLNESSES ARE HARD TO TELL APART

After listening carefully to Juanita describe her pain and discharge, Don Pedro explained that signs often tell us the general kind of health problem someone has. But sometimes several different illnesses can cause the same signs. For example, a change in the amount, color, or smell of a woman's vaginal discharge could be caused by:

- a *sexually transmitted disease (STD).*
- an infection of the vagina that is not an STD.
- *pelvic inflammatory disease (PID),* which is an infection of the *womb* and *tubes,* often caused by an STD.
- *cancer* of the *cervix.*

To get a better idea about which of these problems was causing Juanita's signs, Don Pedro needed to know whether Juanita and her husband used *condoms,* and whether either of them had had other sex partners. Juanita admitted that she suspects her husband has sex with other women, since he is gone for months at a time to work. But they had never discussed it, so she did not know for sure. The last time her husband came home, however, he had complained of some pain when passing urine. He blamed it on the foods he ate at the coast.

With this added information, Don Pedro said he suspected Juanita had an STD, probably gonorrhea or chlamydia. Because it is difficult to tell these diseases apart, it is better to treat both of them.

> *Step 3: Think about all the different illnesses that could be causing the signs.*

> *Step 4: Look for clues that can tell you which answer is most likely.*

> *Step 5: Decide which answer is probably the right one.*

WHAT IS CAUSING THE PROBLEM?

Infectious diseases are those that are spread from one person to another. They can be spread through touching infected people or objects, or through the air or water. The *germs* Don Pedro thinks are causing Juanita's illness are spread through sexual contact.

Non-infectious diseases (not spread between people), may be caused by:

- something that goes wrong in the body, such as weak bones from aging.
- something that harms the body from the outside, such as back problems from carrying heavy loads.
- something the body lacks, such as *nutrition.* By eating too little food or the wrong kinds of food, a person can become malnourished.

But illnesses rarely have just one cause. (To learn more about identifying other causes, see page 26.) Often people's beliefs and cultural practices contribute to disease, as do conditions in their surroundings, and the way that land, wealth, and power are distributed.

What Is the Best Treatment?

IS A TREATMENT HELPFUL OR HARMFUL?

Although Don Pedro was certain that medicines would solve the problem, Juanita wanted more information before deciding on a treatment. She knew, for example, that home remedies had often helped her mother and grandmother when they were ill. Why, then, did the remedies she had tried fail to work? Here is Don Pedro's explanation:

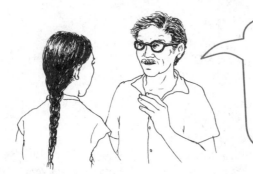

Every community has developed remedies for solving health problems. Home remedies and modern medicine can both be helpful if practiced carefully and correctly. But remember that both home remedies and modern medicines can be helpful, can be harmless, and can also be harmful.

In Juanita's case, she had used all 3 kinds of remedies:

Corn silk tea would have been very **helpful** if Juanita had an infection of the urine system. This is because corn silk tea makes a person pass urine more and so flushes germs out of the body. But these teas probably did not help Juanita because her infection was not in the urine system.

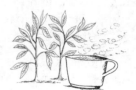

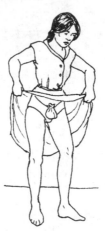

Wrapping *plant medicines* around the belly is a **harmless** remedy. It will not make a health problem worse, because the medicines stay outside the body, but it will not help, either.

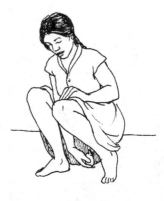

Putting plant medicines into the vagina is **harmful** and should never be done. Plant medicines can irritate the vagina and cause dangerous infections.

Don Pedro told Juanita that she could learn about a particular treatment and how well it works by talking to many different people who have used it. Here are some questions to ask:

- Why do you use this method?
- When do you use it?
- How do you use it?
- What happens when you use it?
- How often does it help the problem?
- Do things ever go wrong?

Think carefully about what different people say about treatments they have used. Then, when you try a remedy yourself, pay attention to what happens to your signs to see if the remedy helps you. Be careful about trying too many remedies at once.

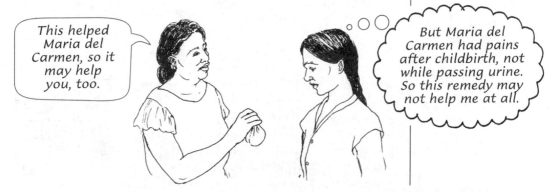

> This helped Maria del Carmen, so it may help you, too.

> But Maria del Carmen had pains after childbirth, not while passing urine. So this remedy may not help me at all.

To decide if a treatment will be helpful, harmless, or harmful, learn all you can about it first. If you are still unsure whether a treatment is harmless or harmful, consider these things:

1. The more remedies there are for any one illness, the less likely it is that any of them works.

2. Foul or disgusting remedies are not likely to help—and are often harmful.

3. Remedies that use animal or human waste rarely do any good, and often cause dangerous infections. Never use them.

4. The more a remedy resembles the sickness it is said to cure, the more likely that its benefits come only from the power of belief. For example, a red plant will not necessarily stop bleeding.

5. Methods that deny people food, exercise, or rest usually make them weaker, not stronger.

6. Methods that blame people for their problems usually add to their suffering and pain.

> *Step 6: Decide on the best treatment. Always remember to think about possible risks and benefits (see below).*

> *Step 7: See if there is some improvement. If there are no results, start over again.*

When Juanita felt satisfied that modern medicines were the best treatment for her health problem, Don Pedro gave Juanita some pills called doxycycline and co-trimoxazole and told her to come back in a week, after she had taken them all. He also explained that her husband, who was away again, must be treated with the medicines when he comes back, and that they must begin to practice safer sex.

When Juanita returned to see Don Pedro the next week, she told him that she had taken all the pills he gave her but her signs had not gone away. She also said her discharge was getting worse and becoming yellow in color. So Don Pedro asked Valeria, a health worker with more training, for help.

Valeria agreed that Juanita had an STD. But because the medicines had not helped, Valeria suspected that Juanita may have a form of gonorrhea that is *resistant* to co-trimoxazole. Valeria explained that many resistant forms of gonorrhea had come from foreign soldiers at the military base on the coast, who have been infecting the local women when they had sex. Valeria recommended that Juanita go to the city where she could get a more complete exam and be tested for gonorrhea, syphilis (another STD), and cancer. She could also get newer, more effective medicines, if needed.

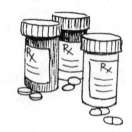

RISKS AND BENEFITS

Juanita went home to think about what to do. She would have to spend most of her family's savings to pay for a trip to the city and the medicine. Since she would be gone at least two days (the trip is almost 6 hours each way by bus and walking), and her husband was still away at the coast, she would also have to find someone to watch her children while she was gone.

Juanita was afraid that her husband would be angry if he came back and found out that she had spent so much money to see a doctor. But she was also scared that if she did not go she would get worse. Valeria told her that without treatment she could pass the infection on to a new baby if she became pregnant. With time she would probably become unable to have more children, would develop severe pain in her lower belly, and would have problems with her urine system and *monthly bleeding*. Her husband could also develop many serious health problems.

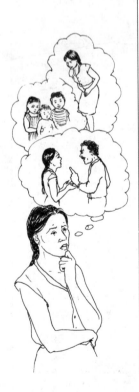

Juanita felt so uncertain about what to do that she went to see Valeria again. When Juanita explained her fears, Valeria suggested thinking about the problem this way:

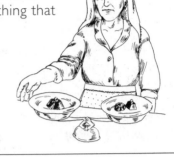

Every treatment has **risks** and **benefits**. A risk is the chance that something may cause harm. A benefit is the good that something may bring. The best choice is to do something that will cause the greatest benefit and the smallest risk.

It may help to think about scales you use to weigh food in the market. When one side weighs more than the other, that side of the scale tilts downward. If the benefits weigh more than the risks, that means the action is worth doing. If the risks weigh more, then the action is not worth doing.

Juanita, you will face these risks if you go to the city:
- *Your husband may be angry when he finds out.*
- *You will spend all your savings, so you may not be able to buy clothes for your children this year.*

These are the benefits if you go to the city:
- *You will feel better and can continue caring for your family.*
- *You will be able to have more children.*
- *You will not pass the infection on to a new baby if you become pregnant.*

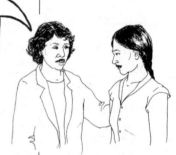

Juanita decided that the benefits of going for treatment weighed more than the risks.

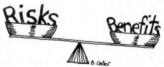

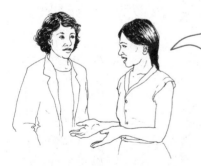

If it were just so I'd feel better, the treatment wouldn't be worth it. But if it's true that I'll get much sicker and cannot have more children, then I must go to the city.

So Juanita went to the city for treatment, where the doctors said it was true that she had gonorrhea and probably chlamydia, but no signs of other STDs or problems. They explained that the medicine she took no longer works in her country. They gave Juanita a newer medicine for both her and her husband.

Working for Change

When Juanita had taken the medicine and was feeling better, it was tempting to think that her health problem had been solved. But she knew this was not true. When her husband returned from the coast, she would get infected again if he did not take the medicine and use condoms. She discussed the problem with Suyapa and other women whose husbands work at the coast, and together they decided to ask Valeria for advice.

LOOKING FOR THE ROOT CAUSES OF HEALTH PROBLEMS

Valeria agreed that Juanita's health problem was not yet solved, because many of the conditions that created the problem still existed. She suggested playing a game called "But why....?" to help everyone identify all the conditions that created the problem.

Valeria gathered the women in a circle, and asked them to try and answer her questions:

Step 8: Look for the root causes of the problem.

Q: Why did Juanita get sick?

A: From gonorrhea and chlamydia.

Q: BUT WHY did she get gonorrhea and chlamydia?

A: Because she was infected by her husband.

Q: BUT WHY did her husband have gonorrhea and chlamydia?

A: Because he had sex with other women.

Q: BUT WHY did he have sex with other women?

A: Because men are taught that they do not need to control their desire, and he was away from his wife for a long time.

Q: But WHY was he away from his wife for so long?

A: Because he does not have enough land to feed his family and must work on the coast for months at a time.

Q: BUT WHY does he have so little land?

A: Because most of the land is owned by big landowners. (A long discussion follows from this answer.)

Q: Why else did Juanita get infected?

A: Because her husband won't use condoms.

Q: BUT WHY won't Juanita's husband use condoms?

A: Because he doesn't know how STDs are spread.

And so on.

When the women had named a long list of causes, Valeria suggested putting the causes in groups. This way it is easier to see the different kinds of conditions that cause health problems:

> Step 9: It may help to group the causes together to think about what can be done to address them.

Physical causes: germs or parasites, or something that goes wrong in the body or that the body lacks

Environmental causes: conditions in the physical surroundings that harm the body, such as cooking smoke, lack of clean water, or crowded living conditions

Social causes: the way people relate to or treat each other, including their attitudes, customs, and beliefs

Political and economic causes: causes having to do with power—who has control and how—and money, land, and resources—who has them and who does not

When the women put the causes of Juanita's problem into these groups, they came up with the following list:

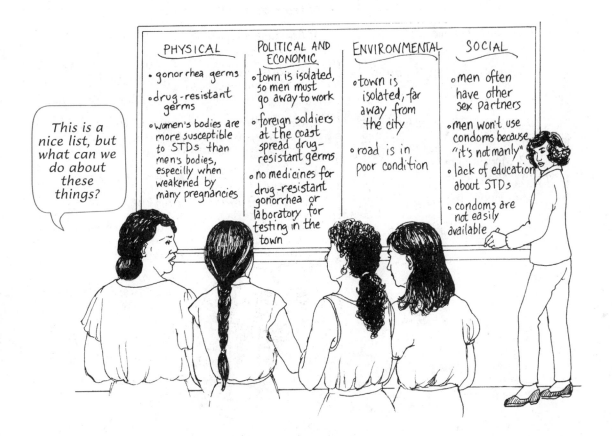

> This is a nice list, but what can we do about these things?

PHYSICAL
- gonorrhea germs
- drug-resistant germs
- women's bodies are more susceptible to STDs than men's bodies, especially when weakened by many pregnancies

POLITICAL AND ECONOMIC
- town is isolated, so men must go away to work
- foreign soldiers at the coast spread drug-resistant germs
- no medicines for drug-resistant gonorrhea or laboratory for testing in the town

ENVIRONMENTAL
- town is isolated, far away from the city
- road is in poor condition

SOCIAL
- men often have other sex partners
- men won't use condoms because "it's not manly"
- lack of education about STDs
- condoms are not easily available

ORGANIZING TO SOLVE COMMUNITY HEALTH PROBLEMS

> **Step 10: Decide which causes you and your community can change.**

The next step, Valeria told the women, is to look at the different causes and decide which ones you and others in the community can change. Then think about what actions must be done to make the changes happen.

> **Step 11: Decide what actions can make those changes happen.**

Juanita and Suyapa thought they could get their husbands to use condoms if their husbands understood more about STDs, and if the condoms were not so costly. The actions they decided to take were:

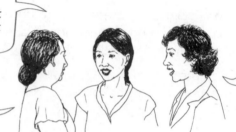

Let's ask Don Pedro to talk with the men about STDs, since they respect him and listen to him.

Let's all meet together to practice talking with our husbands about using condoms.

I'll see if the health center can give out free condoms.

Other members of the group suggested these actions:

- Organize a community group to talk about health problems, and include STDs in the topics discussed.
- While women are washing clothes at the river, talk to them about STDs and how to prevent them.
  - Talk to their sons about STDs before they leave the village to go to the coast.

> **Step 12: Make a plan for carrying out the actions.**

The last step, said Valeria, is to make a plan to carry out each of these ideas for action. The plan, she said, should answer each of these questions:

- What are we going to do? What steps will we take?
- When are we going to do these things?
- Who are we going to do them with?
- What materials will we need?
- Who is responsible for making sure that the plan is carried out?
- How will we evaluate whether the plan is working?

Cause: Men do not use condoms.

Action: Help men learn about how STDs are spread.

What/Who: Don Pedro will talk to the men about STDs and how condoms prevent the spread of STDs.

When: When the men return from the coast

What materials do we need? Condoms.

Who is responsible? Juanita will ask Don Pedro.

How will we evaluate? If men begin to use condoms.

To help you use this method of solving health problems yourself, here is a chart with a list of all of the steps. On the left are the steps and on the right are the parts of Juanita's story that go with each step. Any time you have a health problem you can use this chart to help you remember this method for thinking about and taking action to solve the problem.

The Steps	Juanita's Story
1. Start with doubt.	1. Juanita noticed unusual discharge from her vagina and pain when passing urine. She asked friends and a health worker for help.
2. Find out as much as possible about the problem. Ask questions.	2. Don Pedro asked her questions to find out what could have caused the problem.
3. Think about all the different illnesses that could be causing the signs.	3. Don Pedro thought about all the illnesses with these signs.
4. Look for clues that can tell you which answer is most likely.	4. Don Pedro tried to find out if an STD could have caused Juanita's illness.
5. Decide which answer is probably the right one.	5. Don Pedro decided Juanita probably had an STD.
6. Decide on the best treatment.	6. Don Pedro chose a treatment that works for several STDs.
7. If there are no results, start over again.	7. Juanita took the pills but did not improve and developed new signs. Valeria thought Juanita had a new form of gonorrhea, and that she should go to the city for an examination, tests, and other medicine.
8. Look for the root causes of the problem.	8. Juanita and her friends thought about the reasons why there was this kind of STD in their community.
9. Put the causes into groups to think about what can be done.	9. The women put the causes into physical, environmental, social, political, and economic groups.
10. Decide which causes you and your community can change.	10. Juanita and Suyapa think they can get their partners to use condoms.
11. Decide what actions can make those changes happen.	11. They decided to practice how to talk to their partners about using condoms, to see if the health center will give out free condoms, and to ask Don Pedro to talk with their partners about STDs.
12. Make a plan for carrying out the actions.	12. They made a plan for each action they decided to take.

To the Health Worker

HELPING WOMEN HELP THEMSELVES

In this chapter Don Pedro and Valeria played an important role in helping the women in Juanita's community solve a health problem. The reason that Don Pedro and Valeria were so effective was that they did not tell Juanita and her friends what to do. Rather, Don Pedro and Valeria helped the women learn how to help themselves.

You, too, can help the women in your community by following Don Pedro's and Valeria's example. You can:

- **Share your knowledge.** To help themselves, women need information. Many health problems can be prevented if people know how. But remember that you do not have to have all of the answers to help people. Many times there are no easy answers. It is fine to admit when you do not know something. The people you work with will be glad for your honesty.

➤ *Share your knowledge with other women, other health workers, and with the people who make decisions in the community.*

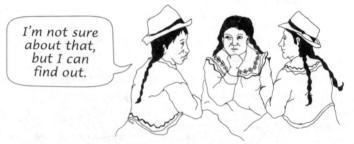

I'm not sure about that, but I can find out.

- **Treat women with respect.** Each person should be treated as someone who is capable of understanding her health problems and of making good decisions about her treatment. Never blame a woman for her problem or for past decisions she has made.

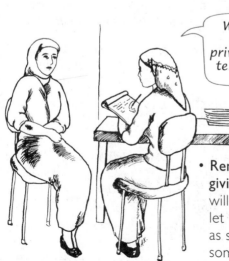

What we have discussed is private. I will not tell anyone else.

- **Keep health problems private.** Health problems should not be discussed where others can hear. Never tell anyone else about a problem someone has unless the person with the problem says it is OK.

- **Remember that listening is more important than giving advice.** A woman often needs someone who will listen to her without judgment. By listening, you let her know you care and that she is important. And as she gets a chance to talk, she may find that she has some of the answers to her problem.

• **Solve problems with others, not for them.** Even when a woman's problems are very large and cannot be solved completely, she usually has some choices she can make. As a health worker, you can help her realize she has choices, and help her find the information she needs to make her own decisions.

• **Learn from the people you help.** Learning how others solve their own problems can help you to better help others (and sometimes yourself, too).

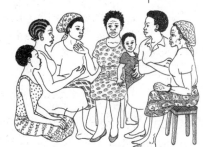

You learn from those you help, and those you help learn from you.

• **Respect your people's traditions and ideas.** Modern science does not have all the answers. And many modern medicines come from studying plant medicines and traditional ways of healing. So it is important to respect and use what is good in both methods—and to realize that both methods can cause harm when used in the wrong way.

• **Find out what people really want to learn about.** It is easy to fall into the trap of giving information without finding out if it will be helpful. This often happens with health workers who give prepared talks. But if you find out exactly what people want to know, they will get knowledge that is useful to them. This also helps them build on their own knowledge.

You must eat red meat to get enough iron.

They are not interested in good nutrition.

We've heard this talk before. We don't have money to buy those foods.

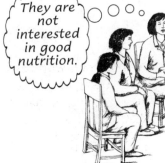

• **Plan with people, not for people.** When you plan your work, be sure to talk first with women and men in your community. Find out how they view the problem you are working to solve. Together, talk about what they think causes the problem and how they would like to solve it. Working together brings the best results!

So, you all know that iron is important. But meat is very expensive. Do you want to talk about other ways to get enough iron?

My aunt Grace grows fresh greens. She says they help make the blood strong.

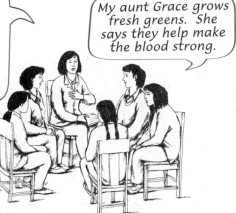

Chapter 3

In this chapter:

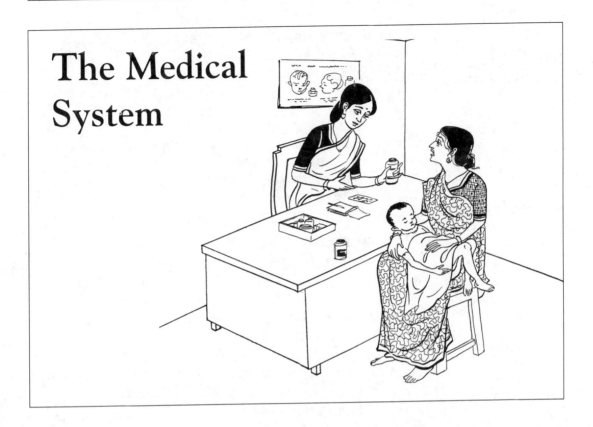

The Medical System

Most people use some combination of modern medicine and traditional remedies to treat their health problems themselves. In many cases, this is all that they need to do. But for some health problems, a woman may need to seek medical advice.

In most areas of the world, there are 4 different levels of health care: community health workers or traditional healers, health posts, health centers, and hospitals. Together, they are called the medical system. A medical system can include health workers, nurses, doctors, and others. They may be in private practice (charge money for their services), or they may be supported by the community, the government, a church, or another organization. Sometimes they are well trained and equipped—and sometimes they are not.

This chapter describes the medical system and how a woman can use it to get help for her health problems. Not every community has each of these 4 levels, and there can be many different combinations of health services that make up the medical system. But no matter what combination of health services is available, women—and all sick people—will get better care if there are good connections between the different levels of health care.

➤ *There are times when you cannot treat a health problem yourself. You may need to seek help from the medical system.*

18

Solving Health Problems

The Medical System

➤ *When health care is provided by trained health workers within the community, everyone can get better care, for less money.*

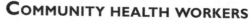

COMMUNITY HEALTH WORKERS

Some communities have well-trained, skilled health workers. These health workers often work out of health posts or centers, but not all do. Community health workers may or may not have formal training. But by working closely with the people in their communities, they can help prevent many common health problems, and help people treat their problems before they become more serious. A health worker can be trained to provide the same services as a health post.

HEALTH POSTS

Many communities have health posts. In some places, this level of care is called a clinic or an MCH (Maternal Child Health). A health post should be able to provide:

- **health information** so that everyone can make better decisions about their health.

- **immunizations or *vaccinations*** that can prevent many diseases, including *tetanus*, measles, diphtheria, whooping cough, polio, *tuberculosis*, rubella, and *hepatitis*.

- **care during pregnancy** (prenatal care) that can help a woman find and treat problems affecting her or her unborn baby before they become serious.

- **family planning** services and supplies. Family planning can save lives by helping women control how many children they have, and the amount of time between births.

- **health exams** to help find and treat problems such as weak blood (anemia), high blood pressure, and sometimes *sexually transmitted diseases (STDs)*.

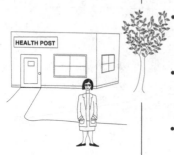

HEALTH CENTERS

Health centers provide a middle level of care. They are usually in larger towns, so people from nearby communities as well as from the town use them. Health centers usually offer all the services a health post offers, and they may also have a few beds where a sick person can stay while being cared for.

Health centers are more likely than health posts to have trained nurses and doctors. They are also more likely to be crowded, and the doctors and nurses may know less about the people they see.

Some health centers have *laboratories* with special equipment. This means they can do tests that give more information about the cause of a health problem (see page 37). Often, however, a person must go to a hospital to have tests done.

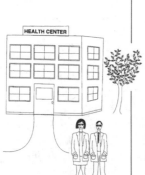

HOSPITALS

Hospitals are usually in large towns or cities, and can be expensive. They usually have many doctors and nurses, and special equipment for treating serious illnesses. A person with a serious illness may need to go to a special hospital that can treat certain problems. A woman might need to go to a hospital for:

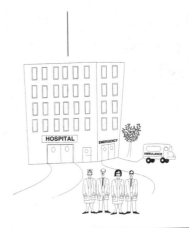

- problems that cannot be treated elsewhere.
- *complications* of childbirth or *abortion*.
- emergencies such as a *pregnancy in the tube*.
- health problems that require an *operation*.

No matter where you go for health care, you should be treated with respect.

All people who care for your health should do their best to provide you with:

1. **Access.** Everyone who needs medical care should be able to have it. It should not matter where you live, how much money you have, what your religion is, how much status you have in the community, the color of your skin, your political beliefs, or what health problem you have.

2. **Information.** You should be told about your problem and about what the different possible treatments mean for you. The person caring for you should make sure you understand what you need to do to get better, and how to prevent the problem from happening again.

3. **Choice.** You should be able to choose whether or not you are treated, and how. Also, you should be able to choose where to go for treatment.

4. **Safety.** You should be given the information you need to avoid harmful side effects or results of treatment. You should also be told how to prevent dangerous health problems in the future.

5. **Respect.** You should always be treated with respect and courtesy.

6. **Privacy.** Things that you say to a doctor, nurse or other health care worker should not be overheard by others or repeated to anyone else. Exams should be given in a way that other people cannot see your body. If there are other people who need to be in the room, you should be told who they are and why they are there. You have the right to tell them to leave if you do not want them there.

Can I come back if I don't get better soon?

7. **Comfort.** You should be made as comfortable as possible during an exam. You should also have a good place to wait and not have to wait too long.

8. **Follow-up care.** If you need more care, you should be able to go back to the same person, or be given a written record of the care you have received to take to a new doctor, nurse, or health worker.

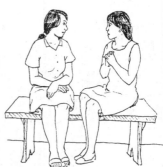

How to Get Better Care

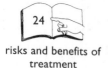

risks and benefits of treatment

There are many decisions to make when you have a health problem. One decision is whether to see a health worker, and what kind of health worker you think you need. If there is more than one way to treat a problem, you will need to consider the *risks* and *benefits* of each kind of treatment before you make a decision. You will be able to make the best decisions—and get the best care—if you can take an active role in working with your doctor, nurse, or health worker to solve your health problem.

KNOW WHAT TO EXPECT

You will be best able to take an active role in your health if you are prepared and know what to expect when you seek medical care.

Questions about your health

It is best to learn as much as you can about your health problem before you use the medical system. Reading this book may help you understand your health problem and the possible causes. For help thinking about health problems, see "Solving Health Problems."

The doctor, nurse, or health worker who sees you should ask about the problem you are having now and about your past health. Try to give complete information, even if you feel uncomfortable, so that the person asking the questions can learn as much as possible about your health. Always tell about any medication you are taking, including aspirin or *family planning methods*.

➤ *It often helps to think of the questions you want to ask before you go for medical care.*

You should also have a chance to ask any questions you may have. It is very important to ask as many questions as you need to make a good decision about how to solve your health problem. If these questions have not already been answered, you may want to ask:

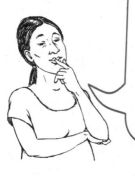

- *What are the different ways this problem can be treated?*
- *What will the treatment do? Are there any dangers?*
- *Will I be cured? Or will the problem come back?*
- *How much will the tests and treatment cost?*
- *When will I get better?*
- *Why did the problem happen and how can I keep it from happening again?*

Many doctors and nurses may not be used to giving good information, or they may be busy and not take the time to answer your questions. Be respectful, but firm! They should answer your questions until you understand. If you do not understand, it is not because you are stupid, but because they are not explaining well.

The exam

In order to know what is wrong with you and how serious your problem is, you may need an examination. Most exams include looking at, listening to, and feeling the part of your body where the problem is. For most problems you need to undress only that part of your body. If you would feel more comfortable, ask a friend or female health care worker to be in the room with you during the exam.

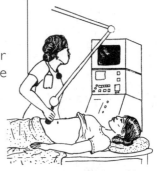

531

pelvic exam

Tests

Tests can give more information about a health problem. Many tests are done by taking a small amount of *urine*, *stool*, or coughed-up *mucus* and sending it to a laboratory. Or, a needle is used to take a small amount of blood from your finger or arm. Other common tests include:

- taking some fluid from your vagina to test for sexually transmitted diseases (STDs).
- scraping *cells* from the opening of your *womb* (*cervix*) to test for *cancer*. (This is called a *Pap test*. See page 378.)
- taking *tissue* from a growth to test for cancer (*biopsy*).
- using *X-rays* or *ultrasound* to see inside your body. **X-rays** may be used to find broken bones, severe lung infections, and some cancers. Try not to be X-rayed during pregnancy. **Ultrasound** can be used during pregnancy to see the baby inside your womb. Neither of these tests causes any pain.

ultrasound machine

➤ *X-rays are safe if they are used properly. A lead apron should be used to protect your reproductive organs.*

Before you have any test, discuss the cost. Ask the doctor, nurse, or health worker to explain what he or she will learn from the test, and what would happen if the test was not done.

BRING A FRIEND OR FAMILY MEMBER

Many people feel worried about seeking medical care—even for illnesses that are not serious. And when a person is sick, it can be even harder for them to demand the care they need. If another person can go along, it can help.

A friend can:

- watch the woman's children.
- help think of questions to ask, remind the woman to ask them, and make sure they are answered.
- answer questions if the woman is too sick to talk.
- keep the woman company while she waits.
- stay with the woman while she is being examined, to support her and make sure the doctor acts in a respectful way.

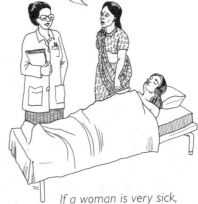

I am her mother. I can answer some of your questions.

If a woman is very sick, someone who can give information should go with her.

If You Need to Go to the Hospital

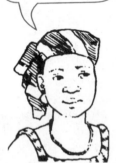

Operations are sometimes done when they are not necessary, or when a medicine could have worked just as well. Get another medical opinion if you are not sure.

If you need to have an operation or you have a serious illness, first find out if it is possible to be treated without having to stay in a hospital. If a hospital is the only place you can get the care you need, this advice may help:

- Bring someone with you who can help you get the attention you need and help you make decisions.
- Different people may examine you. Each one should write down what he or she did on a card that stays with you. This way the next person who cares for you will know what has already been done.
- Before anyone begins a test or treatment, it is very important to ask what they are going to do and why. This way you can decide if you want them to do it and help prevent mistakes.
- Try to make friends with the staff at a hospital. They can help you get better care.
- If you need to have some kind of *operation*, ask if it is possible to have an injection to stop pain only in the area being operated on (local anesthetic). It is safer and you will get better more quickly than if you are given medicine to make you sleep during the surgery (general anesthetic).
- Ask what medicines you are being given and why.
- Ask for a copy of your records when you leave.

Common operations for women

An *operation* is sometimes the only answer to a serious health problem. During many operations, a doctor makes a cut in the skin in order to fix problems inside the body or to change the way the body functions. Here are some of the operations women commonly have:

- **Emptying the womb** by either scraping or suctioning (*D and C, or MVA*, see page 244). Sometimes the lining of the womb must be removed—either during or after an *abortion* or *miscarriage*, or to find the cause of *abnormal bleeding* from the *vagina*.

- **Birth by operation** (cesarean section or c-section). When complications make it dangerous for a woman or her baby to go through normal labor and birth, a cut is made in a woman's belly so her baby can be born. C-sections can be necessary, but too often they are done for the benefit of the doctor, not the woman. See the chapter on "Pregnancy."

- *Sterilization.* During this operation, a woman's *fallopian tubes* are cut and the ends tied. This prevents her eggs from reaching the womb, so a man's sperm will not be able to make her pregnant (see page 223).

- **Removing the womb** (hysterectomy). A hysterectomy is a serious operation, so it should be done only when there is no better way to solve your health problem (see page 381). Ask if you can have your ovaries left in.

Blood transfusions

A *blood transfusion* may be given in an emergency, when you have lost a lot of blood. It can save your life. But if the blood has not been tested properly, it can carry diseases, such as *hepatitis* or *HIV/AIDS*, that are passed through the blood. Avoid blood transfusions except in cases of life or death emergencies.

If you must have an operation that you know about ahead of time, see if it is possible to have some of your own blood taken in advance and stored at the hospital. Then if you need it, you will get your own blood back. If you cannot have your own blood stored, ask a friend or relative to come with you to the hospital. Be sure she has been tested for hepatitis and HIV, and that neither she nor her partner has had a new sex partner in the last 6 months. Her blood must also be tested to make sure that it will work in your body.

If you must receive blood from an unknown person and the hospital does not test its blood for HIV, there is a risk that you might become infected. After the transfusion, protect your partner by practicing safer sex for 6 months and then try to get tested for HIV/AIDS. For more information, see the chapters on "AIDS" and "Sexual Health."

After you have an operation

Before you leave the hospital, ask:

* What should I do to keep the cut clean?
* What should I do about pain?
* How long should I rest?
* When can I have sex again? (If you feel too shy to ask this, perhaps the doctor or health worker can talk to your partner.)
* Do I need to see a doctor again? If so, when?

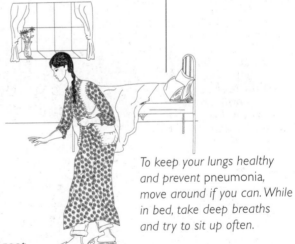

To keep your lungs healthy and prevent pneumonia, *move around if you can. While in bed, take deep breaths and try to sit up often.*

Eat soft, mild foods that are easy to digest.

Rest as much as you can. If you are at home, ask your family to take care of your daily chores. A few days spent taking care of yourself can help you get better faster.

Watch for signs of infection: yellow *discharge* (pus), a bad smell, fever, hot skin near where you were cut, or more pain. See a health worker if you have any of these signs.

If your operation was in the *abdomen*, try not to strain the area that was cut. Press against it gently with a folded cloth, blanket, or pillow whenever you move or cough.

Working for Change

Millions of people throughout the world suffer and die from illnesses that could have been prevented or treated if they had access to good medical care. And even where health services do exist, there are many barriers that keep women, especially poor women, from using them.

But together, health workers and groups of women can change the medical system. They can make it a resource—rather than a barrier—for women as they try to solve their health problems. The medical system will not change on its own, though. It will change only when people demand it, and when they offer creative ways to bring the health care that people need within the reach of all.

A good place to begin changing the medical system is by discussing the health care problems that affect people in your community—including lack of access to good care—with other women and men.

I have to travel very far to get here. If there were a health worker in my area, it would save my family the 2 weeks' wages I spend every time I have to come here.

I wish they didn't run out of family planning supplies. I got pregnant last year because the clinic ran out, and I can't afford to buy a lot all at once when they do have them.

I wish they had mats on the floor like we have at home. These benches are so uncomfortable.

These city doctors look down on us. I would feel better if people from the village helped run the clinic.

I wish they could give us Pap tests here. I can't afford to go to the city and I've heard that they are important.

I want there to be separate rooms where we could be examined without everyone listening.

I don't like having a man examine me. I wish there were women health workers.

I wish they gave us better explanations of what was wrong. This is the 4th time this year I've had pain when I passed urine. Why does this keep happenning to me?

I would like the clinic to be open in the evenings, after I have finished my work.

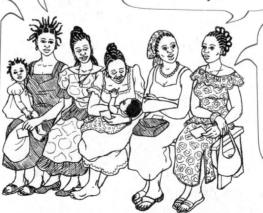

There is always such a long wait. If someone asked right away what each person needed then the really sick people could be treated sooner.

Women can also work together to:
- help every member of the community to learn about women's health problems. For example, you can organize a campaign to explain how important it is that women get good *prenatal* care. If women and their families know about women's health needs, women will be more likely to use the health services that already exist. They will also be more likely to demand that new ones—such as better treatment and screening for cervical and breast cancer—be made available.

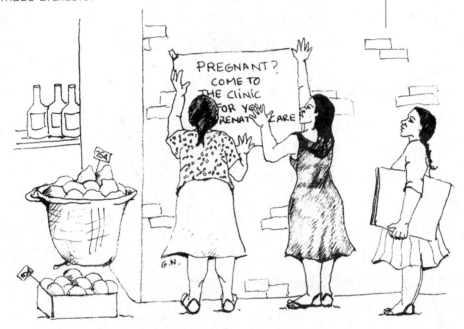

- see how existing health resources can be improved. For example, if there is already a community midwife, how can she get training in new skills?
- find new ways to make health care available. It is important to think about what health services you want to have, and not just what you have now. So, if there is no health worker now, how can one be trained and supported? If there is already a clinic, could it offer new services like workshops or counseling?
- share the knowledge each woman has about health care. Women already do much of the 'health work' in the community. For example, it is usually women who care for the sick, teach children to stay healthy, prepare food, keep the home and community clean and safe, and help other women have babies. Through this work, they have learned many skills that they can use to care for each other and every member of the community.

Chapter 4

In this chapter:

This chapter is about the parts of the body that make up a woman's or a man's sexual and reproductive system. This information will help you to use the rest of this book.

Understanding Our Bodies

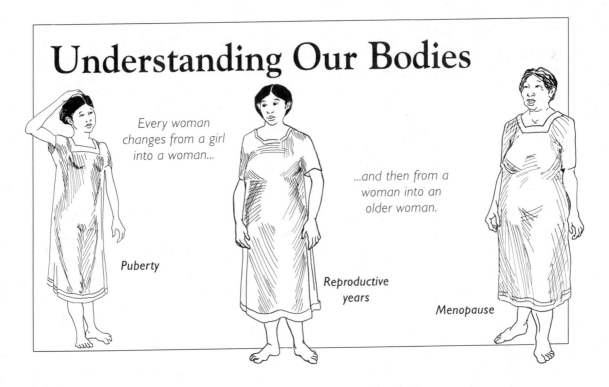

Every woman changes from a girl into a woman...

Puberty

...and then from a woman into an older woman.

Reproductive years

Menopause

In many ways, a woman's body is no different from a man's. For example, women and men both have hearts, *kidneys, lungs,* and other parts that are the same. But one way they are very different is in their sexual or *reproductive* parts. These are the parts that allow a man and a woman to make a baby. Many of women's health problems affect these parts of the body.

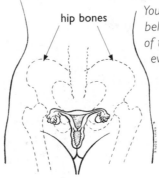

hip bones

You can feel your hip bones just below your waist. They are part of the **pelvis**. The **pelvic area** is everything between the hips. This is where a woman's reproductive parts are.

Sometimes talking about the sexual parts of our bodies can be difficult, especially if you are shy, or do not know what different parts of the body are called. In many places, the reproductive parts of the body are considered 'private'.

But knowing how our bodies work means we can take better care of them. We can recognize problems and their causes and make better decisions about what to do about them. The more we know, the more we will be able to decide for ourselves if the advice that others give us is helpful or harmful.

Since different communities sometimes have their own words for parts of the body, in this book, we often use medical or scientific names. This way, women from many different regions of the world will be able to understand the words.

➤ No one should feel ashamed of any part of his or her body.

➤ The more we know about our bodies, the more we can teach our children how to have better health.

A Woman's Reproductive System

A woman has sexual parts both outside and inside her body. They are called the reproductive organs, or *genitals*. The outside parts are called the *vulva*. Sometimes people may use the word *vagina* for the whole area. But the vagina is the part that begins as an opening in the vulva and leads inside to the *womb*. The vagina is sometimes called the 'birth canal'.

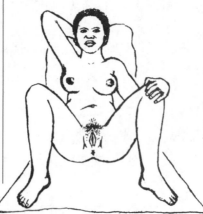

The drawing below shows what the vulva looks like and what the different parts are called. But every woman's body is different. There are differences in the size, shape, and color of the parts, especially of the outer and inner folds.

THE REPRODUCTIVE PARTS ON THE OUTSIDE

Vulva: *All the sexual parts you can see between your legs.*

Outer folds: *The fatty lips that close up when the legs are together. They protect the inner parts.*

Inner folds: *These flaps of skin are soft, without hair, and are sensitive to touch. During sex, the inner lips swell and turn darker.*

Vaginal opening: *The opening of the vagina.*

Hymen: *The thin piece of skin just inside the vaginal opening. A hymen may stretch or tear and bleed a little because of hard work, sports or other activities. This can also happen when a woman has sex for the first time. All hymens are different. Some women do not have a hymen at all.*

Mons: *The hairy, fatty part of the vulva.*

Clitoris: *The clitoris is small and shaped like a flower bud. It is the part of the vulva that is most sensitive to touch. Rubbing it, and the area around it, can make a woman sexually excited and cause* **climax.**

Urinary opening: *The outer opening of the urethra. The urethra is a short tube that carries urine from where it is stored in the bladder to the outside of the body.*

Anus: *The opening of the intestine, where waste (stool) leaves the body.*

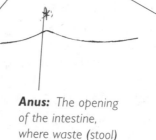

THE BREASTS

Breasts come in all shapes and sizes. They start to grow when a girl is between 10 and 15 years old, when she changes from a girl to a woman (puberty). They make milk for babies after pregnancy. When they are touched during sexual relations, a woman's body responds by making her vagina wet and ready for sex.

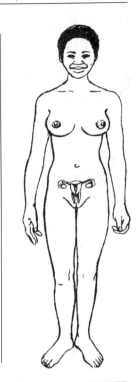

Inside the breasts:

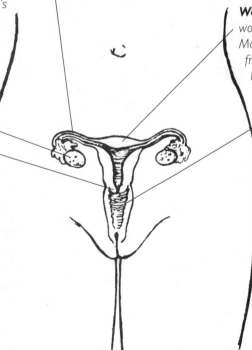

Glands *make the milk.*

Ducts *carry the milk to the nipple.*

Sinuses *store the milk until the baby drinks it.*

The **nipple** *is where milk comes out of the breast. Sometimes they stick out. Sometimes they are flat.*

The **areola** *is the dark and bumpy skin around the nipple. The bumps make an oil that keeps the nipples clean and soft.*

THE REPRODUCTIVE PARTS ON THE INSIDE

Ovaries: *The ovaries release one egg into a woman's fallopian tubes each month. When a man's sperm joins the egg, it can develop into a baby. A woman has 2 ovaries, one on each side of the womb. Each ovary is about the size of an almond or grape.*

Fallopian tubes: *The fallopian tubes connect the womb with the ovaries. When an ovary releases an egg, it travels through the fallopian tubes into the womb.*

Womb *(uterus):* The womb is a hollow muscle. Monthly bleeding comes from the womb. The baby grows here during pregnancy.

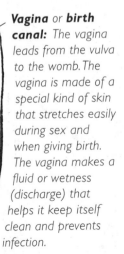

Cervix: *This is the opening or 'mouth' of the womb, where it opens into the vagina. Sperm can enter the womb through the small hole in the cervix, but it protects the womb from other things, like a man's penis. During childbirth, the cervix opens to let the baby come out.*

Vagina *or* **birth canal:** *The vagina leads from the vulva to the womb. The vagina is made of a special kind of skin that stretches easily during sex and when giving birth. The vagina makes a fluid or wetness (discharge) that helps it keep itself clean and prevents infection.*

A Man's Reproductive System

A man's sexual parts are easier to see than a woman's because they are mostly outside the body. The *testicles* (balls) make the main *hormone* in a man's body, called testosterone. When a boy goes through *puberty*, his body begins to make more testosterone. It causes the changes that make a boy look like a man.

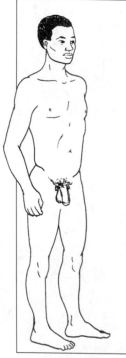

The testicles also make a man's sperm. A man begins to produce sperm during puberty, and makes more every day of his life.

Sperm travel from the testicles through a tube in the penis where they mix with a liquid produced by special *glands*.

This mixture of liquid and sperm is called semen. The semen comes out of the penis when a man climaxes during sex. Each drop of semen has thousands of sperm which are too small to see.

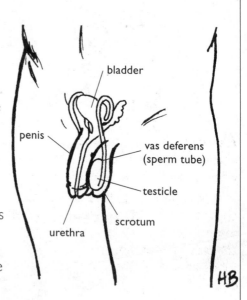

- bladder
- penis
- vas deferens (sperm tube)
- testicle
- scrotum
- urethra

HB

HAVING A BABY—WILL IT BE A BOY OR A GIRL?

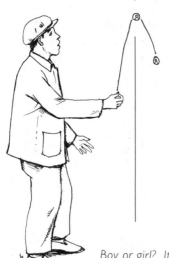

About half of a man's sperm are boy sperm and half are girl sperm. Only one sperm will join with the woman's egg. If it is a boy sperm, the baby will be a boy. If it is a girl sperm, the baby will be a girl.

Because most communities value men more than women, some families would rather have boys than girls. This is unfair because girls should be valued just as much as boys. It is also unfair because in some places a woman is blamed if she does not have any sons. But it is the man's sperm that makes a baby either a boy or a girl!

Boy or girl? It is up to chance—much like flipping a coin.

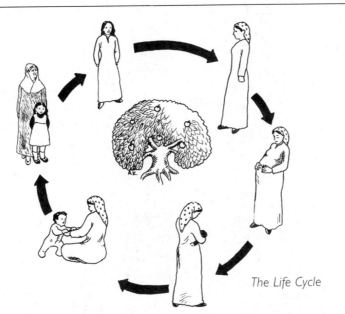

The Life Cycle

How a Woman's Body Changes

A woman's body goes though many important changes during her life—at puberty, during pregnancy and breastfeeding, and when she stops being able to have a baby (*menopause*).

In addition, during the years she can have a baby, her body changes every month—before, during, and after the time of her monthly bleeding. The parts of the body where many of these changes happen are the vagina, womb, ovaries, fallopian tubes, and the breasts, also called the reproductive system. Many of the changes are caused by special chemicals called hormones.

puberty, 54
monthly bleeding, 48
menopause, 124

HORMONES

Hormones are chemicals the body makes that control how and when the body grows. A little while before a girl's monthly bleeding first starts, her body begins to produce more estrogen and progesterone, the main female hormones. These hormones cause the changes in her body known as puberty.

During the years when she can have a baby, hormones cause a woman's body to prepare for possible pregnancy each month. They also tell her ovaries when to release an egg (one egg every month). So hormones determine when a woman can get pregnant. Many *family planning methods* work to prevent pregnancy by controlling the hormones in a woman's body (see page 207). Hormones also cause changes during pregnancy and breastfeeding. For example, hormones keep a pregnant woman from having her monthly bleeding, and after childbirth they also tell the breasts to make milk.

When a woman is near the end of her reproductive years, her body slowly stops producing estrogen and progesterone. Her ovaries stop releasing eggs, her body stops preparing for a pregnancy, and her monthly bleeding stops forever. This is called menopause.

The amount and kind of hormones produced by a woman's body can also affect her moods, sexual feelings, weight, body temperature, hunger, and bone strength.

Monthly Bleeding

About once each month during her reproductive years, a woman has a few days when a bloody fluid leaves her womb and passes through her vagina and out of her body. This is called 'monthly bleeding', the 'monthly period' or 'menstruation'. It is a healthy process and is part of the way the body gets ready for pregnancy.

Around the world, women have many different names for their monthly bleeding.

I see the moon.

My monthly habit is here.

I have a visitor from Russia.

I have my monthly bleeding.

A friend is visiting.

I have my period.

María is crying.

Most women think of their monthly bleeding as a normal part of their lives. But often they do not know why it happens or why it sometimes changes.

THE MONTHLY CYCLE (MENSTRUAL CYCLE)

The monthly cycle is different for each woman. It begins on the first day of a woman's monthly bleeding. Most women bleed every 28 days. But some bleed as often as every 20 days or as little as every 45 days.

The amount of the hormones estrogen and progesterone produced in the ovaries changes throughout the monthly cycle. During the first half of the cycle, the ovaries make mostly estrogen, which causes a thick lining of blood and tissue to grow in the womb. The body makes the lining so a baby would have a soft nest to grow in if the woman became pregnant that month.

In the middle of the cycle, when the soft lining is ready, an egg is released from one of the ovaries. This is called ovulation. The egg then travels down a tube into the womb. At this time a woman is *fertile* and she can become pregnant. If the woman has had sex recently, the man's sperm may join with her egg. This is called fertilization and is the beginning of pregnancy.

During the second half of the cycle—until her next monthly bleeding starts—a woman also produces progesterone. Progesterone causes the lining of the womb to prepare for pregnancy.

Most months, the egg is not fertilized, so the lining inside the womb is not needed. The ovaries stop producing estrogen and progesterone, and the lining begins to break down. When the lining inside the womb leaves the body during the monthly bleeding, the egg comes out too. This is the start of a new monthly cycle. After the monthly bleeding, the ovaries start to make more estrogen again, and another lining begins to grow.

➤ *A woman may find that the time between each monthly bleeding changes as she grows older, after she gives birth, or because of stress.*

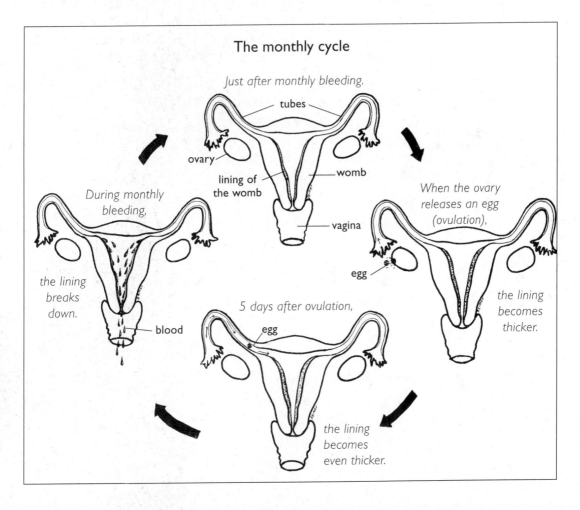

The monthly cycle

Just after monthly bleeding.

tubes

ovary

lining of the womb

womb

vagina

During monthly bleeding,

the lining breaks down.

blood

When the ovary releases an egg (ovulation),

egg

the lining becomes thicker.

5 days after ovulation,

egg

the lining becomes even thicker.

PROBLEMS WITH MONTHLY BLEEDING

If you have problems with your monthly bleeding, try to talk with your mother, sisters or friends. You may find that they have them too and they may be able to help you.

Changes in bleeding

Sometimes the ovary does not release an egg. When this happens, the body makes less progesterone, which can cause changes in how often and how much a woman bleeds. Girls whose monthly bleeding has just begun—or women who have recently stopped breastfeeding—may only bleed every few months, or have very little bleeding, or too much bleeding. Their cycles usually become more regular with time.

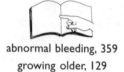

abnormal bleeding, 359
growing older, 129

Women who use *hormonal family planning methods* sometimes have bleeding in the middle of the month. See pages 207 to 215 for more information about changes in bleeding caused by hormonal family planning methods.

Older women who have not yet gone through menopause may have heavier bleeding or bleed more often than when they were younger. As they get closer to menopause, they may stop having monthly bleeding for a few months and then have it again.

Pain with monthly bleeding

During monthly bleeding the womb squeezes in order to push out the lining. The squeezing can cause pain in the lower belly or lower back, sometimes called cramps. The pain may begin before bleeding starts or just after it starts.

What to do:

- Rub your lower belly. This helps the tight muscles relax.
- Fill a plastic bottle or some other container with hot water and place it on your lower belly or lower back. Or use a thick cloth you have soaked in hot water.
- Drink tea made from raspberry leaves, ginger, or chamomile. Women in your community may know of other teas or remedies that work for this kind of pain.
- Keep doing your daily work.
- Try to exercise and walk.
- Take a mild pain medicine. Ibuprofen works very well for the pain that comes with monthly bleeding (see page 482).
- If you also have heavy bleeding and nothing else works, taking a low-dose birth control pill for 6 to 12 months may help (see page 208).

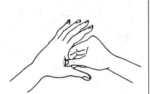

Pressing hard on the tender place between your thumb and first finger can ease many kinds of pain. For other places where pressure can ease pain from monthly bleeding, see page 542.

Pre-menstrual syndrome (PMS)

Some women and girls feel uncomfortable a few days before their monthly bleeding begins. They may have one or more of a group of signs that are known as pre-menstrual syndrome (PMS). Women who have PMS may notice:

- sore breasts
- a full feeling in the lower belly
- constipation (when you cannot pass stool)
- feeling extra tired
- sore muscles, especially in the lower back or belly
- a change in the wetness of the vagina
- oiliness or spots (pimples) on the face
- feelings that are especially strong or harder to control

Many women have at least one of these signs each month and some women may have all of them. A woman may have different signs from one month to the next. For many women, the days before their monthly bleeding starts are a time of unrest. But some women say they feel more creative and better able to get things done.

What to do:

What helps with PMS is different for each woman. To find out what will help, a woman should try different things and notice what makes her feel better. First, try following the suggestions for pain with monthly bleeding (see page 50).

These ideas may also help:

- Eat less salt. Salt makes your body keep extra water inside, which makes the full feeling in your lower belly worse.

- Try to avoid *caffeine* (found in coffee, tea and some soft drinks like cola).

- Try eating whole grains, peanuts, fresh fish, meat and milk, or other foods that are high in *protein*. When your body uses these foods, it also gets rid of any extra water, so your belly feels less full and tight.

- Try *plant medicines*. Ask the older women in your community which ones work.

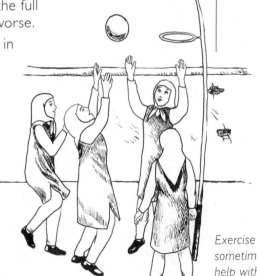

Exercise can sometimes help with the signs of PMS.

Chapter 5

In this Chapter:

Health Concerns of Girls

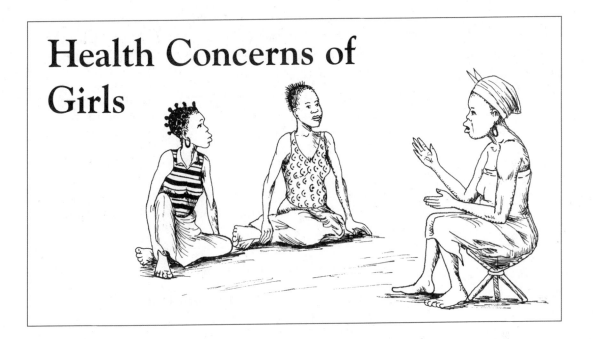

Sometime between the ages of 10 and 15, a girl's body begins to grow and change into an adult body. These can be exciting and difficult years. A young woman may not feel exactly like a girl or a woman—her body is somewhere in between and is doing new things she is not used to. What can make it harder is when no one talks about the changes, and so a girl may not know what to expect. This chapter describes these changes, tells how a girl can stay healthy as she grows, and gives information to help her make the right decisions for a healthy life.

Eating for healthy growth

One of the most important things a girl can do to stay healthy is to eat well. Her body needs to get enough protein, vitamins, and minerals during her years of growth. A girl needs at least as much food as a boy. Getting enough to eat leads to less sickness and more success in school, healthier pregnancies, safer births, and a healthier old age.

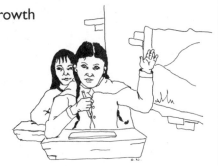

Girls who get enough to eat do better in school.

Girls also need the right kinds of food. When a girl begins her monthly bleeding she will lose some blood each month. To prevent weak blood (*anemia*), she will need to replace the lost blood by eating foods with iron in them. Also, girls and women both need foods with calcium to help their bones grow strong. For complete information on eating well, see page 165.

Changes in Your Body (Puberty)

All girls go through changes in their bodies, but the changes happen differently for each girl. So do not worry if your body does not look exactly like your sister's or friend's.

Growing. Your first change will probably be that you grow fast. You may be taller than all of the boys your age for a while. You will usually stop growing 1 to 3 years after your *monthly bleeding* starts.

Body changes. Besides growing fast, your body will begin to change. There are natural *chemicals* in the body called *hormones* that tell your body to grow and that make these changes happen.

How a girl's body changes in puberty

- You grow taller and rounder.
- Your face gets oily and *pimples* or spots may grow.
- You sweat more.
- Hair grows under your arms and on your *genitals*.
- Your breasts grow as they become able to make milk. As they get larger, it is common for the nipples to hurt sometimes. One breast may begin to grow before the other, but the smaller breast almost always catches up.
- Wetness (*discharge*) starts to come out of your *vagina*.
- Your monthly bleeding starts (*menstruation*).

43 understanding our bodies

➤ *Changes of puberty do not all happen at the same time or in the same order.*

Inside your body. There are other changes that you cannot see. The *womb (uterus)*, *tubes*, *ovaries*, and *vagina* grow and change position.

What you feel. As you go through these changes you become more aware of your body. You may also become more interested in boys, and in your friends. There may be times when your feelings are hard to control. In the days before monthly bleeding, it is even more common to have strong feelings of all kinds—joy, anger, and worry, for example.

Monthly bleeding (period, menstruation)

Monthly bleeding is a sign that your body can become pregnant. No girl can know exactly when she will get her first monthly bleeding. It usually happens after her breasts and the hair on her body start to grow. Several months before her first monthly bleeding, she may notice some wetness coming from the vagina. It may stain her underclothes. This is normal.

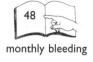

monthly bleeding

Some girls are happy when they have their first monthly bleeding, especially if they know what to expect. Girls who were never told about it often worry when the bleeding starts. It is something that happens to all women, and you can feel accepting and even proud of it. Do not let anyone make you think it is something dirty or shameful.

Caring for yourself during your monthly bleeding

Staying clean. Many girls prefer to make pads of folded cloth or wads of cotton to catch the blood as it leaves the vagina. They stay in place with a belt, pin, or underwear. The pads should be changed several times each day, and washed well with soap and water if they are to be used again.

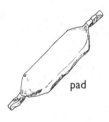

pad

Some women put something inside the vagina that they buy or make from cotton, cloth, or a sponge. These are called tampons. If you use tampons, be sure to change them at least twice each day. Leaving one in for more than a day may cause a serious infection.

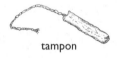

tampon

Wash your outside genitals with water each day to remove any blood that is left. Use a mild soap if you can.

Activities. You can continue all your regular activities.

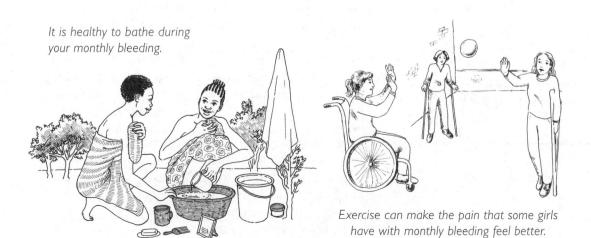

It is healthy to bathe during your monthly bleeding.

Exercise can make the pain that some girls have with monthly bleeding feel better.

Changes that Can Lead to a Better Life

self-esteem

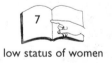

low status of women

The way a woman sees herself forms as she grows. It is important that a girl learn to feel good about herself when she is young, so that she will be able to develop fully and help make her community a better place. A girl is much more likely to learn this when her family and community show her that they value her.

In many places girls are raised to believe they are less important than boys. They are taught to feel shame about their bodies and about being female, and they learn to accept less education, less food, more *abuse,* and more work than their brothers. This not only hurts their health directly, but it makes them feel bad about themselves and less able to make the right decisions for a healthier life in the future. When girls are raised in this way, it shows that their communities do not value them as much as males.

But if a girl's community recognizes the value of each person—whether the person is a man or a woman—she will grow up feeling she can make a better life for herself and for her family and neighbors.

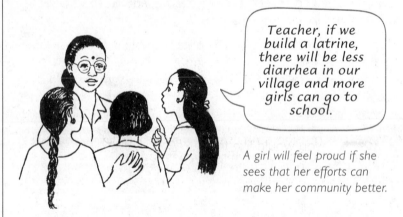

Teacher, if we build a latrine, there will be less diarrhea in our village and more girls can go to school.

A girl will feel proud if she sees that her efforts can make her community better.

The way a community treats females also affects how families treat their girl children. For example, if a community believes that girls should learn skills, a family that lives there is more likely to want their daughter to go to school for as long as she can. But in a community where women are allowed to do only 'women's work' and are not allowed to participate in any public meetings, families are much less likely to believe that their daughters should be educated.

There are many ways to help girls feel better about themselves and to help their families and communities understand that girls' lives can be different. On the next few pages are some ideas.

Ways girls can work for a better life

Find someone to talk to who you think will listen and understand—a friend, a sister, or another female relative. Talk about your fears and problems. Together, you can talk about strong women in your community, your goals, and dreams for the future.

Do things that you and your friends think are important. If you see a problem in your community, get together with your friends to do something to change it. You will all feel proud when you see that your efforts can make your community better.

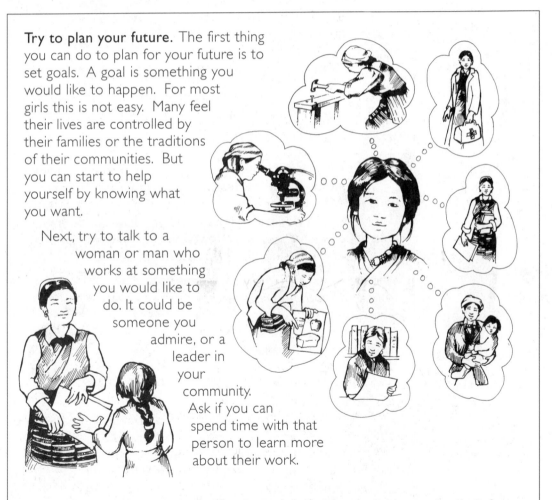

Try to plan your future. The first thing you can do to plan for your future is to set goals. A goal is something you would like to happen. For most girls this is not easy. Many feel their lives are controlled by their families or the traditions of their communities. But you can start to help yourself by knowing what you want.

Next, try to talk to a woman or man who works at something you would like to do. It could be someone you admire, or a leader in your community. Ask if you can spend time with that person to learn more about their work.

Sometimes girls feel frustrated because their dreams and hopes for their future may conflict with the beliefs in their community and family about what a woman should do. It is important to explain your dreams and hopes carefully to adults and to listen to their concerns also. See page 65 for ideas about how to communicate with your family.

Decisions for a better future

There are important decisions that you can make with your family to create new possibilities for your future.

Education and training. Education can help you feel proud of yourself, earn a better living, and live a happier and healthier life. For many girls, education opens the door to a better future. Even if you cannot go to school, there are other ways to learn to read and develop skills. For example you can study at home, join a *literacy* program, or learn a trade from a skilled person (apprenticeship). When you have new skills, you have something special to give to your community, and you can better support yourself and your family. Learning new skills can help you have more choices in your life.

Waiting to get married. Talk with your family about waiting to get married until you feel ready and until you find the right partner. Many girls are able to finish school and find work before starting families. This can help you learn more about yourself and what you want. If you wait, you may even find a partner who feels the same way about life that you do.

Waiting to have children. It is easier to raise a happy and healthy child when you wait until you and your partner feel ready to start a family. If you are thinking about having a baby, these are some things to think about: Will you be able to continue your education? How will you fulfill the child's physical needs—food, clothes, shelter, etc? Are you ready to provide the emotional support a baby needs to grow up into a healthy child? Will your partner commit himself to helping with child raising? How will your family help you?

Parents and girls can work together to organize ways for girls to learn about how the body works, sexuality and prevention of early pregnancy. This can be done at home, and programs can be held in schools, community meeting places, or places of worship.

Decisions about boys and men are difficult. Most young people begin to have loving or sexual feelings as they get older. Thinking about touching or being touched by someone in a sexual way is not unusual. (Girls may even think about another girl or woman in this way.) But people often have these feelings before they are ready to act on them.

Deciding about Boyfriends and Sex

Young women have sex for many different reasons. Some do it because they want to have a baby. Others do it because it makes them feel good or wanted. Some women feel they have very little choice because it is their duty as a wife. Some are forced to trade sex for money or for other things they need to survive, such as food, or clothes for their children, or a place to live.

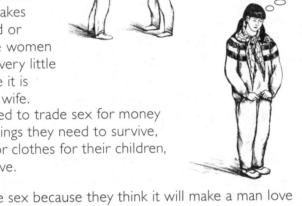

I wonder if he likes me?

➤ Only have sex when you decide that you are ready and know how to protect yourself from harm. Sex can be enjoyed by both people, but not if there is fear or shame.

Others have sex because they think it will make a man love them more. Sometimes a friend or a boyfriend can make a girl feel that she should have sex when she is not ready.

No one should have sex when she does not want to. Only have sex when you decide you are ready. Sex can be enjoyed by both people, but it is difficult to enjoy something when you feel fear or shame.

If you are ready for a sexual relationship, always protect yourself against pregnancy and disease. For more information on how, see the chapters on "Family Planning," "Sexually Transmitted Diseases," "AIDS," and "Sexual Health."

Health risks of early pregnancy

Most girls' bodies are not ready for a safe and healthy birth. Young mothers are more likely to develop toxemia (which causes fits) during pregnancy. Because their bodies may still be too small for a baby to come out, mothers under age 17 are more likely to have long, difficult labors, and blocked births. Without medical help, a woman with any of these problems can die. Blocked births can also damage the vagina, causing *urine* and *stool* to leak (see page 370). Babies born to girls younger than 17 are more likely to be born too small or too soon. If you are already pregnant, try to see a trained midwife or health worker as soon as possible to find out how to have the safest birth. For more information, see page 72.

What girls should know about having sex

- You can get pregnant the first time you have sex.
- You can get pregnant any time you have sex without a *family planning method* (even if it is only once).
- You can get pregnant even if the man thinks he did not let his seed *(sperm)* come out.
- You can get an STD or HIV/AIDS if you do not use a *condom* when you have sex with an infected person. And you cannot always tell by looking at a person if he is infected.
- It is easier for a girl to get a *sexually transmitted disease* (STD) or HIV from a boy or man than it is for her to give these diseases to him. This is because of the way sex works—because she is the 'receiver'. It is also harder to know if a girl has an infection because it is inside her body.

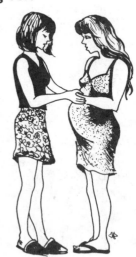

Always use a condom for protection against STDs and HIV/AIDS. But the most certain way to avoid pregnancy, STDs, and HIV/AIDS is to not have sex.

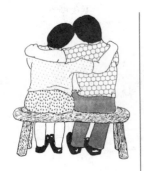

pressure to have sex

Having a relationship with no sex

Building a loving relationship takes time, caring, respect, and trust from both sides. Sex is not the only way of showing someone that you care. Having sex does not mean that you will fall in love.

You can spend personal time together without having sex. By talking and sharing experiences you can learn something more important about each other—how you view life, decisions you would make together, what kind of partner and parent you would each make, and how you feel about each other's plans for life. Touching each other (without *sexual intercourse*) can be satisfying by itself, and is not dangerous as long as it does not lead you to lose control and to have sex when you are not ready.

Talk to your boyfriend. If you are sure he is right for you, but you are not sure you want to have sex, talk about ways to wait. You may find that he is not ready for sex, either. If you respect each other, you will be able to decide together.

Talk to your friends. You may find that some girl friends are facing the same difficult choices. You can help each other find ways to have good relationships without sex. But think twice about advice from a friend who is already having sex. A friend may try to convince you to do something she is doing to make herself feel better about doing it. This is called 'peer pressure'.

PROTECTING YOURSELF IF YOU ARE READY FOR SEX

When you decide you are ready for a sexual relationship, you must protect yourself against pregnancy and disease. There are many ways to make sex safer. This means you have to **plan before you have sex.**

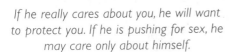

Talk to your boyfriend before you have sex. Let him know how important it is to protect yourself. If you find it hard to discuss, perhaps you can first pretend you are talking about another couple.

If he really cares about you, he will want to protect you. If he is pushing for sex, he may care only about himself.

Many communities have people who are trained to provide condoms and other family planning methods. Talk to them or ask a health worker where to get a method of protection. If you feel embarassed to ask, find someone you trust to help you. Some family planning clinics have special services for teenagers and may have trained teenagers as peer counselors who can give you information.

Since you cannot tell by looking if a man has a sexually transmitted disease or AIDS, sex is safer **only** if you **use a condom every time.** If a man has a discharge coming from his *penis* or a sore somewhere on it, he has an infection and will almost certainly give it to you!

If you had sex and notice a new discharge from your vagina, sores on your genitals, or pain in your lower belly, you could have an STD. See the chapter on "Sexually Transmitted Diseases."

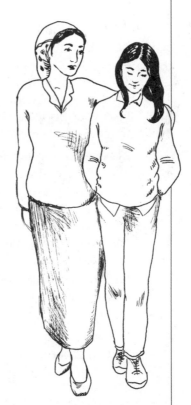

family planning

safer sex

STDs

Pressured or Forced Sex

If someone has forced you to have sex when you do not want it, it is rape.

327
rape

PRESSURE TO HAVE SEX WITH A BOYFRIEND ('DATE RAPE')

All over the world, young girls and women are forced to have sex when they do not want to. Often it is done by boyfriends who claim to love them. In some places this is called 'date rape'. The force is not only physical. You can feel pressure from words or feelings. He may say "please" or somehow make you feel guilty or ashamed if you do not have sex. This is still wrong.

No one should be made to have sex when they do not want to have it.

Prevention:

- If he wants to have sex and you do not, you can tell him you are flattered by his desire for you but that you are not ready. If you are afraid of being alone with the person, bring someone with you, or ask someone else to talk with him.

- **Say "NO" loudly** if you are pushed to have sex. Keep saying "NO" if you have to. Also say no with your body. If you say "NO," but give in with your body, he will think that you really mean "yes."

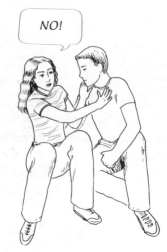

NO!

- **Move away** if you are touched in any way that you do not like. Your feelings are warning you that something worse may happen. **Make a lot of noise and be ready to run if you have to.**

- **Do not drink alcohol or take drugs**. Alcohol and drugs make you less able to use your judgement and control what happens to you.

- **Go out in groups:** In many places, young couples court or date in groups. You can still get to know a boy, but you are less likely to be pushed into having sex because you will not be alone.

- **Go only to safe places** where others can see you.

- **Plan ahead.** Decide how much touching will be too much for you. Do not get caught by your feelings and let things happen to you.

IF SOMEONE IN YOUR FAMILY TRIES TO HAVE SEX WITH YOU (INCEST)

It is never right for someone to touch you if you do not want to be touched. Family members, such as your cousin, uncle, brother, or father should not touch your genitals or any other part of your body in a sexual way. If this happens, **you need to get help.** Even if the man says he will hurt you if you tell, you need to tell an adult you trust as soon as possible. Sometimes it is best to tell someone outside your family such as a woman teacher or religious leader in your community.

327

rape

YOUNG GIRLS AND OLDER MEN

Some girls are attracted to older men. Going with an older man may seem very exciting, especially if he is well known or important in your community, or if he has money and can buy things. In some places a man who buys his girlfriend many presents is called a 'Sugar Daddy'. Often a girl who goes with an older man ends up feeling she was used for sex or treated badly, especially if the man is married or has other women.

Sometimes an older man can make a young woman feel more pressured to have sex than boys her own age can, especially if he has power over her.

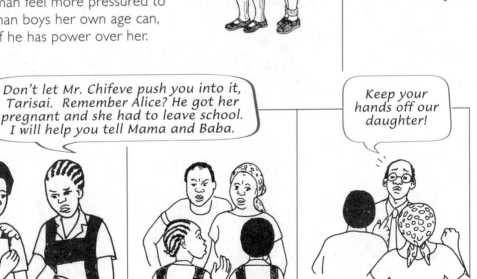

341

sex workers

TRADING GIRLS FOR MONEY OR OTHER NEEDS

Sometimes a poor family will give a young daughter to an older man to pay a family debt. Or they may trade her for money or something the family needs.

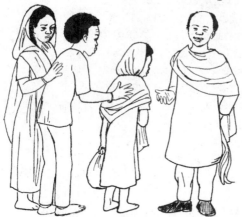

Sometimes the girls are taken away to another town or city. They think they are going to work in factories, or as maids, but they are often forced have sex for money.

If you think that you or another girl in your community is going to be sold into marriage, or sent away to work, try to get help from another adult. Perhaps an older aunt or uncle, or a woman teacher can help.

IF YOU GET PREGNANT AND DID NOT PLAN TO

You may be pregnant if you had sex and your monthly bleeding is late, your breasts hurt, you pass urine often or you feel like vomiting. See a health worker or midwife as soon as you can to find out for sure if you are pregnant.

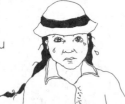

Many young girls get pregnant when they did not want to. Some of them are able to get the support they need from family and friends. For others, it is not so easy.

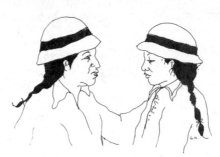

Talk to someone older who you trust.
Your life is too valuable to lose.

241

safe abortion

If you are feeling trapped by a pregnancy you did not plan and you want to end it, **please be careful in the decisions you make**. All over the world, girls and women die from trying to end pregnancies in dangerous ways. There are safe ways to end a pregnancy.

In many communities, a higher number of young women and girls are getting infected with the HIV/AIDS virus than any other group of people. There is more risk for girls who have sex with older men, but it can happen with a man of any age.

Talking with your mother or father can be hard sometimes. Your parents may want you to live by tradition, but you feel that times are changing. You may feel that your parents do not listen or try to understand you. Or you may be afraid they will get angry.

Your family can love you without agreeing with everything you say. They may get angry because they care —not because they do not like you. Try to talk with them respectfully and help them to understand you better.

Getting Help From Adults

Ideas for better communication

- Choose a good time to talk, when your parents are not busy, tired, or worried about something else.

- Share your concerns, worries and goals with them. Ask what they would do in your situation.

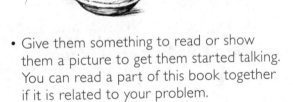

Is this a good time for us to talk?

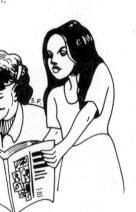

- Give them something to read or show them a picture to get them started talking. You can read a part of this book together if it is related to your problem.

- If you get angry, try not to shout. You can make your parents angry and they may think you do not respect them.

- If you have tried these things and you still cannot talk to your parents, find another older person you can talk to. It could be a teacher, the mother of a friend, an aunt, an older sister, grandmother, someone in your place of worship, or a health worker.

How mothers can help their daughters

You may have grown up in a time when girls were not allowed to have an education, plan their families, or make decisions about their lives. **Life can be different for your daughter**. If you listen to her, share your own experiences, and give her useful information, you can help her make her own good decisions. You can help her to see the good things about being a girl and a woman.

Chapter 6

In this chapter:

Most women in the world today do not get *prenatal* care or trained help during birth. They usually have their babies at home with the help of a local midwife or a family member. This chapter has information for both the pregnant woman and her helpers, about care during pregnancy, and care both during and after the birth.

For more complete information about caring for women in pregnancy and helping them with both normal and difficult births, see the Hesperian Foundation's *A Book for Midwives* (for how to order it, see the last page of this book).

Pregnancy and Childbirth

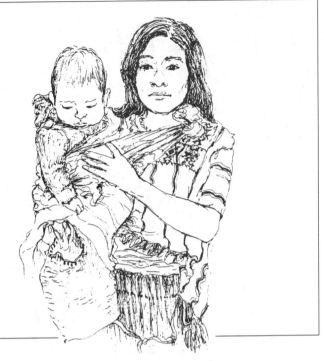

Every pregnant woman needs good health, good food, and the love and support of her family and community. Many women feel very healthy during pregnancy and do not have difficult births. Most babies are born healthy.

At the same time, pregnancy can be one of the main dangers a woman faces in her life. About half a million women die each year from problems of pregnancy and birth (this is also called maternal mortality), mostly in poorer countries.

Most of these deaths could be prevented with basic care. This chapter has information that can help pregnant women care for themselves, or help others care for them.

Without water, the crops would die; and without children, life in the community could not continue.

—Mixtec saying, Mexico

HOW TO TELL IF YOU ARE PREGNANT

- You miss your *monthly bleeding.*
- Your breasts feel sore and grow bigger.
- You feel sick to your *stomach* and sometimes *vomit.*
- You have to pass *urine* more often.
- You feel tired.

HOW TO KNOW WHEN THE BABY IS DUE

Add 9 months plus 7 days to the date when your last normal monthly bleeding began. Your baby will probably be born any time in the 2 weeks before or after this date.

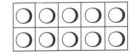

Many women know when their baby will be born by counting the passing of 10 moons.

Staying Healthy during Pregnancy

165

eating for good health

If you can take good care of yourself while pregnant, you are more likely to have a safe pregnancy and birth and a healthy baby.

- Try to **eat enough nutritious foods**. Good *nutrition* gives strength, prevents *infection*, builds a healthy baby, and helps prevent too much bleeding during birth. Remember that you are feeding both yourself and your baby. Use iodized salt to make sure your baby will not suffer from mental slowness.

- **Sleep and rest whenever you can.** If you work standing up, try to sit or lie down several times during the day.

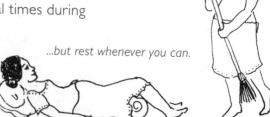

Do your daily work...

...but rest whenever you can.

76

prenatal care

➤ *Read about the 'Danger signs during pregnancy', starting on page 73, to learn when it is important to see a health worker.*

- **Go for prenatal (before-birth) check-ups** to make sure there are no problems, and to find problems before they become serious. If you have never had a *tetanus* immunization, get one as soon as you can. Get at least 2 before the end of the pregnancy.

- **Keep clean.** Bathe or wash regularly and clean your teeth every day.

- **Practice squeezing exercises,** so your *vagina* will be stronger after the birth (see page 371).

- Try to **get daily exercise.** If you sit down at work, try to walk a little every day. But try not to tire yourself.

- **Get treatment if you think you have a *sexually transmitted disease* (STD) or other infection.**

261

STDs

- **Avoid taking modern or *plant medicines,*** unless a health worker who knows you are pregnant says it is OK.

- **Do not drink alcohol or smoke or chew tobacco** during pregnancy. They are bad for the mother and can harm the developing baby.

- **Avoid pesticides, herbicides, or factory chemicals.** They can harm the developing baby. Do not touch or work near them, or breathe in their *fumes.* Never store food or water in their containers.

➤ *If there is malaria where you live, sleep under a bed net to avoid being bitten by mosquitos.*

- **Stay away from a child with a rash all over its body.** It may be caused by *German Measles,* which can harm the baby.

When you are pregnant your body changes and you may have some of the following common problems. But remember, most of these problems are normal in pregnancy.

Common Problems during Pregnancy

SICK STOMACH (NAUSEA)

Although it is often called 'morning sickness', during pregnancy you may feel sick to your stomach at any time during the day or even all day long. It usually goes away by the end of the 3rd or 4th month.

What to do:

- Drink a cup of ginger or cinnamon tea 2 or 3 times a day, before meals.
- Eat small meals often, and avoid foods that are oily or hard to digest.
- Lick a lemon.
- Ask the midwives in your community for good local plant medicines or remedies.

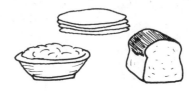

To help with morning sickness...

...try eating a biscuit, a tortilla, a piece of bread, a chapati, or a little rice or porridge when you wake up in the morning.

IMPORTANT *See a health worker if you vomit so much that you cannot keep any food down, or if you are losing weight. Also watch for signs of dehydration (see page 298).*

HEARTBURN OR INDIGESTION

Heartburn causes a burning feeling in the throat and chest. It is most common in later pregnancy, after eating or when lying down.

What to do:

- Eat several small meals instead of one large meal.
- Avoid spicy or oily foods.
- Drink plenty of water and other clear liquids.
- Try not to lie down right after eating.
- Sleep with your head higher than your stomach.
- Take a cup of milk or yogurt, some bicarbonate of soda in a glass of water, or calcium carbonate (antacid).

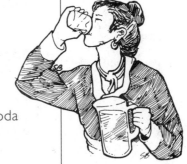

DISCHARGE FROM THE VAGINA

During pregnancy, it is normal to have more white *discharge* than usual from the *vagina*. But if the discharge itches, burns, or has a bad smell, you may have an infection of the genitals, which should be treated. If the discharge is bloody or has mucus in it, or if there is a lot and it looks like water, see a health worker. You may be starting labor too early.

infections of the genitals

SWOLLEN VEINS (VARICOSE VEINS)

Blue swollen *veins* in the legs and around the vagina are called varicose veins. They are caused by the weight of the growing baby. They can become quite large and painful.

What to do:

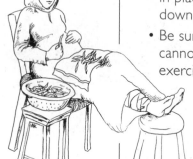

- Try not to stand up for too long. If you have to stand, walk in place or move your feet and legs. When you are sitting down, put your feet up as often as possible.
- Be sure to walk every day. If you have a *disability* and cannot walk, ask someone in your family to help move and exercise your legs.
  - If the problem is severe, wrap your legs with cloths. Begin wrapping at the ankles and work up to just below the knee. The bandage should be tighter around the ankle and looser further up the leg. Take off the bandages at night.

Women with swollen veins should try to put their feet up when they can, and wrap their legs if the swelling is very bad.

CONSTIPATION (DIFFICULTY PASSING STOOL)

Pregnancy makes the *bowels* work more slowly. This can make the *stool* harder, so it is more difficult to pass.

*What to do (these things also help **prevent** constipation):*

- Drink at least 8 glasses of liquid every day.
- Get regular exercise.
- If you are taking *iron* tablets, try taking only one a day with fruit or vegetable juice. Or skip a few days.
- Eat plenty of fruits, vegetables, and foods with fiber—like whole grains and cassava (manioc) root.
- **Do not take *laxatives*.** They only solve the problem for a short while and then you need to take more.

PILES (HEMORRHOIDS)

Hemorrhoids are swollen veins around the anus. They often itch, burn, or bleed. Constipation makes them worse.

What to do:

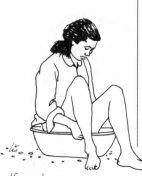

If you have hemorrhoids, sitting in cool water can help with the pain.

- Sit in a basin or pan of cool water to relieve the pain.
- Follow the advice above for preventing constipation.
- Soak some clean cloth in witch hazel (a liquid plant medicine) if you can find it, and put it on the painful area.
- Kneel with your *buttocks* in the air. This can help relieve the pain.

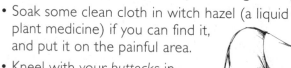

LEG CRAMPS

Pregnant women often get foot or leg *cramps*—especially at night, or when they stretch or point their toes down. Leg cramps may be caused by not enough *calcium* in the diet.

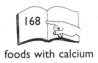

168

foods with calcium

What to do:

- Eat plenty of foods that contain calcium, such as milk, cheese, sesame seeds, and green leafy vegetables.

- If your foot or leg cramps:

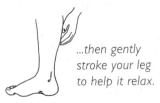

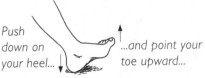

Push down on your heel... ...and point your toe upward...

...then gently stroke your leg to help it relax.

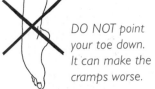

DO NOT point your toe down. It can make the cramps worse.

LOW-BACK PAIN

Low-back pain is caused by the weight of the growing baby.

What to do:

- Ask someone to rub or *massage* your back.
- Ask your family for help with some of the heavy work.
- Take care to stand and sit with your back straight.
- Sleep on your side with a pillow or rolled up cloth between your knees.
- Do the 'angry cat' exercise for a few minutes, 2 times each day, and whenever your back hurts.

398

lifting and carrying heavy loads

Angry cat exercise

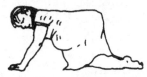 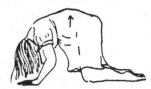 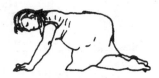

Start on hands and knees with back flat.

Push the lower back up.

Return to flat back. Repeat.

SWELLING OF THE FEET AND LEGS

Some swelling of the feet is normal during pregnancy—especially for women who must stand all day.

What to do:

- Put your feet up as often as you can during the day.
- When resting, lie on your left side.
- If your feet are very swollen, or they are swollen already when you wake up in the morning, or your hands and face also swell, these are signs of danger during pregnancy. See page 74.

74

swelling of the hands and face

Risks and Danger Signs during Pregnancy

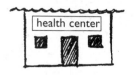

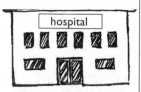

A woman who is likely to have a dangerous birth should plan to have her baby in a health center or hospital.

WOMEN WHO HAVE EXTRA RISKS

Women with any of the following problems can have more dangerous pregnancies and births. They should plan to go to a health center or hospital for the birth. If possible, they should try to get prenatal care during pregnancy.

- **Weak blood** (*anemia*) makes a woman more likely to bleed heavily (hemorrhage) during birth, become ill after childbirth, or even die. For more on anemia, see the next page.
- **Sugar sickness** (*diabetes*) often causes very serious problems for the mother and the baby. The baby can die before birth or sometimes grows very large and gets stuck in the pelvis.
- *High blood pressure* can lead to severe headaches, *fits,* and even death.
- **Older mothers** who have had many babies often have long, difficult labors, and heavy bleeding after the birth.
- **Mothers under the age of 17** are more likely to have *toxemia* (which causes fits), long, difficult labors, babies born too early (premature), and blocked births, which may damage the *bladder,* vagina, and womb (see page 370).
- **Mothers who had problems with past pregnancies**—such as fits, birth by operation, heavy bleeding, a too-early or too-small baby, or a baby born dead—are more likely to have problems in another pregnancy or birth.
- **Women with disabilities**, especially women with a loss of feeling in the body or difficulty walking can have problems during both pregnancy and birth (see page 145.)

Other women who should try to give birth at a health center or hospital

Some women—who have none of the extra risks listed above—are still likely to have dangerous births. These women should also try to give birth at a health center or hospital:

- **A woman with a baby in the wrong position for birth at the end of pregnancy** (see page 75) can have a long, difficult labor. The mother, the baby, or both may die.
- **Women carrying twins** often have one baby in the wrong position for birth. Also, these mothers are more likely to bleed after birth.
- **Women who have been infibulated** can have severe tearing of the *genitals* during the birth. This can cause great pain, heavy blood loss, and *infection* (see the chapter on female circumcision, page 464).

DANGER SIGNS DURING PREGNANCY

In addition to the problems just listed, these danger signs may occur during pregnancy. A woman with any of these signs may be in serious danger and should see a health worker. See the next few pages for more about them.

- feeling very weak or tired
- pain in the belly
- bleeding from the vagina
- fever
- swelling of hands and face, or bad headache and *blurred eyesight*

Feeling very weak or tired (anemia)

If you feel very weak or tired, you could be anemic (see page 172). Women who are very anemic are much more likely to have heavy bleeding after the baby is born.

What to do:

- Eat foods rich in iron—meat, fish, chicken, eggs, beans, peas, and leafy green vegetables.
- Take 325 mg of iron 2 times a day, and 1mg of folic acid once a day, until the baby is born. If you take iron tablets with fruits like oranges, mangoes, or papayas, your body uses the iron better.

167

foods rich in iron

Pain in the lower belly (abdomen)

1. **Strong, constant pain in the first 3 months** may be caused by a pregnancy that is growing outside the womb in the tube (a *tubal* pregnancy). As the tube stretches, it causes pain. If the pregnancy grows large enough, the tube will burst and bleed. **This is very dangerous.** You will bleed inside your abdomen and may die.

   Signs of tubal pregnancy:
   - missed monthly bleeding, **and**
   - pain in the lower *abdomen* on one side, **and**
   - slight bleeding from the vagina
   - feeling dizzy, weak, or faint

   What to do:
   Go to the nearest hospital.

➤ *Strong pain in the abdomen does not always mean something is wrong with a pregnancy. For information about other possible causes, see pages 353 to 357.*

2. **Strong pain that comes and goes (cramping) in the first 6 months** could mean you are losing the pregnancy (having a *miscarriage*). See page 234.

3. **Strong, constant pain in late pregnancy.** This could mean the afterbirth (*placenta*) is coming off the wall of the womb. **This is very dangerous. You could die if you do not get help. Go to the nearest hospital.**

4. **Pain that comes and goes in the 7th or 8th month** could mean you are going into labor too early (see page 75).

TRANSPORT!

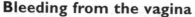

Bleeding from the vagina

1. **Bleeding early in pregnancy.** Light bleeding from the vagina during the first 3 months of pregnancy can be normal. But if you have pain with the light bleeding, it could mean a pregnancy is developing outside the womb, which is very dangerous (see page 73). If the bleeding gets heavier and stronger than a normal monthly bleeding, you are probably losing the pregnancy (having a miscarriage).

234
miscarriage

2. **Bleeding later in pregnancy.** Bleeding after the first 3 months can mean there is something wrong with the afterbirth (*placenta*). **Both you and the baby are in danger.**

What to do:

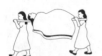

TRANSPORT!

- **Go to the nearest hospital.**
- On the way, lie down with your feet up.
- Do not put anything in your vagina.

Fever

High fever, especially along with shivering, body aches and severe headache, can be caused by *malaria*. Treatment for malaria depends on where you live. See **Where There Is No Doctor** for more information.

Swelling of the hands and face or severe headache and blurred vision (toxemia)

Some swelling in the legs and ankles is normal in pregnancy. But swelling of the hands and face can be a sign of toxemia, especially if you also have headaches, blurred vision, or pains in your abdomen. Toxemia can cause fits, and both you and the baby can die.

What to do:

- Find someone who can check your blood pressure. Go to a health center or hospital if necessary.
- Rest as often as possible, lying down on your left side.
- Try to eat more foods with a lot of protein every day.
- Plan to have the birth in a health center or hospital.

166
foods rich in protein

Danger signs of toxemia

- swollen hands and face
- severe headache
- blurred vision
- dizziness
- sudden, severe pain high in the stomach
- blood pressure 160/100 or higher (see page 528)

TRANSPORT!

IMPORTANT *If a woman has any of the danger signs of toxemia, she needs medical help fast. If she is already having fits, see page 87.*

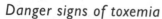
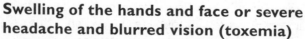

BABY IN THE WRONG POSITION WHEN LABOR STARTS

If the baby is buttocks first (breech) when labor starts, the birth can be more difficult. If the baby is lying sideways when labor starts, the baby cannot be born without an *operation*. (Turn the page to learn how to check the baby's position.)

➤ *If the baby's head is down, the birth is more likely to go well.*

Positions that cause difficult or dangerous births

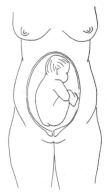

Baby with buttocks first (breech)

If the baby's head is up, *the birth may be more difficult. It may be safer for the mother to give birth in a hospital.*

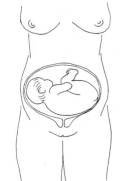

Baby lying sideways

If the baby is lying sideways, *the mother should give birth in a hospital. She and the baby are in danger. Birth may not be possible without an operation.*

During the last month of pregnancy, it may be possible to change the baby's position by lying in this position for 10 minutes, 2 times a day:

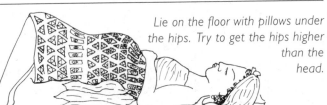

Lie on the floor with pillows under the hips. Try to get the hips higher than the head.

Do this exercise every day with an empty stomach, until the baby changes to a head-down position and then stop. The baby's position should be checked each week.

- If labor starts and the baby is still sideways, the mother must go to a health center or hospital where the baby's position can be changed, or where she can have an operation. Without medical help, the mother and her baby will almost certainly die.
- If labor starts and the baby is still buttocks first, see page 90.

TRANSPORT!

IMPORTANT *DO NOT try to change the baby's position by hand yourself unless you have been trained to do it and have done it before successfully. You can tear the womb and harm both the mother and the baby.*

IF LABOR STARTS TOO EARLY (BEFORE THE 8TH OR 9TH MONTH)

Some babies born too early might not live. A woman may be able to slow or stop labor by lying in bed with her hips raised, and resting until the labor stops (see the picture above). If she can go to a hospital, they may be able to stop the labor. Even if they cannot stop the labor, they can sometimes keep the baby alive. (Also see page 94 for how to care for a baby born too early.)

Prenatal Care (Check-ups during Pregnancy)

➤ *Prenatal check-ups can help you decide the best place to have your baby: at home, or at a health center or hospital.*

Prenatal check-ups are important to find and take care of problems early—before they become dangerous. Good prenatal care is not difficult to give and does not require very expensive equipment. Many birth attendants, midwives and health centers, as well as hospitals, can give this care. It can save many lives.

If you are pregnant, try to have at least 3 check-ups:

1. As soon as you think you are pregnant.
2. Around the 6th month of pregnancy.
3. A month before the baby is due.

A midwife, birth attendant, or health worker will ask about past pregnancies and births, including any problems, such as a lot of bleeding or babies that died. This information can help you both prepare for similar problems in this pregnancy and birth. A midwife may also be able to:

- make sure a woman is eating well enough and suggest ways for her to eat better food, if necessary.
- give iron and folic acid tablets, which help prevent anemia.
- examine the mother, to make sure she is healthy and that the baby is growing well.
- give vaccinations to prevent tetanus, a disease that can kill both mothers and babies (see page 161).
- give medicine to prevent malaria if it is common in the area.
- give tests for *HIV* (see page 288) and *syphilis,* along with other *sexually transmitted diseases* (see page 261).

What to expect at a prenatal check-up

A birth attendant or midwife should do these things at a prenatal check-up:

- Check the eyelids and finger nails for signs of anemia (see page 172).

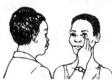

- Check the hands and face for swelling (see page 74).

- Check blood pressure (see page 528).

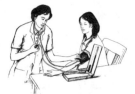

- Check the growth of the baby in the womb. Normally the womb will grow 2 fingers each month. At 4½ months it is usually at the level of the navel. **If the womb seems too small or too big or grows too fast,** it may mean there is a problem.

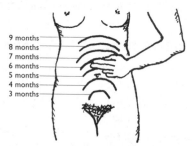

9 months
8 months
7 months
6 months
5 months
4 months
3 months

To check whether the baby is healthy, a midwife may listen for the baby's heartbeat. It may be possible to hear it by putting one ear against the woman's abdomen, but often you cannot tell the baby's heartbeat apart from the mother's. It is easier with a fetoscope. Another sign the baby is healthy is if the mother feels the baby move every day, and if she has felt it move on the day of the check-up.

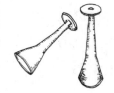

fetoscope

Checking the baby's position

During pregnancy, it is common for a baby to change positions several times in the womb. By the end of the pregnancy, the baby should be lying in the womb with its head down. This is the best position for birth. To make sure the baby is head down, feel for the head like this:

1. Have the mother breathe out all the way. Using both hands, feel the baby.

With the thumb and 2 fingers, push in here, just above the *pubic bone*.

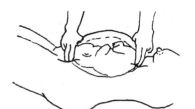

With the other hand, feel the top of the womb.

The baby's bottom is larger and wider...

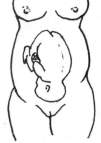

...and its head is harder and more round.

So bottom up feels larger high up...

...and bottom down feels larger low down.

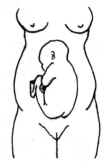

2. Push gently from side to side, first with one hand, then with the other. At the same time, feel what happens to the baby's body with the other hand as you push.

3. Just before birth, a baby will move lower in the womb to get ready for birth. So, late in pregnancy, you may not be able to feel the baby's head move.

If the baby's buttocks are pushed gently sideways, the baby's whole body will also move.

But if the head is pushed gently sideways, it will bend at the neck and the back will not move.

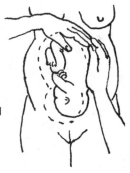

If the baby is still high in the womb, you can move the head a little. But if it has already moved lower, you cannot move it.

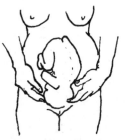

A woman's first baby sometimes moves lower about 2 weeks before labor begins. Second or later babies often do not do this until labor starts.

Preparing for Labor and Birth

THINGS TO HAVE READY BEFORE BIRTH

A pregnant woman should have these things ready by the seventh month of pregnancy:

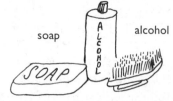

soap

alcohol

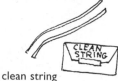

clean string

➤ If you do not have a new razor blade, you can use rust-free scissors or a knife if you boil them for 20 minutes just before cutting the cord.

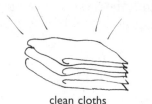

clean cloths

new razor blade

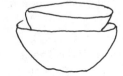

two bowls, one for washing, one for holding the afterbirth

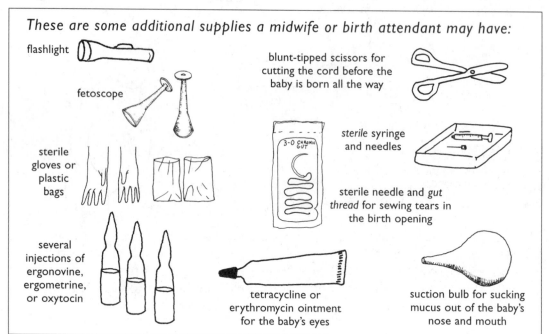

These are some additional supplies a midwife or birth attendant may have:

flashlight

fetoscope

blunt-tipped scissors for cutting the cord before the baby is born all the way

sterile gloves or plastic bags

sterile syringe and needles

sterile needle and *gut thread* for sewing tears in the birth opening

several injections of ergonovine, ergometrine, or oxytocin

tetracycline or erythromycin ointment for the baby's eyes

suction bulb for sucking mucus out of the baby's nose and mouth

---

This is also the time to:

- plan transportation in case you need to go to the hospital.

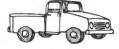

- clean the birth place.

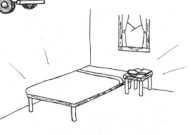

HELPING A WOMAN GIVE BIRTH

If you are pregnant, read this information to know what to expect during *labor* and after the baby is born. It will also make you better able to help other women during birth.

If you are helping a woman give birth, you can make a big difference in helping her have a safe and healthy birth. Remember that most babies are born without problems.

Stay calm and cheerful. Reassure the mother so that she will not be afraid. Let her know that you trust her ability to give birth.

DO

- Keep your nails clean and cut short.
- Wash your hands with soap and clean water. Let them dry in the air.
- Know which women have extra risks and learn the 'Danger Signs during Pregnancy' (see page 73). Make sure the mother gives birth in a health center or hospital if she has any of these risks or danger signs.
- Learn the 'Danger Signs during Labor' (page 85). Take the woman to a hospital if she has any of these signs.
- Treat her with kindness and respect.

preventing infection

➤ *For safe childbirth practice the 3 cleans:*

1. Clean hands

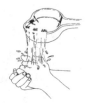

IMPORTANT *Protect yourself from HIV and hepatitis by wearing clean gloves during a birth. If you do not have gloves, use washed plastic bags.*

2. Clean place to give birth

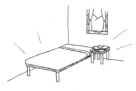

DO NOT

- Do not put your fingers or anything else in the woman's vagina. Checking how much the womb has opened does not help the baby to be born, and may cause a dangerous infection.
- Do not give any medicine to speed up labor or to make labor stronger. These medicines can kill the mother and the baby. (Medicines that cause the womb to contract should only be used to stop bleeding after the baby is born.)
- Do not tell her to push before she is ready. When it is time for the baby to be born, she will feel like she has to pass stool and will start pushing on her own.
- Do not push on the outside of her womb to make the baby come out faster. This can tear her womb or cause the placenta to separate from the womb too soon. Both the mother and the baby can die.

3. Clean tool to cut the cord

Giving Birth

SIGNS THAT LABOR IS NEAR

These 3 signs show that labor is starting or will start soon. They may not all happen, and they can happen in any order.

1. **Clear or pink-colored mucus comes out of the vagina.** During pregnancy, the opening to the womb (*cervix*) is plugged with thick mucus. This protects the baby and womb from infection. When the cervix starts to open, it releases this plug of mucus and also a little blood.

2. **Clear water comes out of the vagina.** The *bag of waters* can break just before labor begins, or at any time during labor.

3. **Pains *(contractions)* begin.** At first contractions may come 10 or 20 minutes apart or more. Real labor does not begin until contractions become regular (have about the same amount of time between each one).

When any one of these signs occurs, it is time to get ready for the birth. Here is a list of things you can do:

- Let your midwife know that labor is starting.

- Make sure that the supplies for the birth are ready.

- Wash yourself, especially your genitals.

- Continue to eat small meals and drink whenever you are thirsty.

- Rest while you can.

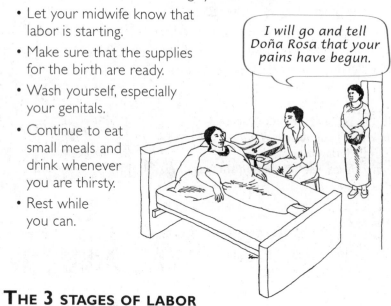

I will go and tell Doña Rosa that your pains have begun.

THE 3 STAGES OF LABOR

Every birth has these 3 parts.

Stage 1 begins when contractions start to open the cervix and ends when the cervix is fully open. When it is the mother's first birth, this stage usually lasts 10 to 20 hours or more. In later births, it often lasts from 7 to 10 hours. It can vary a lot.

Stage 2 begins when the cervix is open and ends when the baby is born. This stage is usually easier than Stage 1, and should not take more than about 2 hours.

Stage 3 begins when the baby is born and ends when the placenta comes out.

Stage 1: The cervix opens

To make sure that labor is going well, check:

1. **How long has the woman been having contractions and how often do they come?** At first, they may come every 10 or 20 minutes and last for a minute or less. After some time they will come more quickly—about every 2 to 5 minutes—and each one will last longer, about a minute and a half, until the baby is born. If she has had a contraction every 10 minutes or faster for more than 1 day and 1 night (24 hours) and the baby is not ready to be born, see 'Too long labor', page 86.

2. **Have her waters broken?** If they have, ask when. If it has been more than a day, see 'Waters break and labor does not start in a few hours', page 85. If the waters are green or brown, see 'Green or brown waters', page 86.

3. **Is the baby in a head-down position?** Feel the mother's abdomen (see page 77). If the baby is sideways or breech, you must take her to a health center or hospital.

too long labor, 86

waters break and labor does not start, 85

green or brown waters, 86

checking the baby's position, 77

You can also help the mother by reassuring her that she is doing well and by encouraging her to:

- stay active.
- eat light foods, not heavy or oily foods.
- drink as much sweet liquid and warm tea as she wants.
- pass urine often.
- take deep, slow breaths during contractions, and to breathe normally between them.
- not push until she feels a strong need to push (see page 82).

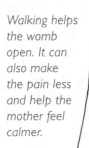

Walking helps the womb open. It can also make the pain less and help the mother feel calmer.

During labor, let the woman choose the most comfortable positions. For many years, doctors and some midwives asked women to lie on their backs, but this is often a difficult position for going through labor and giving birth. Encourage a woman in labor to try different positions. Most women find it easier to push the baby out when they are kneeling, squatting or sitting propped up.

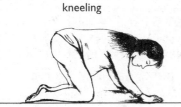

kneeling

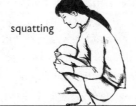

squatting

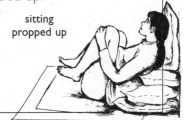

sitting propped up

Stage 2: Pushing the baby out

Signs that it is time to push (this means the cervix is fully open):

- The mother feels a strong need to push. It may feel like needing to pass stool.
- During contractions, you can see the mother's bottom bulging and you may see the baby's head at the opening of the vagina. At first, the baby's head moves back inside between contractions.

What to do:

- Stay with the mother all the time and reassure her that she and the baby are doing well.
- Each contraction will come with a very strong urge to push. When the mother feels like pushing, have her take a deep breath and push as if she were passing stool, but with all her strength. Many women find it helpful to moan or groan in a deep voice with the pushes.
- Make sure that everything is going well and is ready for the birth. If the woman has been pushing for more than 2 hours, see 'Too-long labor,' page 86.

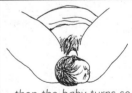

86

too-long labor

Birth of the head

When the baby's head stays at the opening of the vagina, even between contractions, it is time for the head to be born:

1. Tell the mother not to push hard, but to give little grunts or little pushes.
2. Allow the head to come out slowly, between contractions. This will help to prevent the mother's skin from tearing.
3. After the head is born, wipe the baby's mouth and nose with a clean cloth.

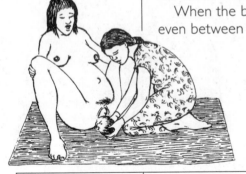

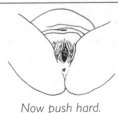

Now push hard.	*Now do not push hard.*	*The head usually comes out face down...*	*...then the baby turns so the shoulders can be born.*

Birth of the shoulders

To help the shoulders come out:

1. Gently hold the baby's head and guide it toward the mother's back (away from her abdomen). This lets the front shoulder be born first. **Never pull or twist the head.**
2. The rest of the baby will then come out easily. **Be ready!** Hold the baby so it does not fall.

Care of the baby at birth

A healthy baby will start breathing, move its arms and legs, and start crying right away. To care for the baby:

- Wipe its mouth and nose with a clean cloth. To help the *mucus* drain, keep the baby's head lower than its body. If there is a lot of fluid or mucus, remove it with a suction bulb (see page 86).

- Give the baby to the mother right away. Put a clean cloth around both of them. Do this as soon as possible so the baby stays warm.

- Put the baby to the mother's breast immediately. When the baby sucks, the mother's womb tightens and stops the bleeding. This will also help the *placenta* come out more quickly.

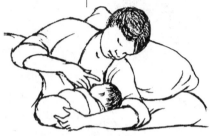

- Tie and cut the *cord* only when it turns white and stops pulsing. To prevent tetanus, a serious disease that kills many babies, cut the cord close to the baby's body.

To cut the cord:

1. When the cord stops pulsing, put 2 clean ties around it, using square knots. Put one tie about 2 finger widths from the baby and put the other one about 2 more finger widths farther from the baby.

The first loop of a square knot...

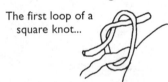

...the second loop of a square knot.

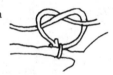

2. Cut the cord between these 2 ties with a new razor blade. If you must use something else to cut the cord, make sure it has been boiled for 20 minutes.

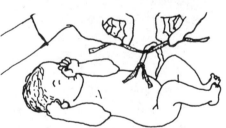

Tie the cord in 2 places before cutting. The chance of a baby getting tetanus is greater when the cord is cut far from its body

IMPORTANT *To avoid tetanus and other infections, the cord and anything that touches it must be very clean. Never put dirt or animal dung on the cord stump.*

Care of the eyes

To prevent infection from gonorrhea, put 1% tetracycline, erythromycin, or chloramphenicol eye ointment in each eye within an hour of birth.

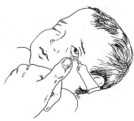

Pull down the lower lid to put a little bit of ointment inside. Putting ointment outside the eye does no good.

274

problems in newborn babies

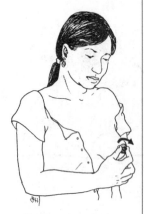

Rolling the nipples can help the womb contract and stop bleeding.

➤ *When the placenta is out, put it in a bowl and check it to make sure it is all there.*

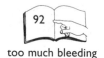

too much bleeding

Stage 3: The placenta comes out

When the baby is wrapped and at the mother's breast, it is time for the placenta to come out.

Watch the vagina to see when the cord gets longer. This means the placenta is separating from the womb. Also watch to make sure there is no heavy bleeding. When the cord lengthens, tell the mother to push out the placenta. **Do not pull on the cord.**

If the placenta does not come out right away and there is no bleeding, it is OK to wait up to 1 hour.

To help the placenta come out:

- Have the mother squat and push. If she cannot push, have her blow into a bottle, sneeze, or cough.
- Ask the mother to pass urine.
- Encourage the baby to nurse, or have someone roll the mother's nipples. This will help make her womb contract.
- If nothing else works, give her an injection of 10 milligrams of oxytocin in her hip or thigh.
- If the mother starts to bleed, see page 92.

Check the Placenta

Usually the placenta comes out whole, but sometimes a piece gets left inside. This could cause bleeding or infection later. To see if everything has come out, check the top and bottom of the placenta, and the membranes from the bag of waters.

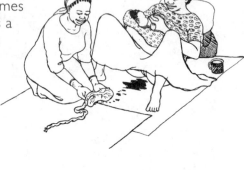

If the mother is bleeding, or there seems to be a piece of the placenta or membranes missing, follow the instructions on page 92 for too much bleeding.

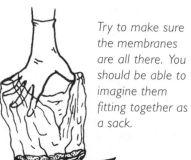

Try to make sure the membranes are all there. You should be able to imagine them fitting together as a sack.

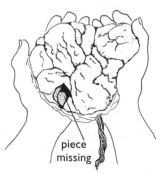

piece missing

DANGER SIGNS DURING LABOR

- waters break but labor does not start
- baby lying sideways
- bleeding before the baby is born
- too long labor
- green or brown waters
- fever
- fits or convulsions

Waters break but labor does not start

Most women will start labor within 24 hours after their waters break. If labor has not started after 1 day and 1 night, the woman and her baby could get a serious infection.

What to do:

- The mother must not put anything in her vagina. She should not have sex. This could cause an infection.

- If she has a fever or there is a bad smell in the vagina, an infection is starting. She needs *intravenous (IV) antibiotics.* Even if labor starts, the woman and her baby could die. **Go to a health center or hospital**.

- Try to get labor started. The woman should swallow 2 tablespoons of castor oil, roll her nipples, or have someone suck them for awhile every few hours until labor starts. There may also be special local teas that women use to start labor. If labor still does not start after a few more hours, she should go to a health center or hospital.

DANGER!! Do not use injections to start labor. They can cause contractions that are so strong that they can kill the woman or the baby.

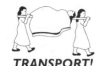

TRANSPORT!

Baby lying sideways (transverse)

If labor has started and the baby's arm comes out first, it almost always means the baby is sideways. Check the baby's position (see pages 75 and 77). A baby lying sideways cannot be born without an operation. Do not try to change the position of the baby once labor has started. This can tear the womb or separate the placenta from the womb wall.

What to do:

Take the mother to the hospital.

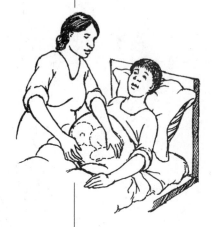

Bleeding before the baby is born

Some light, pink-colored fluid, or mucus and brown blood during labor is normal. But if the mother is bleeding bright red blood, it could mean that the placenta is separating from the womb wall or is covering the opening of the womb. **This is very dangerous.**

What to do:

Take the mother to the hospital right away. If possible, start an IV and give her IV fluids.

TRANSPORT!

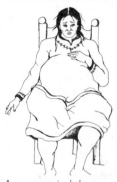

A woman in labor should not see the sun rise twice.
—Proverb from Niger

TRANSPORT!

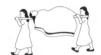

TRANSPORT!

➤ *A woman who is only a little warm may just need to drink more fluids.*

TRANSPORT!

Too-long labor

If the mother has been in good strong labor for more than 1 day and 1 night, or she has been pushing for more than 2 hours without any signs that the baby will be born soon, there may be a problem.

What to do:

If her contractions are not coming every 2 or 3 minutes and lasting for a full minute, she may not be in good labor yet. Encourage her to sleep. If she cannot sleep, ask her to roll her nipples and walk between contractions to help labor get stronger. Encourage her to drink and eat light foods. Fruit juices or tea with sugar can give her energy.

If the mother is getting *exhausted* and she has been in labor for more than 24 hours, or has been pushing for more than 2 hours, take her to a health center or hospital. She may need medicines to help her labor or an operation for the baby to be born.

Green or brown waters

Brown or green waters can mean that the baby is in trouble.

What to do:

If it is still early in labor or if the mother has not started pushing, it is best for this baby to be born in a hospital.

If the mother is in Stage 2 of labor and the baby is going to be born soon, have the mother push as hard as she can and get the baby out quickly. As soon as the baby's head is born, wipe its mouth and nose with a clean cloth or use a suction bulb to suck the mucus out. Keep the baby's head lower than its body to help the mucus come out.

Fever

Fever is usually a sign of infection.

What to do:

Touch the woman's forehead with the back of one of your hands, and touch your own forehead with your other hand. (See page 526 for taking *temperature* with a thermometer if you have one.) If she feels a little warmer than you, she may just need fluids. Give her plenty of water, tea, juice, or soda pop. Remind her to pass urine every few hours.

If she feels very hot to touch and she has chills, take her to a health center or hospital. She needs antibiotics right away. Give ampicillin, 500 mg by mouth every 6 hours, or inject 1.2 million Units of procaine penicillin into her buttock or thigh, every 12 hours until you can get to a hospital.

Fits, or very swollen hands and face (toxemia)

If the mother starts to have a fit:

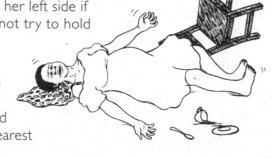

- Put something under her head to protect it, and put her on her left side if possible. But do not try to hold her down.
- Keep her cool.
- Send someone to get emergency transportation and take her to the nearest hospital.

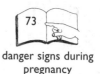

danger signs during pregnancy

TRANSPORT!

➤ *For more information about these medicines, see the "Green Pages."*

If possible, give one of the following medicines:

- magnesium sulfate, 50% solution. Inject 10 ml into each buttock muscle once. Repeat after 4 hours if needed.
- diazepam.

How to give diazepam

A woman having fits cannot swallow pills, and diazepam may not work well when injected into a muscle during a fit. So it is usually best to put either liquid (injectable) diazepam or diazepam pills that have been crushed and mixed with water into the mother's *rectum*.

Liquid diazepam. Give 20 mg after the first convulsion. If there are other convulsions, give 15 mg after each one.

To give liquid diazepam, first load a syringe and then **TAKE OFF the needle**.

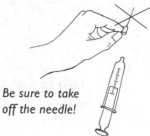

Be sure to take off the needle!

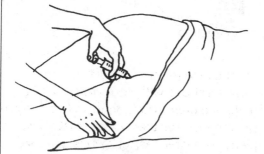

Put the barrel of the syringe gently into the rectum about 2 inches and empty it inside. Hold the barrel of the syringe in place for at least 5 minutes. It will act as a plug to keep the medicine from coming out. If some fluid leaks out of the anus, it is OK to give 5 mg more.

Diazepam pills. If you only have diazepam pills, you can crush them and mix them with water. The pills will not completely dissolve. Crush 20 mg of pills.

To give the pills, draw the water and pill mixture up into a syringe with the needle already removed, and put it into the rectum—the same as above.

Difficult Births

Cord comes out before the baby

If the cord comes out before the baby's head, the cord gets squeezed when the head comes down. The baby can die or get brain damage from too little *oxygen*.

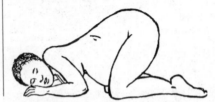

cord showing at opening of vagina

What to do:

If the baby is coming very fast and is almost born, have the mother push as hard as she can in a squatting position and get the baby out.

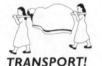

TRANSPORT!

If the baby is not coming quickly, put the mother in the knee-chest position, help her to stop pushing, and get her to a hospital. The baby needs to be born by operation.

Baby's shoulders get stuck

If a baby is very big, the shoulders can sometimes get stuck after the head is born. The baby can die or be harmed if it is not born soon.

What to do:

1. Have the mother get on her hands and knees, and push. The stuck shoulder will usually slip out and the baby can be born.

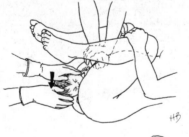

2. If the hands-and-knees position does not work, bring the mother's bottom to the edge of the bed. Ask her to pull her knees back as far as she can while someone else pushes straight down just above the mother's pubic bone. Have the mother push as hard as she can during her next contraction.

DO NOT try to pull the baby out. This can hurt or kill the baby.

3. If the baby still does not come out, slide your hand along the baby's neck until your fingers are touching the baby's back. Push the baby's upper shoulder forward at the same time the mother pushes with a contraction.

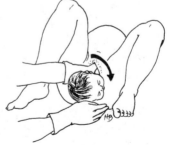

IMPORTANT *DO NOT let anyone push on the TOP of the mother's womb. This can make the baby more stuck and can tear the mother's womb.*

Twins

When a mother is carrying more than one baby, it is best for her to give birth in a health center or hospital. It is more likely that one baby will be in a wrong position, or that there will be heavy bleeding after the birth. But if you must help a woman give birth to twins here is what to do:

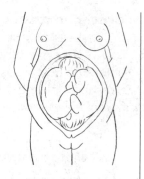

What to do:

1. Deliver the first baby just as you would any single baby.

2. When you cut the first baby's cord, carefully tie the end that is coming out of the mother. If you do not, the second baby could die.

3. DO NOT give any injections.

4. Give the first baby to the mother to begin breastfeeding. This will help get the second baby born.

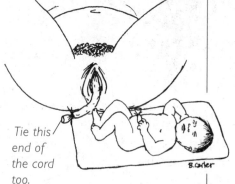

Tie this end of the cord too.

cutting the cord

5. The second baby should be born within 15 to 20 minutes. Feel for its position. If the second baby is sideways, you can gently try to turn it. If it will not turn easily, you must go to the hospital.

TRANSPORT!

Cord around the baby's neck

Sometimes the cord is wrapped around the baby's neck. Usually you can just loosen the cord and slip it over the baby's head or shoulder.

If the cord is very tight and seems to be holding the baby back, you may have to tie the cord in 2 places and then cut it. Use clean string and clean scissors. Be careful not to cut the baby or the mother.

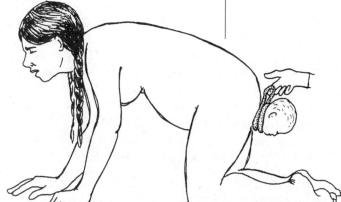

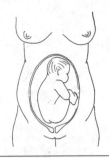

Breech birth

A breech birth is when the baby comes out buttocks first. (See page 77 for how to check the baby's position before birth.) If this is a first baby, it may be best for the woman to have the baby in the hospital. If she stays at home, try to have an experienced midwife or doctor there to help her.

What to do for breech birth:

1. Help the mother keep from pushing until you see the baby's bottom at the vagina. It is very important for the cervix to be fully open.

2. Have the mother get into a standing squat position.

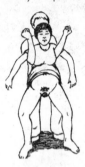

Or if the mother is unable to squat, help move her bottom to the edge of the bed as soon as the baby's legs or bottom come out.

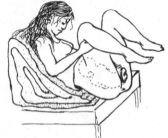

3. Encourage her to push the rest of the baby's body out slowly. The legs usually fall out but you may need to put your fingers inside the mother to bring them out.

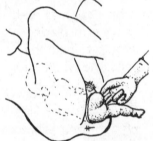

4. Gently loosen the cord a little so it does not get pulled tight later. If the cord is still under the mother's pubic bone, move the cord to the side where the flesh is softer.

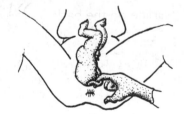

5. Wrap the baby's body in a dry warm cloth. This will help you hold the baby better and will keep the baby from trying to breathe before the head is born. (In the rest of the pictures, we will not draw the towel. This is so that you can see better. But in a real birth, keep the baby wrapped while you deliver it.)

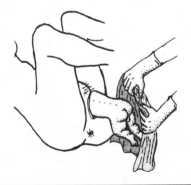

6. Have a helper put pressure on the mother's pubic bone (not her abdomen). This is to keep the baby's head tucked to its chest, not to push the baby out. Carefully guide the baby's body down to deliver the top shoulder. Hold the baby by the hips or legs. **Be careful! Pressure on the baby's back or abdomen can injure its insides!**

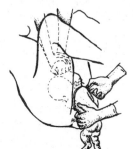

   You may need to put your fingers inside the mother to bring the arms out. Try to grasp the arms by following them down from the shoulder. Bring the arm across the chest by gently pulling on the elbow. Deliver the top shoulder.

7. Carefully lift the baby to deliver the back shoulder.

8. The baby now needs to turn so it faces down towards the mother's bottom. You may wish to support its body with your arm, placing your finger in the baby's mouth to help the head stay tucked. This is because when the baby's chin is tucked to its chest, it passes more easily through the hip bones.

9. Lower the baby until you can see the hairline on the back of the neck. **Do not pull the baby! Do not bend the neck or it may break!**

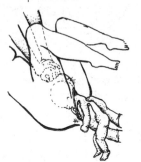

10. Keep the baby's head tucked in while you raise the body to deliver the face. Let the back of the head stay inside the mother.

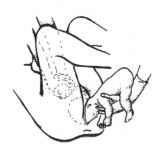

11. The mother should relax, stop pushing, and 'breathe' the baby out. The back of the head should be born slowly. If it comes too fast, the baby could bleed in the brain and die or be damaged.

Too much bleeding (hemorrhage)

It is normal for a woman to bleed a little after childbirth. **But bleeding is a serious problem if it does not stop within an hour after birth, or if there is a lot of blood—more than 2 cupfuls, or enough to soak through 2 thick rags in an hour.**

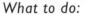

What to do:

1. Send for emergency help.
2. While you are waiting do the following.

For too much bleeding before the placenta comes out:

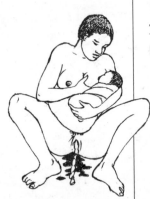

- Ask the mother to squat and push the placenta out.
- Ask her to pass urine.
- Put the baby to the mother's breast to start suckling. If the baby will not suckle, have the mother roll her nipples or have someone else suck on her breasts. This will help her womb contract and push the placenta out.
- If you have it, you can also give 10 mg oxytocin by injection in the buttock or thigh.

If the mother is too weak to deliver the placenta herself or if she is bleeding so heavily she becomes faint, you may need to help guide the placenta out. Only do this if you you believe the woman's life is in danger. First look for signs that the placenta has separated.

1. Mark the cord by tying a clean string around it about a hand's width from the opening of the vagina.
2. Put one hand on the mother's abdomen just above her pubic bone. Wait until her womb feels hard and then push upward toward her head.
3. If the string you tied to the cord moves toward the mother, the placenta is probably still attached to the womb. **Take the mother to the nearest hospital.**

   If the string on the cord does not move, the placenta may be lying in the vagina and you can try to help guide it out.
4. With your other hand, hold the cut end of the cord (a dry cloth will help), and pull slowly and firmly. Do not pull hard. If you do not feel the placenta moving down, **STOP**.
5. When the placenta comes out, rub the top of the womb with one hand until it stays very hard. At the same time, push the bottom of the womb upward with your other hand.
6. Give fluids either in the vein (IV) or in the rectum (see page 537).

If the placenta does not come out and the mother continues to bleed, take her to a health center or hospital.

If the bleeding starts after the placenta comes out:

- Ask the mother to pass urine.

- Keep the mother lying down and put the baby to her breast. If the baby will not suckle, try rolling the mother's nipples. This will make the womb contract and stop bleeding.

- Firmly rub the top of her womb at the level of her navel until the womb becomes hard. Keep rubbing until the bleeding has stopped.

- If the womb does not become hard after a few minutes of rubbing, or if bleeding continues, give ergometrine, 0.2 mg by mouth, or 0.5 mg by injection in her buttock or thigh (see page 538). If she is still bleeding after 10 minutes, give the same amount of ergometrine again.

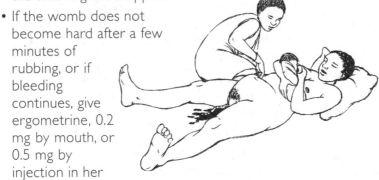

If the mother continues to bleed, take her to the health center or hospital. Send 2 family members with her to give blood if needed. In the meantime, watch her for signs of *shock*. See page 254 for signs of shock and how to treat it.

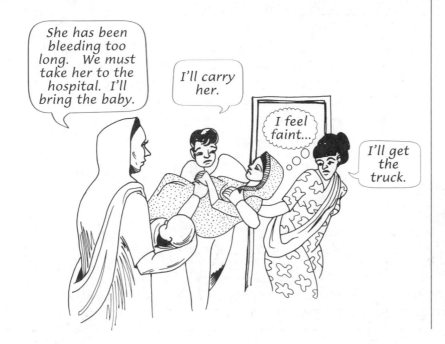

She has been bleeding too long. We must take her to the hospital. I'll bring the baby.

I'll carry her.

I feel faint...

I'll get the truck.

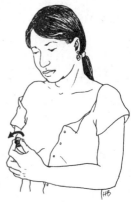

Rolling the nipples can help the womb contract and stop bleeding.

483

medicines for heavy bleeding from the vagina after childbirth

TRANSPORT!

254

shock

Danger Signs for the Baby at Birth

breastfeeding

Baby born too early or too small

A baby born before 9 months is born too early. A baby that weighs less than 2500 grams or 5 pounds is born too small. These babies need special care.

Treatment:

1. Dry the baby with a warm, clean cloth immediately after birth.

2. Put the naked baby against the mother's body. Cover the baby with many warm cloths or blankets. Make sure the head is covered and the room is warm.

3. Put the baby to the mother's breast. Small babies need to nurse at least every 2 hours.

4. DO NOT bathe the baby. It must stay warm.

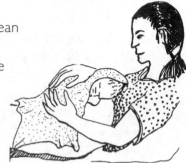

Keep baby warm and dry.

Baby does not breathe

A baby must begin to breathe on its own within 2 to 3 minutes after the cord becomes white or the placenta separates from the womb wall. If the baby does not start to breathe, it can suffer serious brain damage or die.

What to do:

Clear the baby's mouth and nose, and firmly rub its back and feet. If the baby still does not start to breathe, **do rescue breathing:**

1. Lay the baby on a hard surface, like a table or the floor.

2. Open the baby's throat by tilting her head back slightly.

3. Put your mouth over the baby's mouth and nose, and gently blow little puffs of air into the baby. Blow about 30 puffs per minute (which is a little faster than you breathe when resting). Let the baby breathe out between puffs.

4. The baby's belly and chest will rise and fall with each breath. If the belly stays up, it means that air is going into the baby's stomach, not its *lungs.* Try changing the position of the head. Make sure nothing is blocking the throat.

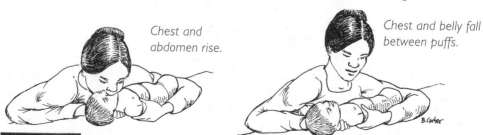

Chest and abdomen rise.

Chest and belly fall between puffs.

IMPORTANT *The new baby's lungs are very delicate. If you blow too hard, you will damage them. Blow little puffs of air from your cheeks and not from your chest.*

CARING FOR THE MOTHER JUST AFTER THE BIRTH

Encourage the mother to breastfeed her baby, which will help her to stop bleeding sooner. Also:

- Feel the top of the mother's womb. It should be hard and rounded, at about the level of her navel. If the womb feels soft, ask the mother to pass urine, then rub her womb until it gets hard. Keep checking the womb to see if it gets soft again. Check for bleeding. Teach the mother how to feel her womb and rub it if it gets soft.
- Look at the mother's vagina. If she has a long, deep tear, or a tear that will not stop bleeding, she should have it stitched by someone who knows how.
- Give her plenty to drink and eat if she is hungry.

BABY CARE

Make sure the mother knows that breastfeeding is the best food for her baby. Keep the baby with the mother so it can suck the breast and stay warm. Encourage the mother to keep the baby warm and clean and to let it suckle as often as it likes.

Babies often have a little yellowish mucus coming from their eyes in the first weeks after birth. You can wash out the eye with breast milk or cool, boiled water and a clean cloth. If the baby's eyes get red, swollen, and have a lot of pus in them, the baby should be seen by a health worker.

Care of the cord

Keep the cord stump on the baby clean and dry. If possible, clean it with alcohol and a clean cloth with every diaper (nappy) change. It will turn black and fall off during the first week. You do not need to cover it with anything unless there are flies or dust. Then you can use a very clean piece of *gauze* or cloth to cover it loosely.

If you notice redness or pus around the cord, the baby may have an infection. The baby should be seen by a health worker and be given antibiotics right away.

Tetanus of the newborn

Danger signs of tetanus in the newborn		
• fever	• baby cries all the time	• baby's body gets stiff
• baby cannot suckle the breast	• fast breathing	

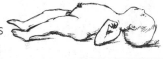

What to do:

Take the baby to a health center or hospital right away.
If the hospital is more than 2 hours away and you know how, first inject the baby with 100,000 units of benzylpenicillin.

Caring for the Mother and Baby after Birth

breastfeeding

TRANSPORT!

IN THE FIRST WEEKS AFTER BIRTH

Caring for a new mother

Mothers need care after birth just as the baby does. People are often so busy looking after the baby that the mother's needs may be forgotten.

- To **prevent infection** the mother should not have sex or put anything in her vagina until her bleeding stops.

- She should get a lot of **rest** for at least 6 weeks.

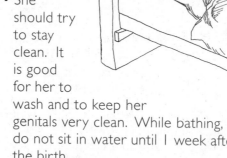

- She should try to stay clean. It is good for her to wash and to keep her genitals very clean. While bathing, do not sit in water until 1 week after the birth.

- A new mother needs to eat more food than usual. She can eat any kind of food: fish, meat, beans, grains, vegetables, and fruit will all help her heal from the birth and have energy to be a good mother.

- She should drink plenty of fluids.

breastfeeding

- If she is breastfeeding her baby and giving no other milk, the breastfeeding can protect her from getting pregnant again too soon. For full protection, see the directions on page 218.

- If she has a tear at the opening of her vagina, she should keep it clean. She can apply a hot, damp cloth and honey to the tear to help it feel better and to heal more quickly. If the tear causes burning, she can pour water over her genitals while she passes urine.

  Any plant medicines used to help her genitals heal should be clean (boiled is best). **Do not put plant medicines inside the vagina.**

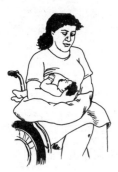

- She should start a **family planning** method soon, especially if she ever feeds her baby something other than breast milk. For her good health, she should start using a family planning method before she has sex again, or she could become pregnant too soon.

family planning

DANGER SIGNS IN THE FIRST FEW DAYS AFTER BIRTH

Bleeding

Bleeding that starts more than a day after the baby is born is usually caused by pieces of the placenta that have been left in the womb.

> *Danger signs of too much bleeding:*
> * soaks more than 2 pads or thick rags an hour in the first day after birth
> * soaks more than 1 pad or thick rag an hour after the first day
> * has a continuous small flow of blood

What to do:

1. Rub the top of her womb until it gets very hard and the bleeding stops. Have the baby suck on her breasts, or have someone roll her nipples.

2. Inject 0.5 mg of ergometrine in a large muscle, or give 0.2 mg of ergonovine by mouth every 6 hours for 4 to 7 days.

3. **If the bleeding will not stop, get medical help.** Continue to rub her womb as you take her to the hospital.

4. If she has signs of infection, give the same antibiotics as for womb infection described below.

TRANSPORT!

Womb infection

Infection of the womb is **very dangerous. It must be treated or the woman can become infertile or die.**

> *Danger signs of womb infection:*
> * fever and chills
> * pain and tenderness in the belly
> * bad-smelling fluid from the vagina

Treatment:

1. If these signs are present, give **one** of these combinations of medicines:
   * **1st choice:** amoxicillin, 1 g (1000 mg) by mouth, 3 times a day for 10 days, **plus** metronidazole, 500 mg by mouth 2 times a day for 10 days.
   * **2nd choice:** procaine penicillin, 800,000 Units by injection in the buttock 2 times a day for 7 days, **or** penicillin tablets, 400,000 Units (250 mg) by mouth 4 times a day for 7 days, **plus** chloramphenicol, 1 g by mouth the first time, then 500 mg 4 times a day for 7 days.

2. Encourage her to drink a lot of fluids. If she does not start to feel better by the next day, take her to the nearest hospital.

➤ *If the mother complains that she does not feel well, watch her carefully for signs of infection.*

TRANSPORT!

Women with Special Needs

LOSS OF A PREGNANCY (MISCARRIAGE)

A miscarriage is a pregnancy that ends by itself before the baby is fully developed. It is often the body's way of ending a pregnancy when the unformed baby has a serious problem that would have kept it from developing well. Most miscarriages happen in the first 3 months of pregnancy. After a miscarriage, a woman can still become pregnant again and have a normal pregnancy and a healthy baby.

The signs of miscarriage are pain and bleeding. (For more information on other possible causes, see page 234.) The bleeding and pain usually begin like normal monthly bleeding and then get heavier and stronger. There may also be some *tissue* or clots with the blood.

If the bleeding and pain continue for more than a few days, if the bleeding is much heavier than normal monthly bleeding, or if a woman gets a fever or has a bad-smelling fluid from her vagina, part of the pregnancy may still be inside the womb. This is called an *incomplete miscarriage*. It can lead to heavy blood loss, a dangerous infection, or even death. The woman should go to a health center or hospital where a trained health worker can empty the womb.

If a woman has strong, constant pain in her lower abdomen, she may have a pregnancy in the tube. This is very dangerous (see page 73).

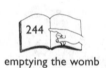

244
emptying the womb

353
pain

After a miscarriage a woman should rest and avoid heavy work or lifting for 2 weeks. She should not douche or wash inside her vagina. Also she should avoid sex until all bleeding stops because her womb is still open and could get infected.

Many women feel very sad after a miscarriage. Some do not. This is all normal. Some women may find it helpful to talk with other women who have lost a pregnancy.

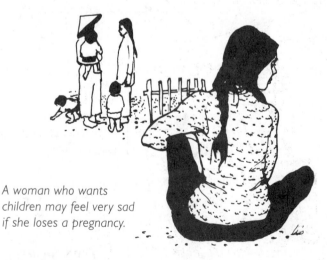

A woman who wants children may feel very sad if she loses a pregnancy.

HELPING WOMEN WHO HAVE TROUBLE CARING FOR THEMSELVES AND THEIR BABIES

Some women are more likely to have difficult births and problems following birth, and their babies are more likely to be unhealthy. Mothers who are alone, very poor, very young, mentally slow, or who already have poorly nourished or sick children may have a harder time caring for themselves and their babies.

If someone takes special interest in these mothers, and helps them get the food, care, and companionship they need, it can often make a great difference in the well-being of both the mothers and their babies.

IF THE BABY DIES

Most women have healthy pregnancies and give birth to healthy babies. But sometimes, no matter what anyone does, the baby dies.

This is always a hard time for a mother. She feels great sadness and loss. At the same time, she has been through a pregnancy and birth and she needs to rest and get her strength back, just like a mother with a new baby.

The following advice may also help:

• Her breasts will probably be sore, especially around the 3rd day after the birth when her milk comes in. Cloths soaked in cool, clean water may reduce the soreness.

She should:

• not squeeze out either the first yellow milk (colostrum) or the regular breast milk. Removing milk will cause the body to make more.

• watch for signs of breast infection and treat if necessary (see page 117).

• wait for at least 3 months before trying to get pregnant again. A woman's body needs time to heal.

• start using a family planning method as soon as possible. She can become pregnant again too soon.

For many women, this is a death like any death of somone she is close to, and she will need to mourn her loss. She needs special care, kindness, and support.

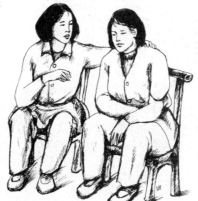

Do not wait for those in need to come to you. Go to them.

197
family planning

➤ *A woman needs extra care and support when her baby dies.*

To the Father

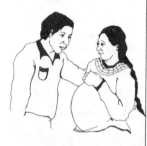

> ➤ *Throughout pregnancy, childbirth and after, be alert for danger signs in the mother and baby. Seek help if you think there is a problem.*

PREGNANCY

Showing your wife that you care about her can help her both physically and emotionally. Make sure she has help with her work. If you cannot do some of the work yourself, try to get someone else to help. Make sure she eats healthy foods and goes for prenatal care (see page 68).

CHILDBIRTH

You can help your wife feel strong and safe during labor and childbirth by:

- making sure there is enough water and food in the house.
- bringing her midwife or health worker to the house to help with the birth.
- taking care of the other children.

If you stay with her during the birth, you can help by giving her both emotional and physical support. Encourage her and tell her she is doing well. Give her water to drink. Help her walk or squat during contractions or rub her back.

AFTER BIRTH

The first 6 weeks after birth are the most important time for a woman to feel strong and healthy again. During this time she needs a lot of healthy foods and plenty of rest. You can help her rest more by doing some of her work—like fetching

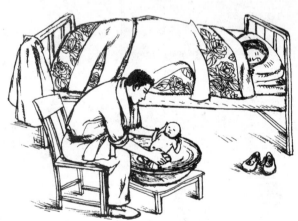

water or fire wood, taking care of your other children, or preparing some of the meals. If you cannot help, try to find someone else who can.

If you take time to hold and care for your baby, your wife will have a chance to sleep and you can be close to your new child.

Do not have sex until the bleeding stops to prevent an infection in her womb.

FAMILY PLANNING

family planning

To have healthy mothers and babies, it is best to wait at least 2 years between pregnancies. One of the most important ways you can help your family be more healthy is by using family planning. Visit the family planning clinic with your wife and decide together which method will work best. Then share the responsibility for using it.

Throughout the world, millions of women die needlessly from problems during pregnancy and childbirth. Many of these deaths happen because a woman or her family wait too long to get help for emergencies.

Here is the story of a group of women who worked in their community to understand and solve some of these problems.

Working for Change

During the last rainy season, my friend Ekwefi was pregnant. When it was time for her to give birth, her husband had gone away on a trip. Several wise women were there to help her. But the labor was too long and Ekwfi started bleeding. I said that we needed to take her to the health center. No one could decide what to do. Her husband was gone and he was the one who should decide. Soon after we realized that Ekwefi and the baby would not survive, they both died in front of us.

This made me very sad. Ekwefi was my friend, and we could not help her. I started talking with other women in my village. We had to do something about this problem. Ekwefi was not the first woman to die while she was giving birth. Many other women lost their babies during birth. Some women said this is how things are in our small village and we should accept it. But we said no, we can do something to solve this problem.

We decided to have a meeting to learn more about the problem of women and babies dying during birth. During our meeting we decided to talk to the families with this problem. Six women in our group agreed to visit families where a woman had died from a difficult birth during the past two years, or where a woman was still recovering from one.

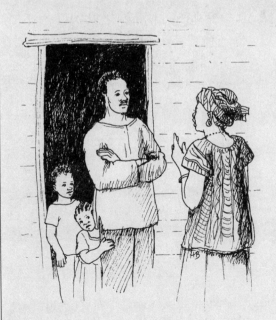

We learned several important things. Everyone agreed that the biggest problem was that women wait a very long time before they call a doctor or go to the health center. Sometimes a woman cannot ask for help without her husband's permission. Many times, like with my friend Ekwefi, the husband is not in the village when the woman needs to ask his permission to get help. The neighbors are afraid to give help, because they do not want the husband to be angry or offended. We also learned that most husbands do not know about the many risks women face during labor.

We decided to walk the 7 miles to the health center to talk to the midwife. We told her what we had learned and asked her to help us find ways to solve this problem. The midwife was very happy to help us. She talked to the head of our village and asked for a meeting with the elders. During the meeting, the midwife talked to the elders about the health risks of a long labor. She also told them what

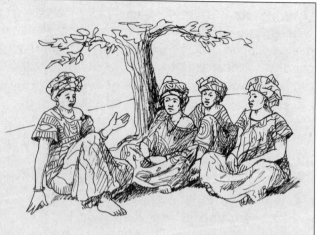

we had learned about women dying while giving birth in our village. The elders all agreed that this was a very serious problem for the whole village. They asked the midwife how this problem could be solved. The midwife told the elders that this was not just a problem in our village but in many villages in Nigeria. She suggested that the village pick 12 men and 12 women to go to a five-day training on *reproductive health* and family planning. These villagers would become reproductive health workers, and would work to teach and motivate the rest of the village.

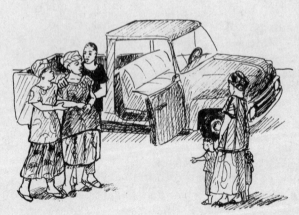

After the training, the men who had gone realized that they had to be actively involved in solving this serious problem. They decided to work hard to teach the other men in the village about the risks of labor and how to help women in labor. They also decided to have a transportation committee to help women get to the health center when they needed it.

We all worked very hard to solve this health problem in our village. In the beginning, many people said that women often die giving birth and there was nothing we could do about it. But we did not get discouraged. By working together with the women, the midwife, the elders, and the men of the community, we came up with a solution that works in our village. And the answer to our problem wasn't more money or a new technology. The answer was in our time and effort. All of us from the village of Lado encourage you to work together to improve the life and health of your community.

To learn more about thinking about and solving health problems, read the chapter on "Solving Health Problems."

How to help save more childbearing women's lives

Most deaths and injuries from pregnancy and birth could be prevented through better nutrition, child spacing (with family planning), access to safe *abortion,* good care during pregnancy and birth, good transportation, and good blood services. To reduce these deaths:

- learn the danger signs during pregnancy, birth, and after birth.

- plan how to get help before it is needed.

- when problems arise, get help early.

- try to organize your community so that emergency transportation, money, and blood donations will be ready when difficult births happen.

- work with local leaders to build small houses near a hospital where women from remote areas can stay until it is time to give birth.

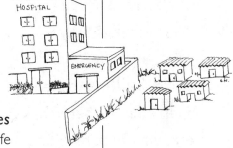

How health workers can help save women's lives

- Offer family planning services to prevent unsafe abortions and to help women avoid having births too close together.

- Offer STD treatment and prevention to all women and girls old enough to have children.

- Make tetanus vaccines available to all women, even if they are not pregnant.

- Learn how to detect problems during pregnancy, birth, and after birth.

- Refer women with problems in a pregnancy (now or in the past) to a health center that has emergency transportation.

- Teach birth attendants and midwives how to prevent infection and how to watch for and treat danger signs during pregnancy and birth.

- Encourage all women to breastfeed for at least 2 years.

- Have a medicine box that includes:
    - oxytocin, ergometrine, and local plants to prevent and control severe bleeding after the birth.
    - antibiotics to treat infection.
    - equipment to do injections in the muscle (IM) and the vein (IV).
    - medicines to treat toxemia (see page 87).
    - gloves or clean plastic bags.
    - new razor blades.
    - enema bag or can for rectal fluids.

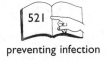

preventing infection

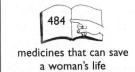

medicines that can save a woman's life

Chapter 7

In this chapter:

It is possible to breastfeed your child for as long as you like and never have any problems. But if you have a problem, there are many ways you can help yourself and continue to breastfeed. This chapter has information on healthy breastfeeding practices and help for common problems.

Breastfeeding

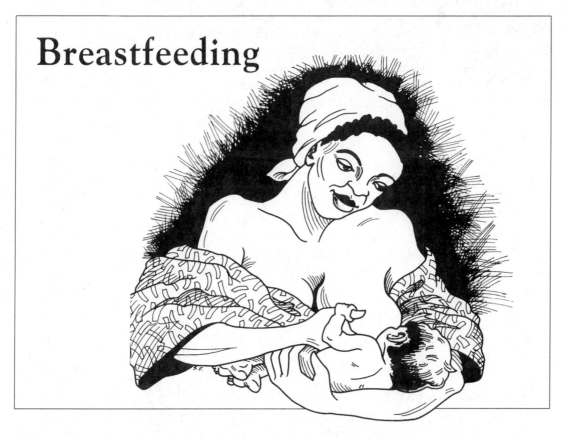

Breastfeeding is one of the oldest and healthiest practices in the world. But as the world changes, women sometimes need information and support to keep breastfeeding their babies.

Breastfeeding is important because:

- **Breast milk is the only perfect food** to help a baby grow healthy and strong.
- Breastfeeding helps the womb stop bleeding after birth.
- Breast milk protects the baby against illnesses and *infections* like *diabetes, cancer, diarrhea,* and *pneumonia.* The mother's defenses against illness are passed on to the baby through her milk.
- Breastfeeding helps protect the mother against diseases like *cancer* and weak or brittle bones *(osteoporosis).*
- When a woman breastfeeds her baby, the milk is always clean, always ready, and always the right temperature.
- Breastfeeding helps the mother and baby feel close and secure.
- For some women, giving their babies nothing but breast milk can help protect them from becoming pregnant again too soon.
- Breastfeeding is free.

Why Breast Is Best

➤ *It is best to give your baby nothing but breast milk for about the first 6 months.*

Why Other Feeding Can Be Harmful

Companies that make artificial milk (infant formula) want mothers to feed their babies formula instead of breast milk so that the companies can make money. Using bottles or giving formula is often very unsafe. Millions of babies fed with bottles or formula have become malnourished or sick, or have died.

- Formula and other milks, such as tinned milk or the milk of animals, do not protect babies from disease.

- Formula and other milks can cause sickness and death. If the bottle, nipple, or water used to make the formula is not boiled long enough, the baby will swallow harmful *germs* and get diarrhea.

➤ *More than 1 million babies die each year because their mothers were discouraged from breastfeeding.*

- When babies drink from the breast, they use their tongue to 'milk' the breast. This is called *suckling*. It is very different from what a baby's mouth does when sucking on a bottle. By sucking on a bottle or rubber teat (pacifier, dummy), the baby may forget how to suckle well on the breast because the bottle teaches it a different kind of sucking. And if the baby does not suckle on the breast enough, the mother's milk supply will decrease, and the baby will stop feeding from the breast completely.

- Bottle-feeding costs a lot of money. For one baby, a family would need 40 kg of formula powder in the first year. Buying a day's worth of formula and enough fuel to boil water can cost more than the family earns in a week—or even a month.

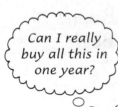

Can I really buy all this in one year?

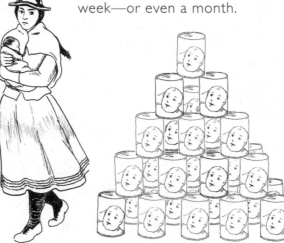

Some parents try to make the milk or formula last longer by using less powder or more water. This makes a baby malnourished, grow more slowly, and get sick more often.

FOR THE NEW BABY

After birth, **a mother should breastfeed during the first hour**. It will help her womb to stop bleeding and return to normal. Skin-to-skin contact between mother and baby, and the baby's suckling will help her milk to start flowing.

Newborn babies need the first yellow-colored breast milk (*colostrum*) that comes out of the breasts for the first 2 or 3 days after birth. Colostrum has all the nutrition that a new baby needs, and it protects against disease. Colostrum also cleans the baby's gut. There is no need to give herbs or teas to do this.

FOR ANY BABY

Feed from both breasts, but **let the baby finish one breast first** before offering the other. The whiter milk that comes after the baby has been feeding for a few minutes is richer in fat than the first milk. The baby needs this fat, so it is important to let the baby finish one breast before offering the other. The baby will let go when it is ready to stop or switch. If the baby takes only one breast at a feeding, begin the next feed on the other breast.

Feed your baby whenever it is hungry, day and night. Many new babies will suckle about every 1 to 3 hours, especially in the first months. Let the baby suckle as long and as often as it wants. The more it suckles, the more milk you will make.

You do not need to give cereals, other milk, or sugar water—even in hot climates. These can make the baby take less breast milk and may be harmful before 4 to 6 months.

How to Breastfeed

➤ *Babies want to suckle when they are hungry, thirsty, fighting off a sickness, growing a lot, or need comfort. If you are not sure what your baby wants, try breastfeeding.*

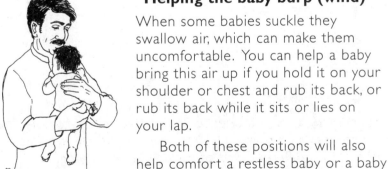

Mothers who keep their babies close by at night can breastfeed more easily. If she sleeps with the baby, the mother can breastfeed and sleep at the same time.

Helping the baby burp (wind)

When some babies suckle they swallow air, which can make them uncomfortable. You can help a baby bring this air up if you hold it on your shoulder or chest and rub its back, or rub its back while it sits or lies on your lap.

Both of these positions will also help comfort a restless baby or a baby that cries more than usual.

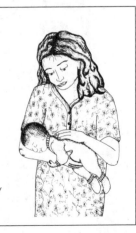

How to hold the baby

When breastfeeding, it is important to hold the baby so it can suckle and swallow easily. The mother should also be in a relaxed, comfortable position so that her milk can flow well.

➤ *Do not pinch the nipple when giving the breast to the baby.*

Support the baby's head with your hand or arm. Its head and body should be in a straight line. Wait until its mouth is open wide. Bring the baby close to the breast and tickle its lower lip with the nipple. Then move the baby onto your breast. The baby should have a big mouthful of the breast, with the nipple deep inside its mouth.

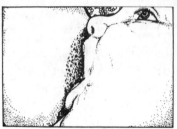

This baby has a good mouthful of breast.

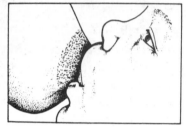

This baby does not have enough breast in its mouth.

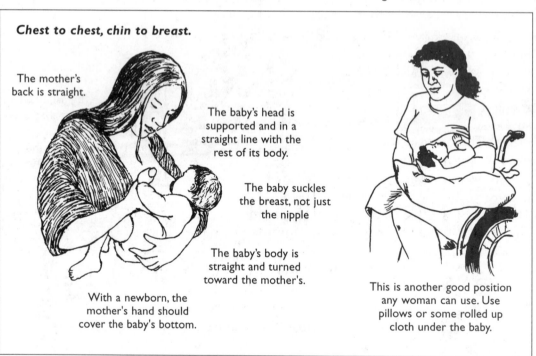

Chest to chest, chin to breast.

The mother's back is straight.

The baby's head is supported and in a straight line with the rest of its body.

The baby suckles the breast, not just the nipple

The baby's body is straight and turned toward the mother's.

With a newborn, the mother's hand should cover the baby's bottom.

This is another good position any woman can use. Use pillows or some rolled up cloth under the baby.

If you are having trouble breastfeeding, get help from a woman who has experience. She can often help more than some health workers. Do not use a bottle. It will teach the baby a different kind of sucking. **Keep trying.** Sometimes it takes practice for you to find good positions for your baby, or for a baby to learn to suckle well.

These are signs that something may be wrong with how you are holding the baby, or how much breast the baby has in its mouth:

- If the baby is restless, cries, or does not want to feed, it may be in an uncomfortable position.
- If the baby's body does not face yours; for example it might be lying on its back and turning its head to reach the breast.
- If you see a lot of the brown part around the nipple (areola), it might mean the nipple is not far back enough in the baby's mouth.
- If the suckling is very fast and noisy, the baby might need a bigger mouthful of the breast. After the first few minutes, the baby should suckle slowly and deeply, and swallow well.
- If you feel pain, or get a cracked nipple, you may need to help the baby get the nipple farther back in its mouth.

Mother's diet while breastfeeding

Mothers need to eat well to recover from pregnancy, to care for their babies, and for all the other work they do. They need plenty of foods rich in protein, fats, and lots of fruits and vegetables. They also need to drink plenty of liquid—clean water, milk, herb teas, and fruit juices. But no matter how a woman eats and drinks, her body will make good breast milk.

Breastfeeding saves money. If she can, a mother should use some of that savings to improve her own diet, especially with extra foods with protein like beans, nuts, eggs, milk, yogurt, cheese, fish or meat.

Some people believe that new mothers should not eat certain foods. But if a mother does not get a balanced diet (see page 166), it can lead to *malnutrition*, weak blood *(anemia)*, and other sickness.

Sometimes women are given special foods during breastfeeding. These practices are good, especially if the foods are nutritious. Good foods help a woman's body to grow healthy and strong more quickly after childbirth.

A woman needs extra food if:

- she is breastfeeding 2 young children.
- she is breastfeeding one child and is also pregnant.
- her children are spaced closer than every 2 years.
- she is sick or weak.

Advice for the Mother

165

eating for good health

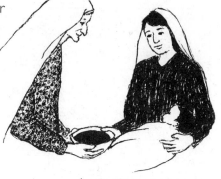

➤ *Eat and drink enough to satisfy hunger and thirst. Avoid alcohol, tobacco, drugs and unnecessary medicines. Clean water, fruit and vegetable juices, and milk and herb teas are better than coffee and sodas.*

Breastfeeding and child-spacing

Child-spacing means having babies at least 2 or 3 years apart. This allows a woman's body to get strong before another pregnancy. For some women, breastfeeding helps them space their children. For more information, see page 218.

Giving other foods

If a baby does not seem happy with breastfeeding, and it is between 4 and 6 months old, it may simply need to suckle more so that the mother's breasts will make more milk. The mother should breastfeed the baby as often as the baby wants for about 5 days. If the baby is still unhappy, then she should try other foods.

A baby is ready for other feedings when:
- it is about six months old, or older.
- it starts to grab food from the family or from the table.
- it does not push food out with its tongue.

Between 6 months and 1 year, give breast milk whenever the baby wants it. Even if it is eating other foods, it still needs as much breast milk as before. Follow breastfeeding with other foods, 2 or 3 times a day at first. Begin with a soft, mild food, like cereal or porridge. Some women mix these with breast milk. You do not need expensive baby cereals.

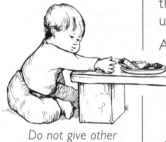

Do not give other foods before 4 months.

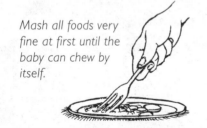

Mash all foods very fine at first until the baby can chew by itself.

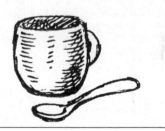

Use a cup or bowl and spoon to feed the baby.

➤ *Add new foods one at a time. By about 9 months to 1 year, a baby can eat most family foods if they are cut up and made easy to eat.*

➤ *Even in the second year, breast milk continues to protect your child against infection and other health problems.*

Babies need to eat often—about 5 times a day. Each day, they should have some main food (porridge, maize, wheat, rice, millet, potato, cassava), mixed with a body building food (beans, finely ground nuts, eggs, cheese, meat or fish), brightly colored vegetables and fruits, and an energy-rich food (finely ground nuts, spoonful of oil, margarine or cooking fat). You do not have to cook 5 times a day. Some meals can be given as a cold snack.

If you can, keep breastfeeding until the child is at least 2 years old, even if you have another baby. Most babies will slowly stop breastfeeding on their own.

Many women now work away from their homes. This can make it hard for a mother to give her baby nothing but breast milk during the first 6 months.

Working mothers need help. Some jobs allow a mother to bring her baby for a few months. This makes breastfeeding the easiest. Or maybe the person caring for a woman's children can bring the baby to the mother at feeding time. If a mother has child care nearby, she might be able to breastfeed during the day, on her breaks. Some employers organize child-care centers so that parents can have their children close by.

But he could get sick without my milk.

When the Mother Works Outside the Home

➤ *A working mother should not have to choose between her work and her child's health.*

Here are some ways to make sure your baby gets only breast milk while you are at work:

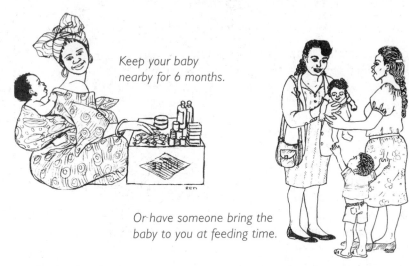

Keep your baby nearby for 6 months.

Or have someone bring the baby to you at feeding time.

When you are with your baby, feed it only from your breasts. If you sleep with the baby at night, it may feed more, and this will help you to make enough milk.

Some women ask a friend or a relative, like the baby's grandmother, to breastfeed their baby. If you want another woman to breastfeed your baby, it should be someone you know is healthy and has no risk of getting *HIV/AIDS*.

AIDS, 284
breastfeeding and AIDS, 293

Removing Milk by Hand

Another way a woman can give her baby breast milk during the day is if she can have time at work to remove the milk from her breasts. Then someone else can feed the baby for her.

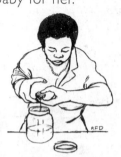

You can remove your milk by hand 2 or 3 times each day...

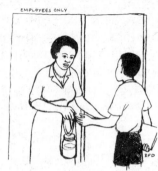

...then send or store the milk for someone to feed your baby.

➤ *If a mother removes more milk than her baby needs, she can give it to another baby whose mother is sick, or whose milk has not come in yet.*

You may also need to remove your milk by hand if your breasts are too full, or if your baby cannot breastfeed for some reason, and you want to keep a good milk supply.

How to remove your milk by hand

1. Wash and rinse a wide-mouth jar and lid with soap and clean water, and leave them in the sun to dry. Just before using them, pour boiling water, that has boiled for 20 minutes, into them and let the water sit for a few minutes. Then pour the water out.

2. Wash your hands well before touching the jar or your breasts.

3. Find a quiet place if you can. Think about the baby as you remove your milk. Be patient and try to relax. Massage the breasts lightly with your finger tips or fist, moving toward the nipples.

4. To make the milk come out, place your fingers and thumb at the back edge of the areola (the darker part), and press in toward the chest. (Do not squeeze the nipple. The milk comes from behind the areola.) Then relax your fingers. Continue to press and relax your fingers, moving them all the way around the areola. You should not feel any pain.

   Press back, do not pinch.

5. Repeat several times on each breast. At first, not much milk will come out. With practice you will remove more. Plan to remove about half a cup of your milk as often as your baby eats, or at least 3 times each day. (The person who gives your milk to the baby can let you know if there was enough.) If you start to practice 2 weeks before you return to work, you will be able to remove enough milk by the time you must be separated from your baby.

How to store the milk

Keep your milk in a clean, closed container (see steps 1 and 2 on page 112). You can store milk in the same jar used to remove the milk. Keep the milk in a cool place away from sunlight. The milk can be used for up to 8 hours. Or you can bury the closed container in wet sand, or keep it wrapped in a cloth that is kept wet all the time, and it will keep for about 12 hours.

➤ *Breast milk can change color. The color comes from what you eat. No matter what color it is, your milk is good for your baby.*

The container can be stored longer in a cool place such as a clay pot with water in it.

Milk can be kept in a glass jar in a refrigerator for 2 or 3 days. The cream (fat) in the milk will separate, so before giving it to the baby, shake the container to mix the milk. Heat it gently in warm water. Test the milk to make sure it is not too hot by shaking a few drops onto your arm.

Warm bottle method

This method may work best if the breasts are too full or very painful. This may happen right after birth, or if a woman gets a cracked nipple or breast infection (see pages 115 and 117).

1. Clean a large glass bottle that has a 3 to 4 cm-wide mouth. Warm it by filling it with hot water. Fill it slowly so the bottle does not break. Wait a few minutes and then pour the water out.

   3 to 4 cm wide

2. Cool the mouth and neck of the bottle with clean, cool water so that it does not burn you.

3. Fasten the bottle mouth over your nipple so that it makes a seal. Hold it firmly in place for several minutes. As it cools, it will gently pull the milk out.

4. When the milk flow slows down, use your finger to loosen the seal around the breast.

5. Repeat on the other breast if it is also painfully full. Now you can comfortably breastfeed your baby.

Sometimes a woman may not want to save the milk to give her baby—for example, when she is just softening her breast to make it easier for the baby to suckle. In that case, since she is throwing the milk away, she does not need to clean the container for the milk with boiling water.

Common Concerns and Problems

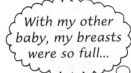

With my other baby, my breasts were so full...

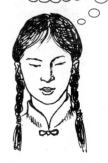

➤ *A baby older than 2 weeks may not pass stool every day. If the baby is feeding well, wetting, and seems content, the stool will come.*

➤ *The size and shape of your nipple is not important—the baby suckles from the breast, not just the nipple.*

FEAR THERE IS NOT ENOUGH MILK, OR THAT MILK IS NOT GOOD ENOUGH

Many women think they do not have enough milk. This is almost never true. Even mothers who do not have enough to eat can generally make enough milk for their babies.

The amount of milk your breasts make (your milk supply) depends on how much the baby suckles. The more the baby suckles, the more milk you will make. If you skip a feeding and give a bottle instead of breast milk, your body will make less milk.

Some days it may seem like the baby is always wanting to breastfeed. If you feed your baby whenever it is hungry, your milk supply will increase. In a few days the baby will probably seem satisfied again. Night feeding helps to build up a mother's milk supply. Try not to believe anyone—even a health worker—who says that you do not have enough milk.

Breasts do not have to feel full to make milk. The more babies a woman has breastfed, the less full her breasts will feel. Small breasts can make as much milk as large breasts.

A baby is getting enough milk if:

• it is growing well, and seems happy and healthy.
• it wets 6 or more times and dirties the diaper (nappy) about 1 to 3 times in a day and night. You can usually tell this after the baby is 5 days old, when the baby will start to pass *urine* and *stool* more regularly.

Because breast milk looks different from other milks, some women fear that it is not good milk. But breast milk gives babies everything they need.

NIPPLE CONCERNS AND PROBLEMS

Flat or pushed-in (inverted) nipples

Most women with nipples that are flat or pushed-in can breastfeed without a problem. This is because the baby suckles on the breast, not just the nipple. You do not need to do anything to prepare your nipples during pregnancy.

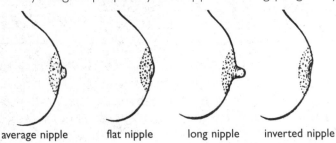

average nipple   flat nipple   long nipple   inverted nipple

These ideas may make it easier for your baby to suckle:

- Start breastfeeding right after birth, before your breasts become full. Make sure your baby takes a good mouthful of breast (see page 108).

- If your breasts become too full, remove some milk by hand to make them softer. This will make it easier for the baby to get more breast in its mouth.

- Lightly touch or roll your nipple before you feed. Do not squeeze it.

- Try cupping your hand around the breast and pushing back to make your nipple stick out as much as possible.

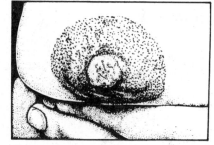

Offer the whole breast. This helps the baby get a good mouthful of the breast.

Sore or cracked nipples

If you feel pain from breastfeeding, the baby probably does not have enough of your breast in its mouth. If the baby suckles only on the nipples, they will soon become painful or cracked. A cracked nipple makes it easier for a woman to get an infection. You can teach your baby to take more breast in his mouth. Here are some suggestions.

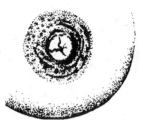

Prevention and treatment:

- Be sure to hold the baby so it can get a good mouthful of the breast (see page 108).

- Do not pull your breast out of the baby's mouth. Let the baby feed as long as it wants. When it is done, it will let go of the breast itself. If you need to stop before the baby is ready, pull down on its chin or gently put the tip of a clean finger into its mouth.

- Soothe sore nipples with breast milk at the end of a feed. When the baby has stopped feeding, squeeze out a few drops of milk and rub them on the sore places. Do not use soap or cream on your breasts. The body makes a natural oil that keeps the nipples clean and soft.

- Avoid rough or tight clothing.

- To help sore nipples heal, leave your breasts open to the air and sun, if possible.

- Continue to feed from both breasts. If a nipple is very sore or cracked, start on the less painful breast and then switch to the other breast when the milk is flowing.

- If the pain is too great when the baby suckles, remove the milk by hand and feed the baby with a cup or spoon (see page 119). The sore should heal in 2 days.

breast infection

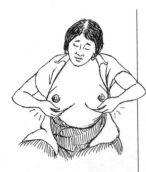

PAIN AND SWELLING IN THE BREASTS

A woman's breasts are too full (engorgement)

When the milk first comes in, the breasts often feel swollen and hard. This can make it difficult for the baby to suckle, and the nipples may get sore. If you breastfeed less because of the pain, your milk supply will be less.

Prevention and treatment:

- Start breastfeeding within the first hour after birth.
- Make sure you are holding the baby well (see page 108).
- Feed the baby often, at least every 1 to 3 hours, and on both breasts. Sleep with the baby nearby so you can breastfeed easily during the night.
- If the baby cannot suckle well, remove some milk by hand—just enough to soften the breast—and then let the baby suckle.
- After feeding, apply fresh cabbage leaves or cool wet cloths to the breasts.

After 2 or 3 days, the swelling should go down. Engorgement that does not improve can become *mastitis* (a hot, painful swelling of the breast).

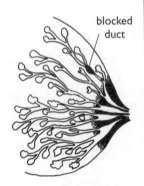

blocked duct

Blocked duct, mastitis

If a painful lump forms in the breast, it may mean that a duct is blocked by thick milk. When milk flow stops in part of the breast, it can also cause mastitis. If a woman has a fever and part of her breast is hot, swollen and painful, she probably has mastitis. **It is important to continue breastfeeding** so that the duct can empty and the breast does not get infected. The milk is still safe for the baby.

Treatment for blocked duct and mastitis:

- Apply warm wet cloths to the painful breast before you breastfeed.
- Continue to feed the baby often, especially from the painful breast. Make sure the baby is holding the breast well in its mouth (see page 108).
- As the baby feeds, gently massage the lump, moving your fingers from the lump toward the nipple. This will help to clear the blocked duct.
- Change feeding positions to help the milk flow from all parts of the breast.
- If you cannot breastfeed, remove your milk by hand or use the warm-bottle method. The milk must be kept flowing from the breast to clear the blocked duct.
- Wear loose-fitting clothing, and rest as much as you can.

Most mastitis clears up in 24 hours. If you have fever for more than 24 hours, you need treatment for breast infection.

Breast infection *(mastitis with infection)*

If you have had signs of mastitis with no improvement after 24 hours, or severe pain, or a crack in the skin where germs can enter, **you must get treatment for breast infection right away.**

Treatment:

The most important part of treatment is to continue breastfeeding often. Your milk is still safe for the baby. Medicines and rest are necessary too. If you can, take time off from work and get help with your household work. Also follow the treatment for blocked duct and mastitis. If needed to keep the milk flowing, you can milk your breast by hand or use the warm bottle method.

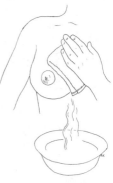

Warm, wet cloths can help with blocked ducts or mastitis.

Medicine for Breast Infection		
Medicine	**How much to take**	**When and how to take**
For infection take:		
dicloxicillin	250 mg	4 times a day for 10 days. Take at least 30 minutes before food.
If you cannot find this or are allergic to penicillin, take:		
erythromycin	500 mg	4 times a day for 10 days.
Before taking medicines, see the "Green Pages."		
For fever and pain, take:		
paracetamol (acetaminophen) or aspirin until the pain goes away (see pages 511 and 492 in the "Green Pages").		

Important: If a breast infection is not treated early, it will get worse. The hot and painful swelling will feel as if it is filled with liquid (abscess). If this happens, follow the treatment described here AND see a health worker who has been trained to drain an abscess using sterile equipment.

Thrush (yeast)

If you are holding the baby so it is comfortable and feeding well, and the pain in your nipples lasts for more than a week, it may be caused by thrush in the baby's mouth. Thrush can feel like an itchy, stabbing or burning pain, moving through the breast. You may see white spots or redness on your nipple and in the baby's mouth.

Treatment:

Mix Gentian Violet with clean water to a strength of 0.25% and paint on the nipples and on the white patches in the baby's mouth once every day for 5 days, or until 3 days after healing is complete. Use a clean cloth or finger to apply. If it does not get better, see the "Green Pages" for other medicines. You can continue to breastfeed. The medicine will not hurt you, your milk or the baby.

How to mix Gentian Violet with clean water to make a 0.25% solution:

If your Gentian Violet says...	Use
0.5% . . .	1 part Gentian Violet plus 1 part water
1% . . .	1 part Gentian Violet plus 3 parts water
2% . . .	1 part Gentian Violet plus 7 parts water

Special Situations

BABIES WITH SPECIAL NEEDS CAN BREASTFEED

Small baby. If a small baby cannot suckle strongly enough to feed itself, you will need to remove your milk by hand and feed the baby with a cup and spoon. Begin right after birth, and continue even when the baby can suckle some by itself. This will help your breasts make more milk. If your baby weighs less than 1½ kilos or 3½ pounds, it may need special medical care, including a tube that goes through the nose and down to the stomach. Your milk can be given through that tube. Talk with a health worker about this.

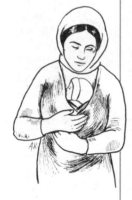

Baby born too early. Babies born too early need warmth. Place the baby naked, with a hat and a diaper or nappy, upright inside your clothing, against your skin and between your breasts. (It helps to wear a loose blouse, sweater, or wrap tied at the waist.) In some places this is called 'Kangaroo Care'. Keep skin-to-skin contact inside your clothing day and night, and breastfeed often. If the baby suckles weakly, also give milk you have removed by hand.

Cleft lip or *cleft palate*. These babies may need special help to learn how to suckle. If the baby has only a cleft lip, it can still suckle well. (To help make a seal, use your finger to cover the cleft.) If the roof of the mouth is also open, try to hold the baby up straight while keeping a good feeding position. You may need to get special help. You can remove your milk by hand to keep up a good supply while the baby is learning to suckle.

Yellow baby (jaundice). A yellow baby needs plenty of sunlight and breast milk to get the jaundice out of its body. Some babies with jaundice are very sleepy. If a baby is too sleepy to take the breast, remove milk by hand and give it with a cup and spoon, at least 10 times in 24 hours. Put the baby in the sun in the early morning and late afternoon. Or keep the baby in a bright room.

Most jaundice does not start until after the first 3 days of life and clears up by the 10th day. If the baby has jaundice or very yellow eyes at any other time, or if a jaundiced baby was also born very early, or if the yellow or sleepiness gets worse, the baby could have a serious illness. If possible, take the baby to a health center or hospital.

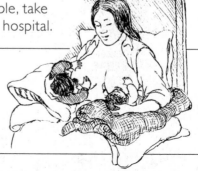

Twins. Sometimes one twin is smaller or weaker. Be sure that each baby gets plenty of your milk. You have enough milk for both babies.

When your baby is sick

- If your baby is sick you should not stop breastfeeding. Your baby will get better more quickly if it is breastfed.

- Diarrhea is especially dangerous in babies. Often no medicine is needed, but special care must be taken because a baby can die very quickly of *dehydration*.

- For diarrhea, breastfeed more often and also give sips of Rehydration Drink.

rehydration drink

- Breastfeed more often if the baby is weak. If the baby is too weak to breastfeed, remove the milk by hand and give the milk with a spoon. Take the baby to a health worker.

- For vomiting, give shorter feeds more often, and also give Rehydration Drink in small sips with a cup or spoon every 5 to 10 minutes. If you can, see a health worker—dehydration can lead to death.

- Keep breastfeeding your baby even if the baby needs to go to the hospital. If you cannot stay at the hospital, remove your milk by hand and get someone to give it to the baby with a cup or spoon.

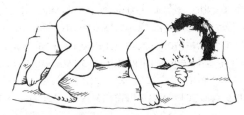

How to feed a baby with a cup or spoon (first clean the cup and spoon with soap and water if boiling is not possible).

1. Hold the baby upright or almost upright on your lap.

2. Hold a spoon or small cup of milk to the baby's mouth. Tip the cup or spoon so the milk just reaches the baby's lips. If you are using a cup, rest it lightly on the baby's lower lip and let the edges of the cup touch the baby's upper lip.

3. Do not pour the milk into the baby's mouth. Let the baby take the milk into its mouth from the cup or spoon. For very small or ill babies, it may be better to use a spoon.

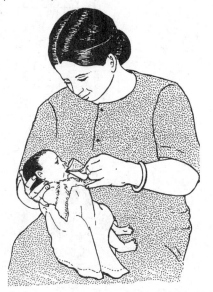

WHEN THE MOTHER IS SICK

If she can, it is almost always better for a sick mother to breastfeed her baby than to feed other foods too soon. If you have a high fever and sweat a lot, you may make less milk. To prevent this, you should:

- drink plenty of liquid.
- continue to breastfeed often.
- breastfeed in the lying-down position (see page 107).
- remove the milk by hand (if necessary someone can help you).

To prevent passing any infection to the baby, wash your hands well with soap and water before touching your baby or breasts.

When the mother needs medicine

Most medicines pass into breast milk in very small and weak amounts, so they do not harm the baby. It is usually more harmful to the baby to stop breastfeeding.

There are a few drugs that cause side effects. In this book we have marked these medicines with a warning and suggest other medicines that will be safer (see the "Green Pages").

If a health worker tells you to take a medicine, remind her that you are breastfeeding so that a safe one can be selected.

HIV/AIDS AND BREASTFEEDING

A woman with the HIV virus or AIDS must make a decision about feeding her baby. For more information on making this decision and on other ways to feed your baby, see the chapter on "AIDS."

WHEN A WOMAN BECOMES PREGNANT OR GIVES BIRTH TO ANOTHER CHILD

If a nursing mother becomes pregnant, she can continue to breastfeed. Since breastfeeding and pregnancy take a lot from her own body, she should eat plenty of good foods.

It is safe to continue breastfeeding an older child when a woman has a new baby. The new baby should be fed before the older child.

➤ *Get treatment right away for any serious disease caused by infection, like TB, typhoid or cholera, so it does not get passed on to the baby.*

293

HIV/AIDS and breastfeeding

165

eating for good health

A woman with a new baby and an older baby can safely breastfeed both of them.

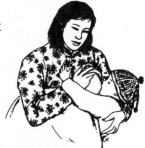

It is safe to breastfeed when you are pregnant.

If you are a health worker, it is not enough to talk about breastfeeding. Women need information and support. Teach women to give nothing but breast milk for the first 6 months. Teach them that other kinds of feedings may harm the baby.

Support women with breastfeeding before problems start. Help women feel confident that they have enough milk. Mother-to-mother support is the best help for common problems. Try starting a breastfeeding group in your community led by women who have breastfed exclusively, and whose children are growing well.

Learn how to make your health center friendly to breastfeeding. Help mothers to breastfeed within the first hour after birth. Allow babies to sleep with or near their mothers. When a mother is sick, let the baby stay with her.

If you are a mother yourself, breastfeed your own baby to show other working mothers they can work and breastfeed too.

Remove any posters or educational materials that promote artificial milks. Do not pass on samples or gifts from the infant formula companies and do not let representatives from these companies come to the clinic.

Working for Change

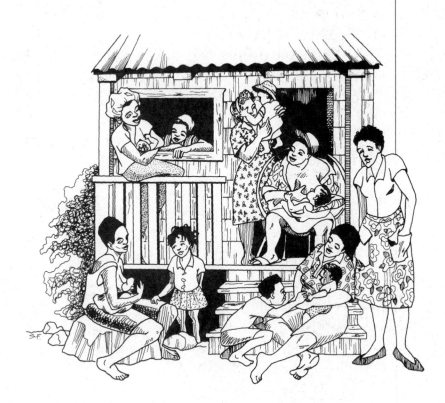

Chapter 8

In this Chapter:

Growing Older

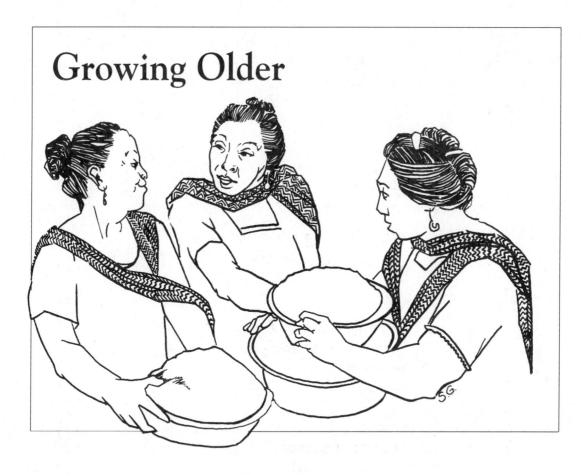

Today more and more people are living longer. Cleaner living conditions, *vaccinations* and better *nutrition* help prevent many diseases and modern medicines cure others.

But longer life has also brought difficulties. First, older people tend to have more health problems than younger people. Although most of these problems are not caused by age itself, the changes age makes in a person's body can make the problems more serious or difficult to treat.

Second, as the world changes and younger family members move away from their communities to earn a living, many older people are left to care for themselves. Or, if they do live with their children, older people may feel like a burden in a family or community that no longer values and respects age.

Older women are more likely to face these problems than older men, because women usually live longer and often reach old age without a partner. So in this chapter we describe how older women can take care of their health, treat common health problems of aging, and work to improve the difficult conditions under which many older women live.

➤ *Everyone is the age of their heart.*
—Guatemalan proverb

The End of Monthly Bleeding (Menopause)

One of the main signs of growing older is that a woman's *monthly bleeding* ends. It may end suddenly, or it may stop gradually over 1 to 2 years. For most women this change happens between the age of 45 and 55.

Signs:

- Your monthly bleeding changes. It may just stop, or you may bleed more often for a while. Or you may stop bleeding for a few months and then bleed again.
- At times you may suddenly feel very hot or sweaty (this is also called having 'hot flashes'). This can wake you up at night.
- Your vagina becomes less wet and smaller.
- Your feelings change easily.

These signs happen because a woman's *ovaries* stop making eggs, and her body makes less of the hormones *estrogen* and *progesterone*. The signs will start to go away as her body gets used to less estrogen.

How a woman feels about the end of her monthly bleeding sometimes depends on how she is affected by the changes in her body. It also depends on how her community thinks about and treats older women. She may be relieved not to have her monthly bleeding every month. But she may also feel sad that she cannot have any more children.

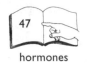

47

hormones

What to do during menopause:

If you are having signs that make you uncomfortable, try the following:

- Dress in clothes that you can take off easily when you begin to sweat.

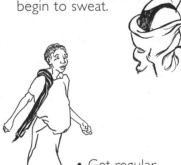

- Get regular exercise.

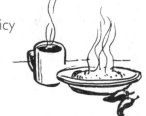

- Avoid hot or spicy foods or drinks. They can cause hot flashes.

- Do not drink much coffee or tea. They contain *caffeine*, which can make you feel nervous and prevent you from sleeping.

Medicines for problems during menopause

If a woman's signs of menopause are so severe that they stop her from doing her daily work or keep her from sleeping at night, she can try taking medicine for a few months to see if she feels better. This is called 'hormone replacement therapy', or HRT. The most common medicine is made from estrogen and progesterone. If a woman decides to take HRT, she should always take both hormones, unless she has had her womb removed by surgery. Estrogen taken by itself can cause *cancer* of the womb.

HRT can stop hot flashes and make the vagina more wet. If taken for a long time, HRT may also help reduce other health risks, such as weak bones and heart disease, which come from having less estrogen in the body. But HRT can be costly, and may cause an increased risk of *gallbladder* disease. The medicine may also cause *side effects*, such as bleeding from the *vagina*, *cramping* pains, *nausea*, tender breasts, weight gain, and *depression*.

Before taking HRT, a woman needs to think about its *risks* and *benefits*. HRT is usually not recommended for women who have had trouble with *blood clots*, breast cancer, or liver or gallbladder disease. Be sure to talk to a health worker about the right dose.

A woman can stop taking the medicine at any time, but she should do so slowly—or her signs may come back.

➤ *Although women sometimes feel uncomfortable during menopause, **only a few need medical treatment**.*

problems of the womb, 380

depression, 419

breast cancer, 382

➤*Taking hormones does not cause breast cancer. But if a woman already has cancer, hormones can make it worse.*

➤ *Always take the lowest possible dose of the medicines.*

• If you drink alcohol, drink only small amounts. Alcohol can increase bleeding and hot flashes.

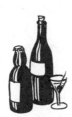

• Stop smoking or chewing tobacco. It can cause unusual bleeding and make problems with weak bones (see page 133) much worse.

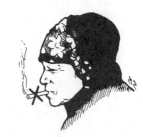

• Explain to your family that your feelings may change easily. It may also help to discuss how you feel with other women who are going through menopause.

• Ask about the use of traditional remedies in your community. Often women who have already been through menopause will know ways to help you feel better.

Taking Care of Your Health

eating for good health, 165

calcium-rich foods, 168

Just as a girl's body changes when she becomes a woman, so a woman's body changes when her childbearing years end. Menopause and aging cause changes in bone strength, muscle and joint strength and flexibility, and overall well-being.

A woman can make a big difference in living her later years with energy and good health by:

Eating well. As a woman grows older she still needs *nutritious* food to keep her body strong and to fight disease. Her need for certain kinds of food also increases. Because her body makes less estrogen, it helps to eat foods high in plant estrogens, such as soy beans, tofu (bean curd), lentils, and other beans. Since her bones become less dense as she ages, it helps to eat foods high in *calcium*, a *mineral* that makes strong bones.

Sometimes older people feel less like eating than they used to. This may be caused by changes in taste and smell, which make eating less pleasurable. Or changes in the body that come from aging can make a person quickly feel full after starting to eat. But this does not mean that older people need less nutritious food. They need encouragement to continue to eat well, and to eat a variety of foods.

Drinking a lot of liquids. As a person ages, the amount of water in the body decreases. Also, some older people drink less to avoid having to pass *urine* during the night or because they are afraid of leaking urine. All these things can cause *dehydration*. To prevent this, drink 8 glasses or cups of liquid every day. To avoid getting up at night to pass urine, try not to drink anything for 2 to 3 hours before going to sleep.

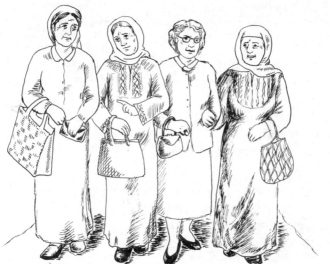

Getting regular exercise. Everyday activities, such as walking, playing with grandchildren, going to the market, cooking, and farming can all help keep a woman's muscles and bones strong, and prevent stiff joints. Regular exercise will help maintain weight and prevent heart disease.

Treating illness early. Some people think that getting older means being sick much of the time. But this is not true. If a woman does not feel well, she may have an illness that can be treated, and that has nothing to do with age. She needs treatment as soon as possible.

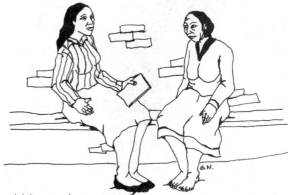

Staying active. A woman will stay healthier and happier if she is active and productive. Try to take up an activity, join a group, or work on a community project. This may be a good time for a woman to work for better conditions in the community. Here is an example:

➤ *Try to see a health worker if you feel ill and have been unable to treat the problem yourself.*

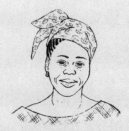

Louise Waithira Nganga is a coffee farmer in Kandara town, in Kenya. In 1991, as a member of an organization planting trees in Kenya, she met a group of women farmers who complained about a coffee factory upstream. The fertilizers and chemicals the factory used to make coffee were getting into the river, and the women's cows were getting sick and dying from drinking the dirty water.

Soon many of the women began meeting to talk with Louise. They became aware of how the river also affected their health and their children's health. They decided to put pressure on the district officers to force the factory to keep waste out of the river.

Louise, however, always insisted that rights and responsibilities go together. So she also helped the women realize how their own habits affected other people down the river. For example, when they cleaned their fertilizing machines or washed their clothes in the river, it was harmful for the health of the people downstream. As Louise said, "We must first be responsible ourselves so that we may, in clear conscience, demand our rights."

In 1993, Louise and her women farmers created an organization called Rural Women's Sanitation. Whenever the river is in danger from polluting factories, Louise is able to organize as many as 100 women, who 'pay a visit' to the local authorities, and inform them of the problem. Besides taking care of the river, the group is building latrines and demanding that local governments reclaim public wells that have been taken over by private owners.

Louise has stopped planting trees, but has no regrets. "There were more pressing problems that were part of Kandara soil itself." She tells her fellow women, "God will not come to earth to solve your problems. The government cannot know what your problems are. Only you can make sure they get solved."

Sexual Relations

➤ *There is no reason based on age alone that a woman cannot enjoy sex for as long as she lives.*

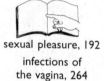

sexual pleasure, 192

infections of
the vagina, 264

infections of the urine
system, 366

➤ *Do not use petroleum gel or oils that contain perfumes to increase wetness in the vagina. These can cause irritation.*

190

dry sex

For some women, menopause means freedom from the sexual demands of marriage. Other women become more interested in sex because they no longer fear an unwanted pregnancy. All women, though, continue to need love and affection.

As a woman grows older, some of the changes in her body may affect her sexual relations:

• She may take longer to become excited during sex (this also happens to men).

• Her *vagina* may be more dry, which can make sex uncomfortable, or make her get an *infection* of the vagina or the urine system more easily.

What to do:

• Try to take more time before having sex, so your vagina can make its natural wetness. You can also use spit (saliva), oils made from vegetables (peanut oil, corn oil, olive oil), or other lubricants like spermicides during sex.

IMPORTANT *Do not use oils for wetness if you are using condoms. Oil will weaken the condom and it may break.*

• If it is difficult for your partner to get or keep his *penis* hard (erection), try to learn what he likes. Touching him may help make him excited.

• To prevent urine problems, do not try to make the vagina dry before having sex. Pass urine as soon as possible after sex to flush out *germs*.

Protecting yourself against pregnancy and sexually transmitted diseases (STDs)

You can still become pregnant until your monthy bleeding has stopped for one full year. To prevent unwanted pregnancy, you should continue to use a family planning method during that time (see page 197).

If you are using a *hormonal method of family planning* (the pill, injections, or implants), stop using it around the age of 50 to see if you are still having monthly bleeding. Use another method of family planning until you have no monthly bleeding for one whole year (12 months).

Unless you are certain neither you nor your partner has an STD, including HIV/AIDS, be sure to use a condom each time you have sex—even if you can no longer become pregnant (see page 188).

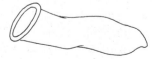

The following pages describe some of the most common health problems of older women. For other problems, like gallbladder problems, heart trouble, *stroke*, *thyroid gland* problems, sores on the legs from poor blood flow, and difficulty sleeping, see *Where There Is No Doctor* or another general medical book. For information on *diabetes*, see page 174.

WEAK BLOOD (ANEMIA)

Although many people think that anemia is a problem only of young women, it also affects many older women—most often because of poor nutrition or heavy monthly bleeding. For more about anemia, see page 172.

HEAVY MONTHLY BLEEDING OR BLEEDING IN THE MIDDLE OF THE MONTH

Between the ages of 40 and 50, many women have changes in their monthly bleeding. Some have heavier bleeding, or bleeding that lasts longer. Heavy bleeding that goes on for months or years can cause anemia.

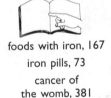

The most common causes of heavy monthly bleeding and bleeding that lasts longer are:

- hormone changes
- growths in the *womb* (*fibroids* or *polyps*)

Treatment:

- Eat foods every day that are rich in *iron*, or take iron pills.
- Take 10 mg medoxyprogesterone acetate once a day for 10 days. If bleeding has not stopped at the end of 10 days, take the medicine for another 10 days. If you are still bleeding, see a health worker.
- Try to see a health worker for heavy bleeding that has lasted for more than 3 months, for bleeding in the middle of the month, or for bleeding that starts 12 months or more after menopause. A trained health worker will need to scrape out the inside of the womb (*D and C*) or do a *biopsy* and send the tissue to a laboratory to be checked for cancer.

If you have had pain and heavy monthly bleeding for years, see the chapter on "Cancer and Growths."

BREAST LUMPS

Older women often find lumps in their breasts. Most breast lumps are not dangerous, but some may be a sign of cancer (see page 382). The best way to find lumps in your breasts is to examine your breasts yourself (see page 162).

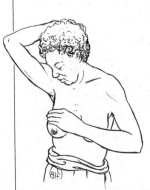

HIGH BLOOD PRESSURE

High *blood pressure* can cause many problems, like heart disease, kidney disease, and strokes.

Signs of dangerously high blood pressure:

- frequent headaches
- dizziness
- ringing sound in the ears

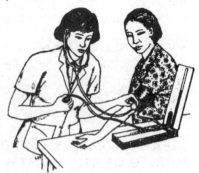

➤ *All these signs can also be caused by other diseases. For more information, see* **Where There Is No Doctor** *or another general medical book.*

If you are visiting a health worker for any reason, try to have your blood pressure checked at the same time.

528

blood pressure

IMPORTANT *High blood pressure at first causes no signs. It should be lowered before danger signs develop. People who are overweight or who think they might have high blood pressure should have their blood pressure checked regularly.*

Treatment and prevention:

- Get some exercise every day.
- If you are overweight, try to lose weight.
- Avoid foods with a lot of fat, sugar, or salt.
- If you smoke or chew tobacco, try to stop.

If your blood pressure is very high, you may also need to take medicine.

losing weight, 174
eating for good health, 165

PROBLEMS PASSING URINE AND STOOL

Many older women have problems with leaking urine or have difficulty passing *stool*. They may be too embarrassed to speak about these problems, especially to a male doctor. So they suffer alone.

Urine problems are often caused by a weakness in the muscle inside the vagina. The 'squeezing exercise' helps strengthen this muscle. Also, to help push the stool out during a bowel movement, a woman can put 2 fingers into her vagina and push toward her back.

leaking urine, 370
squeezing exercise, 371

An older woman may also have trouble passing stool because her intestines work more slowly as she ages. It helps to drink a lot of liquids, to eat foods with a lot of fiber (like whole grain breads or vegetables), and to get regular exercise.

FALLEN WOMB (PROLAPSED UTERUS)

Sometimes, as a woman gets older, the muscles that hold up her womb become weak. The womb can fall down into her vagina and part of it may even stick out between the folds of the *vulva*. In very bad cases, the whole womb can fall outside the vulva when a woman passes stool, coughs, sneezes, or lifts heavy things.

A fallen womb is usually caused by damage during childbirth—especially if the woman has had many babies or babies born close together. It can also happen if the woman pushed too early during her labor, or if the birth attendant pushed on the mother's belly from the outside. But both aging and lifting heavy things can make it worse. The signs often appear after menopause, when the muscles become weaker.

161 preventing fallen womb

Signs:

- You need to pass urine often, or it is difficult to pass urine, or urine leaks out of your body.
- You have pain in your lower back.
- You feel as though something is coming out of your vagina.
- All of the above signs disappear when you lie down.

Treatment:

The 'squeezing exercise' can make the muscles around the womb and vagina stronger. If you have been doing this exercise every day for 3 or 4 months and it does not help, talk to a health worker. You may need a vaginal pessary (a piece of rubber shaped like a ring) that you put in the vagina to keep the womb in place. If this does not work, you may need an operation.

371 squeezing exercise

Kinds of Vaginal Pessaries

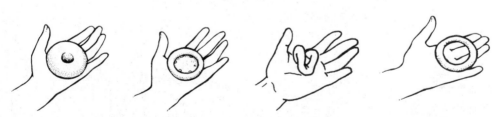

Put the pessary high up in your vagina to hold your womb in place.

If pessaries are not available where you live, ask older women in your community what they use for this problem.

SWOLLEN VEINS IN THE LEGS (VARICOSE VEINS)

Varicose veins are veins that are swollen and often painful. Older women who have had many children are most likely to suffer from this problem.

Treatment:

There is no medicine for varicose veins, but the following can help:

This woman is keeping her leg up as she sews.

- Try to walk or move your legs at least 20 minutes every day.
- Try not to spend much time standing or sitting with your feet down, or with your legs crossed.
- If you have to sit or stand for a long time, try to take breaks to lie down with your feet above the level of your heart. Do this as often as possible during the day.
- When you have to stand for a long time, try to walk in place.
- Sleep with your feet up on pillows or on a bundle of cloth.
- To help hold in the veins, use elastic stockings, elastic bandages, or cloth that is not wrapped too tightly. But be sure to take them off at night.

BACK PAIN

Back pain in older women is often caused by a lifetime of heavy lifting and carrying.

It can often be helped by:
- exercising every day to strengthen and stretch the muscles in the back. It may be more enjoyable if you organize a group of women to exercise together.
- asking younger members of your family to help you, if you must continue to do hard work.

400

back exercises

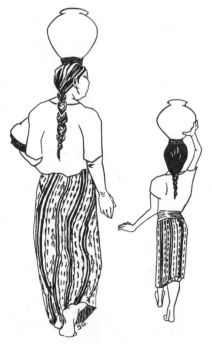

JOINT PAIN (ARTHRITIS)

Many older women suffer from *joint* pain caused by arthritis. Usually it cannot be cured completely, but the following treatment may help.

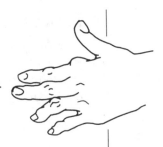

Treatment:

- Rest the place that hurts.
- Soak cloths in hot water and place them on the painful areas. Be careful not to burn your skin. (Some people with joint pain lose their sense of feeling from the skin on the painful areas.)
- Keep your joints moving by gently rubbing and stretching them every day.
- Take a mild pain medicine. Aspirin works best for arthritis. For very bad pain, take 600 to 1000 mg of aspirin up to 6 times a day, with food, milk, or a large glass of water. Ibuprofen also works well. Take 400 mg 4 to 6 times a day.

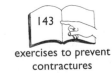

143 exercises to prevent contractures

482 medicines for pain

IMPORTANT *If your ears start to ring or you start to bruise easily, take less aspirin. Also, if you are having a lot of bleeding from your vagina, you should not take aspirin.*

WEAK BONES (OSTEOPOROSIS)

After menopause, a woman's body starts to make less estrogen, and her bones become weaker. Weak bones break easily and heal slowly.

A woman is more likely to get weak bones if she:

- is over 70 years old.
- is thin.
- does not exercise.
- does not eat enough foods rich in calcium.
- has been pregnant many times.
- drinks a lot of alcohol.
- smokes or chews tobacco.

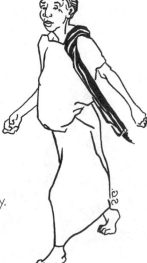

➤ *Weak bones are a major cause of disability for older women.*

➤ *Both exercise and calcium make the bones stronger.*

Treatment:

- Walk for 20 to 30 minutes every day.
- Eat foods rich in calcium.

It may also help to take hormone medicines (HRT, see page 125).

168 calcium-rich foods

PROBLEMS WITH SEEING AND HEARING

As they get older, many women are not able to see and hear as well as they used to. Women with seeing or hearing problems are more likely to have accidents, and less likely to work outside the home or to take part in community life.

Problems with Seeing

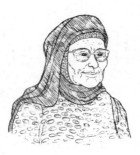

After the age of 40, it is common to have problems seeing close objects clearly. This is called being *farsighted*. Often eye glasses will help.

A woman should also watch for signs of too much pressure from fluid in the eye (glaucoma), which can damage the inside of her eye and lead to blindness. *Acute* glaucoma starts suddenly, with severe headache or pain in the eye. The eye will also feel hard to the touch. *Chronic* glaucoma usually is not painful, but a woman slowly starts to lose vision to the side. If possible, older women should get their eyes checked at a health center for these problems. For more information, see **Where There Is No Doctor** or another general medical book.

Problems with Hearing

Many women over the age of 50 have hearing loss. Other people may overlook the problem since they cannot see it. Or they may start to leave the person out of conversations and social activites.

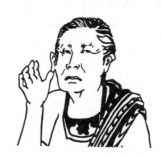

If you notice that you are losing your hearing, here are some things you can do:

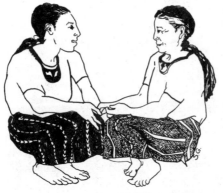

- Sit facing the person you are talking to.
- Ask family members and friends to speak slowly and clearly. But tell them not to shout. Shouting can make words even more difficult to understand.
- Turn off radios or televisions when participating in conversations.
- Ask a health worker if your hearing loss can be treated with medicines, surgery, or by using a hearing aid.

ANXIETY AND DEPRESSION

Older women sometimes feel anxious or depressed because their role in the family and community has changed, because they feel alone or worried about the future, or because they have health problems that cause pain and discomfort. For more information on anxiety and depression, see the chapter on "Mental Health."

MENTAL CONFUSION (DEMENTIA)

Some older people have difficulty remembering things and thinking clearly. When these problems become severe, it is called *dementia.*

Signs:

- difficulty concentrating, or getting lost in the middle of a conversation.
- repeating the same thing over and over. The person will not remember having said the same thing before.
- difficulty with daily tasks. The person may have trouble knowing how to dress or prepare food.
- behavior changes. The person may become irritable, angry, or do sudden, unexpected things.

These signs are caused by changes in the brain, and usually develop over a long period of time. If the signs begin suddenly, the problem probably has other causes, such as too much medicine in the body (toxicity), a serious infection, *malnutrition*, or severe depression. The confusion will often go away if these problems are treated.

Treatment:

There is no special treatment or cure for dementia. Caring for someone who is confused can be very hard on family members. It helps to share the responsibility of care and get support from people outside the family when possible.

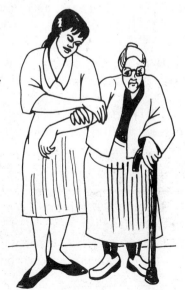

To help the person with dementia, try to:

- make her surroundings as safe as possible.
- keep daily routines regular so she knows what to expect.
- keep familiar objects around the house.
- talk to her in a calm, slow voice. Give her plenty of time to answer.
- set clear limits without a lot of choices. Ask questions that can be answered "yes" or "no."

Working for Change

It is traditional in most places for families to live together and for young people to care for their elders. But now many women and men work away from their communities, often traveling far from their homes to earn money to support their families. Older people are now often left to care for themselves.

Older women are more likely than men to live alone. Women usually live longer than men and often marry older men. In many places women whose partners have died are considered less important than married women. When an older woman lives in a community that no longer values elders, she—as well as her family—may feel that her health problems are not worthy of treatment. Or services to treat her health problems may not exist.

When an older woman is also very poor, the problems she faces are much worse. She may not have the money to pay for health care and medicines, to buy healthy foods, or to pay for a healthy place to live.

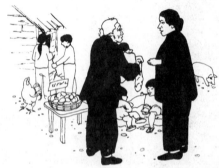

Income earning projects. One way that older women can improve their situation is by finding ways to earn money to support themselves and even help their families, such as:

* raising animals, like chickens, goats, or cows, and then selling the eggs, milk, cheese, or meat.
* making bread or other food to sell.
* making traditional crafts or sewing things to sell.

Six widows living in a small community in El Salvador decided they wanted to earn some money by raising chickens to sell for meat. None of them had ever raised chickens before, but they asked a group that supports cooperatives to help show them how.

After a local community association loaned them money, the group started to work. At night the women took turns sleeping in the chicken coop to keep animals and people from stealing the chickens. At dawn the women rose to kill and clean chickens. Every day the women walked for miles to other communities to sell the chickens, carrying them in baskets on their heads.

Men from their community—and even a specialist who worked with an agency—all told them their project would not be successful. But the women earned enough money to cover their costs, buy new chickens, and pay themselves each about $45 a month. Although it was not much money, it was more than any of them had ever earned before. And they gained respect in their community because they had a successful business. As one of them said, "We never imagined that we could run our own business. Now look at us. We are the bosses!"

Community services for older women. By working together, older women can encourage their communities to:
- create less costly housing for older women, or form groups that live together to cut down on living expenses.
- include older women in nutrition programs.
- train health workers in the special health needs of older women.

Older women can teach others. Older women are the main keepers of traditional healing practices, and only they can pass on this knowledge to the next generation. To preserve these practices and remind others that older women have important skills, women can teach these practices to their children and grandchildren. Older women can also help health workers learn traditional healing practices, so that health workers can use the best methods of both traditional and modern medicine.

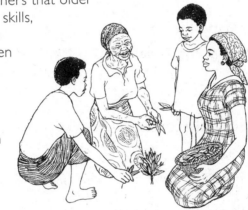

Changing government policies and laws. Many governments provide monthly income (pensions), housing, and health care for older people. If your government does not, try to work together with other women to change these laws. This kind of change takes time. But even if a woman does not see the changes herself, she will know she has worked toward a better life for her daughters and grand-daughters.

➤ *Older women have much wisdom and experience. Working together can make them very powerful.*

Accepting Death

Every culture has a system of beliefs about death and ideas about life after death. These ideas, beliefs, and traditions may comfort a person facing death. But she also needs support, kindness, and honesty from her loved ones.

You can help a dying person most by listening to her feelings and needs. If she wants to die at home—surrounded by the people she loves—rather than in a hospital, try to respect her wishes. If she wants to talk about death, try to be honest. Anyone who is dying usually knows it, partly by what her body tells her, and partly by the reactions she sees in those she loves. Let her talk openly about her fears, and about the joys and sorrows in her life. This way, when death comes, she may more easily accept it as the natural end of life.

Chapter 9

In this Chapter:

In this chapter we use the word 'women with disabilities' rather than 'disabled women.' We do this to remind people that although a disability can prevent a woman from doing certain things, in other ways she is just like other women. She is a woman first.

No matter what causes a woman's disability, she can be just as productive as a woman without a disability. She just needs the opportunity to develop her skills to their fullest.

For more complete information on health care and disabilities, see the Hesperian Foundation book, *Disabled Village Children*. For information about ordering, see the last page of this book.

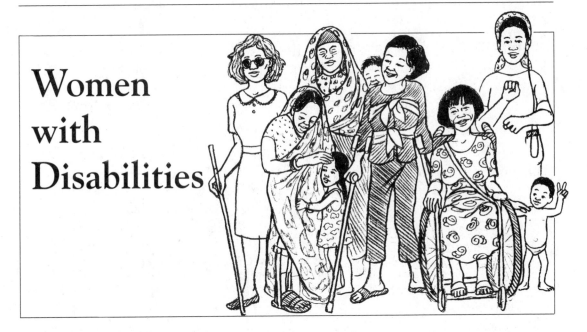

Women with Disabilities

About 1 out of every 10 women has a disability that affects daily living. She may have difficulties with walking, lifting, seeing, hearing or using her mind. Yet many of these women are never seen or heard. They are often hidden away and do not take part in community activities because they are thought of as less useful and of less value than women without disabilities.

WHAT CAUSES DISABILITY?

Local customs and beliefs often give people false ideas about disability. For example, people may think a woman has a disability because she did something bad in a former life and is now being punished. Or they may think her disability is 'catching' (contagious), so they are afraid to be around her.

But disabilities are not caused by anything a person does wrong. In poor countries, many disabilities are caused by poverty, and sometimes by wars, which few people can control. For example:

- If a mother does not get enough to eat when she is pregnant, her child may be born with a disability (birth defect).

- If a baby or young child does not get enough good food to eat she or he may become blind or mentally slow.

- Poor *sanitation* and crowded living conditions, together with poor food and a lack of basic health services and *vaccinations*, can lead to many disabilities.

- In today's wars, more women and children are killed or disabled than are soldiers or other men.

But even if these reasons for disability are eliminated, there will always be persons with disabilities—it is a natural part of life.

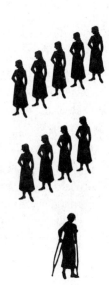

1 out of every 10 women has a disability that affects daily living.

Self-Esteem

The following letter came from a group of women with disabilities in Ghana, West Africa. But it could have come from any community, because all over the world, women—and especially women with disabilities—are taught not to value themselves.

Our Association was formed in 1989 by women with disabilities to help promote the welfare of the woman with a disability. We have 21 members with various disabilities (sight, hearing, speech, and movement). We hold a meeting once a month to talk about our problems and to try to find solutions.

We all agree that women with disabilities are often *discriminated* against because:

- we are women.
- we have disabilities.
- we are mostly poor.

We are rejected as suitable marriage partners or regarded as the 'wrong' image in the work place. Girls and women with disabilities are not often able to get an education, even when education is available. For example, even in special schools for children with disabilities, boys usually receive priority.

We are unlikely to receive training for any kind of work. We experience abuse—physically, emotionally, and sexually. Unlike all men and women without disabilities, we are seldom allowed to make decisions at home or in the community.

But for each of us in the Association, the biggest problem is lack of self-esteem. We are taught by society not to value ourselves. We are generally considered to be incapable of keeping a man and bearing children, and unable to do meaningful work. Therefore we are considered worthless. Even our extended families only want us if we prove valuable to them.

—*Dormaa Ahenkro, Ghana*

If a woman grows up with the support of her family, school and community to live the best life she can, her feelings of self-worth will be very high, whether or not she has a disability. But if a woman grows up feeling she is worth less than others because she has a disability, she has to work hard to learn to value herself. This process is never easy, but it can be done by taking small steps.

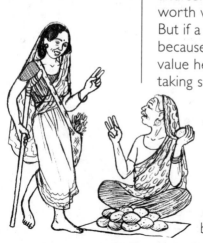

The first step is to meet other people. If you are a woman with a disability, you might try sitting at the door of your home and greeting your neighbors. Then, if you are able, go to the market and talk to people there. As they get to know you, they will find out that women with and without disabilities are not really very different from each other. Each time you go out it will become easier to meet and talk with others.

A second step is to start or join a group for women.
Talking with others can help you begin to learn about your
strengths and weaknesses. A group can provide a safe place for
women to speak freely—if you all agree not to speak outside
the group about anything that is said inside the group.

support groups

You can also join or start a group for women with disabilities
and share your thoughts and experiences about the special
challenges that come from having a disability. You can all
support each other during both happy and difficult times.

You can support each other in learning how to become
independent, too. All over the world women with disabilities
are working as doctors, nurses, shop keepers, writers, teachers,
farmers, and community organizers. With each other's help, you
can begin to prepare for the future, just as any woman would.

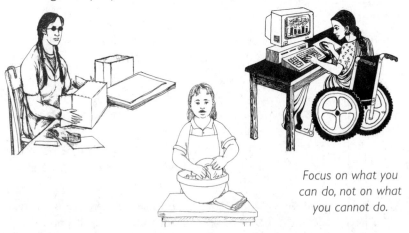

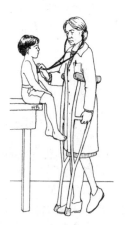

*Focus on what you
can do, not on what
you cannot do.*

If you have a disability, most of your health problems are
probably no different from those of other women, and you can
find information about them in other chapters in this book. But
the following issues can be of special concern for women with
disabilities, especially women with a loss of feeling in the body.

**Taking
Care of
Your
Health**

KNOWING WHEN YOU ARE SICK

Some women with disabilities may find it it difficult to tell
when they have a health problem. For example, a woman who
has an *infection* in her *womb* may not be able to feel pain from
it. But she may notice an unusual *discharge* or smell from her
vagina that an infection can cause.

As a woman, you know and understand your body better
than anyone else. So if you have an unusual feeling, or body
reaction, or a pain somewhere, try to find out as soon as
possible what might be causing it. If necessary, ask a family
member, friend, or health worker to help.

➤ *Pressure sores are one of the main causes of death in persons with spinal cord injury.*

SKIN CARE

If you sit or lie down all or most of the time, you can develop pressure sores. These sores start when the skin over the bony parts of the body is pressed against a chair or bed. The blood vessels get squeezed shut, so that not enough blood can get to the skin.

If too much time passes without moving, a dark or red patch appears on the skin. If the pressure continues, an open sore can develop and work its way deeper into the body. Or the sore can start deep inside near the bone and gradually grow out to the surface. Without treatment, the skin can die.

wound care

Treatment:

For information on how to treat pressure sores, see page 306.

Prevention:

- Try to move at least every 2 hours. If you lie down all the time, have someone help you change position.

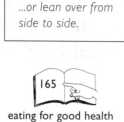
If you sit all day...

...lift your bottom by pushing yourself up with your hands...

...or lean over from side to side.

- Lie or sit on a soft surface that reduces pressure on bony areas. A cushion or sleeping pad that has hollowed-out areas around the bony parts will help. Or make a simple cushion or sleeping pad from a plastic bag filled with uncooked beans and rice. It must be refilled with new rice and beans once a month.

- Examine your whole body carefully every day. You can use a mirror to look at your back. If you notice a dark or red place, try to avoid any pressure on this area until your skin returns to normal.

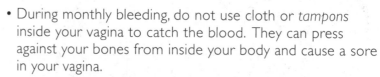
Examine your skin every day.

eating for good health

- Try to eat plenty of fruits, vegetables, and foods rich in *protein*.

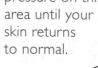

monthly bleeding

- During monthly bleeding, do not use cloth or *tampons* inside your vagina to catch the blood. They can press against your bones from inside your body and cause a sore in your vagina.

165
eating for good health

48
monthly bleeding

149
staying healthy

- Try to bathe every day. Pat your skin dry, but do not rub it. Avoid lotions or oils, because they can make your skin soft and weaker. And **never** use alcohol on your skin.

EXERCISE

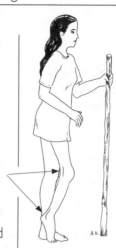

Some women—for example, those who suffer from *arthritis* or *strokes*, or who are in bed because of *AIDS* or old age—have difficulty moving their arms and legs enough to keep their *joints* flexible. When this happens, and an arm or a leg is kept bent for a long time, some of the muscles become shorter and the limb cannot fully straighten. Or short muscles may hold a joint straight so that it cannot bend. This is called a 'contracture'. Sometimes contractures cause pain.

To prevent contractures and keep your muscles strong, you need to find someone who can help you exercise your arms and legs every day. Try to make sure that every part of your body is moved. If you have had contractures for many years, it will be difficult to completely straighten your joints. But these exercises will prevent the contractures from getting worse and can make your joints a little less stiff and keep your muscles strong.

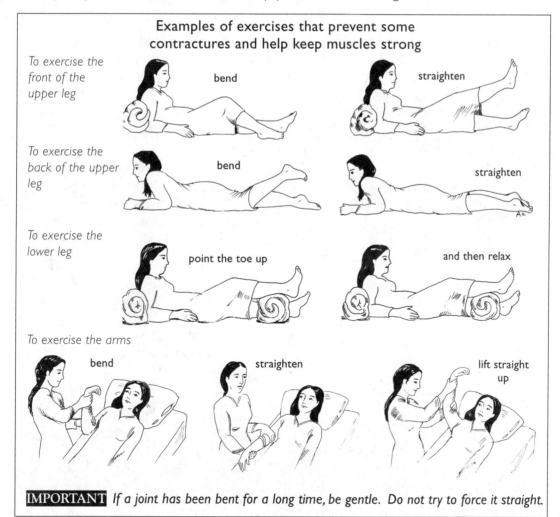

Examples of exercises that prevent some contractures and help keep muscles strong

To exercise the front of the upper leg

bend

straighten

To exercise the back of the upper leg

bend

straighten

To exercise the lower leg

point the toe up

and then relax

To exercise the arms

bend

straighten

lift straight up

IMPORTANT *If a joint has been bent for a long time, be gentle. Do not try to force it straight.*

Sexuality and Sexual Health

➤ *Be careful not to let other people take advantage of you. It can be difficult to protect yourself against violence and abuse.*

313 👉
violence

181 👉
sexual health

Many people believe that women with disabilities cannot have, or should not have, sexual feelings. They are not expected to want to have close, loving relationships or to become parents. But women with disabilities do have a desire for closeness and sexual relations just like anyone else.

If you were born with a disability, or it happened when you were very young, you may have a hard time believing you are sexually attractive. Talking with other women who have disabilities about their own fears, and how they overcame them, is often the best way to learn to feel differently about yourself. But remember to have patience. It takes time to change beliefs you have held for a long time.

If you are a woman with a new disability, you may already be used to thinking of yourself as a sexual person. But you may not realize that you can continue to enjoy sex. You may think you are not sexually attractive any more and feel sad that sex may be different now.

All women with disabilities can be helped by reading the same information about sexuality that women who are not disabled read. Try to talk about sexuality with them and with trusted teachers, health care workers, and other women with disabilities.

You and your partner will both need to experiment with how to please each other. For example, if you have no feeling in your hands or genitals, during sex you can find other body parts that will create sexual feeling, such as an ear, or breast, or neck. This can also help if a disability has made sex in the vagina uncomfortable. You can also try different positions, like lying on your side, or sitting on the edge of a chair. If you and your partner can talk together honestly, a satisfying sexual relationship can happen. But remember that you do not have to settle for less than you would like. You do not have to have sex with someone who does not care about you.

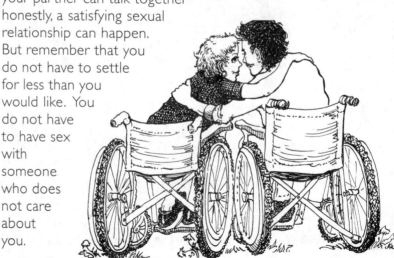

Family planning

Many girls with disabilities grow up with no information about sex or *family planning*. Yet most women with disabilities can become pregnant—even those with no feeling in the lower body. So if you plan to have sex and do not want to become pregnant, you will need to use a family planning method.

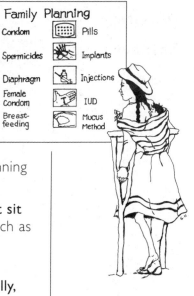

Family Planning

Condom		Pills	
Spermicides		Implants	
Diaphragm		Injections	
Female Condom		IUD	
Breast-feeding		Mucus Method	

Here are some guidelines for deciding which family planning method might be best for you:

If you have had a stroke, or cannot walk and you must sit or lie down all the time, do not use *hormonal methods*, such as birth control pills, injections, or implants. They can cause problems with blood clots.

If you have no feeling or only a little feeling in your belly, do not use an *intra-uterine device* (IUD). If it is not put in correctly, or if there is a possibility you might get a *sexually transmitted disease*, it can cause an infection. Without feeling you may not be able to tell that you are infected.

➤ *Condoms will help prevent both pregnancy and STDs, including HIV/AIDS.*

If you cannot use your hands well, it may be difficult for you to use *barrier methods*, such as the diaphragm, the female condom, or foam. If you feel comfortable asking your partner, he may be able to put them in for you.

197

family planning

If your disability changes over time, you may need to change your family planning method as your disability progresses.

Pregnancy and disability

A woman with a disability can become pregnant and have a healthy baby. Here are some things to consider, especially if you cannot move your body very much, or if you use a walking aid:

- As your belly gets larger, your balance changes. Some women can use a stick or crutch to prevent falls. Some women may want to use a wheelchair while pregnant.

- Since many pregnant women have trouble with hard stools (constipation), you may need to do your 'bowel program' to remove the stool more often (see page 372).

- During labor, you may not be able to feel the birth pains (*contractions*). Instead, watch for the shape of your belly to change, and use this to count the time between contractions.

- To prevent stiff joints (*contractures*) and to keep your muscles strong, exercise as much as you can. Try to do the exercises on page 143.

- For more general information on pregnancy and birth, see page 67.

Personal Safety

332

self defense

Since a woman with a disability may be less able to protect herself, she is more at risk for violent attack and abuse than a woman without a disability. But there are things a woman can do to defend herself. It may help to practice some of these things with a group of women with disabilities:

- If you are in a public place and someone tries to hurt or abuse you, shout as loudly as you can.

- Do something he might find disgusting, such as drooling spit (saliva), or trying to vomit, or acting as though you are 'crazy'.

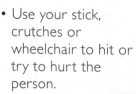

- Use your stick, crutches or wheelchair to hit or try to hurt the person.

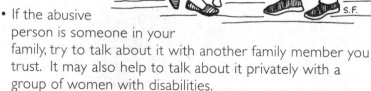

- If the abusive person is someone in your family, try to talk about it with another family member you trust. It may also help to talk about it privately with a group of women with disabilities.

Special care for women who have mental disabilities

Women and girls who have problems with understanding or learning (mental disabilities) may need special care, as it can be even more difficult for them to defend themselves.

If there is a girl or woman in your family with these problems, it is important to talk openly with her about abusive or harmful people. Talk about when it is OK for someone to touch another person in a sexual way and when it is not, and about what is safe and unsafe in public and private situations. Let her know it is OK to tell you if anything she does not like happens to her. Help her learn how to say "No." Teach her how to defend herself.

It is also a good idea to talk with persons with mental disabilities about sexually transmitted diseases (STDs) and pregnancy, and to give them what they need to protect themselves (see pages 263 and 226). But be careful not to treat girls and women with mental disabilities like prisoners. When it is safe, let them go outside, or to the market, or to work in the fields.

Working for Change

To build a better life, women with disabilities need health, education, and the ability to move around independently and earn a living. The first step toward achieving these things may be to form a group with other women with disabilities. Together you can decide what things in your community can be changed, in order to make life better for you all.

Here are some suggestions:
- Start a *literacy* class for the women who cannot read or write.
- Try to get funds—either as a low-interest loan or through a donation—to begin an income-earning project so you can all make your own living.
- As a group, go to the local authorities and ask them to:
  - make the village water supply, schools, and health centers easier to get to, and easier for people who are blind and deaf to use.
  - help you start a library, and to find more information about disabilities.
  - work with you to make disability aids and equipment available.

➤ *The particular tasks your group chooses are not as important as just working together. Start with what you as a group feel is most important, and work from there.*

To give you an idea of what a group working together can do, here is the rest of the letter from the women in Ghana:

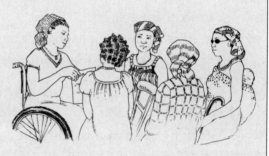

Being in this Association gives us a new value, a way to be a part of something which counts, and a chance to organize ourselves for our rights.

Most members have learned skills such as weaving, sewing, candle making, shoe repairs, basket making, and typing. Some of our other activities are:

- Involving women with disabilities in community activities.
- Meeting with teachers and parents to choose materials with positive images of disability.
- Finding ways to support ourselves financially so we can obtain working tools, disability aids, and wheelchairs for our members.

Friendship and trust between women with disabilities gives rise to many new ideas. We run the Association by and for ourselves, and we are encouraged in our efforts. This helps to raise the image of all women with disabilities.

Just like the women in Ghana, working with others can help you achieve an independent, productive life. You do not have to stay inside your house unless you want to. Go after your dream, whether it is a job, a relationship, or motherhood!

Chapter 10

In this chapter:

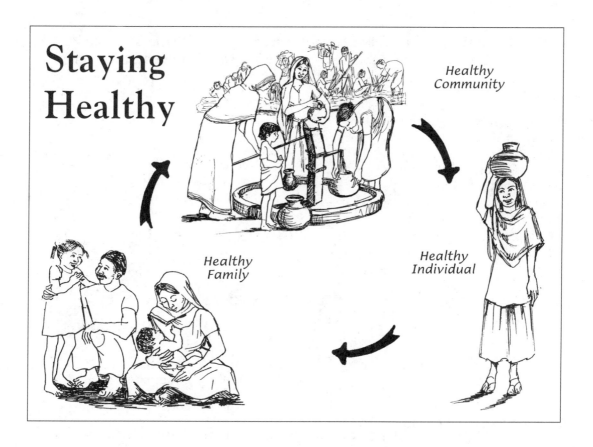

Staying Healthy

Healthy Community

Healthy Family

Healthy Individual

Most of this book describes health problems and what to do about them. But many of these problems can be prevented (stopped before they start) by better *nutrition*, cleanliness, rest, and by meeting women's special health needs. So in this chapter we describe some of the things a woman, her family, and her community can do to prevent illness.

It is not always easy for women to prevent illness. Although they do a lot to keep their families and communities healthy, many women have difficulty finding the time, energy, and money to pay attention to their own health needs. Since women are often taught to put the needs of others first, they have little time left for themselves after caring for their families. And the family's limited resources are often spent on the children and men first.

Yet, in the long run, it saves a lot of pain and *stress* to prevent health problems before they start rather than treating them later. Some of these things do not take much time or money. Others take some extra time, effort, and money—at least in the beginning. But since prevention builds the health and strength of a woman, her family, and her community, life will be easier and better later on.

➤ *Healthy communities help women stay healthy. Healthy women can care for their families. Healthy families can contribute more to the community.*

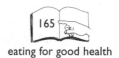

eating for good health

Cleanliness

➤ *Different germs are spread in different ways. For example, tuberculosis (TB) germs are spread through the air. Lice and scabies are spread through clothes and bed covers.*

Many illnesses are spread by *germs* that pass from one person to another. Here are some of the most common ways that germs are spread:

- by touching an infected person.

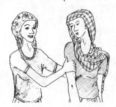

- through the air. For example, when someone coughs, germs in small drops of spit (saliva) can spread to other people or objects.

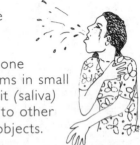

- through clothes, cloths, or bed covers.

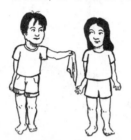

- by eating *contaminated* food.

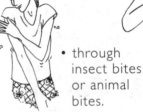

- through insect bites or animal bites.

Cleanliness in the community (sanitation), cleanliness in the home, and personal cleanliness are all important to prevent these sicknesses by stopping the spread of germs. For example:

1. A man infected with parasites has diarrhea outside.

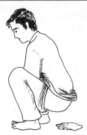

2. A pig eats the man's stool.

3. One of the man's children plays with the pig and gets stool on himself.

4. Later, the child starts to cry and his mother comforts him and cleans his fingers with her skirt. She also gets stool on her hands.

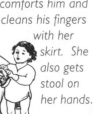

5. The mother prepares food for the family, forgetting to wash her hands first. She uses her soiled skirt to keep from burning her hands.

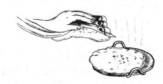

6. The family eats the food. Soon everyone has diarrhea.

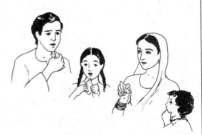

What could have prevented the family's illness?

If the family had used any of these precautions, the spread of illness could have been prevented:

- if the man had used a latrine or toilet.
- if the pig had not been allowed to run free.
- if the mother had not used her skirt to wipe the child's hands and then touch the food.
- if the mother had washed her hands after touching her child and before preparing food.

CLEANLINESS IN THE COMMUNITY (SANITATION)

Many common health problems are best solved in the community. When the community works together to improve sanitation, everybody benefits. For example:

Work together to develop a source of clean water for drinking and cooking. The source should be close enough to the community for people to get water easily.

To keep drinking and cooking water clean:

- do not let animals go near the water source. If necessary, build a fence to keep them out.
- do not bathe, or wash clothes, cooking pots, or eating utensils near the water source.
- do not pass stool or throw garbage (rubbish) near the water source.

Clean drinking water can help prevent diarrhea and parasites.

Get rid of garbage in a safe way. If possible, bury, *compost*, or burn garbage. If you bury it, make sure the pit is deep enough to keep animals and bugs away. If the garbage is above ground, fence off the dump and cover the garbage with dirt to reduce flies. Also, find safe ways to get rid of dangerous and *toxic* materials. For example, do not burn plastic near the house, because the *fumes* can be toxic, especially to children, old people, and sick people.

➤ *Use composted food waste to fertilize your crops.*

Drain standing water in washing areas, and in puddles, tires, and open containers. *Malaria* and *dengue fever* are spread by mosquitos, which breed in water that is not flowing. If possible, use mosquito nets when sleeping.

Organize your community to build latrines (see the next page for how to build a latrine).

➤ *For more information about building latrines, see* **Where There Is No Doctor**.

➤ *After using the latrine, throw a little lime, dirt, or ash in the hole to reduce the smell and keep flies away.*

How to build a latrine

1. Dig a pit about ½ meter wide, 1½ meters long, and 3 meters deep.

2. Cover the pit, leaving a hole about 20 by 30 centimeters.

3. Build a shelter and roof out of local building materials.

To be safe, a latrine should be at least 20 meters from all houses, wells, springs, rivers, or streams. If it must be anywhere near a place people go for water, be sure to put the latrine downstream.

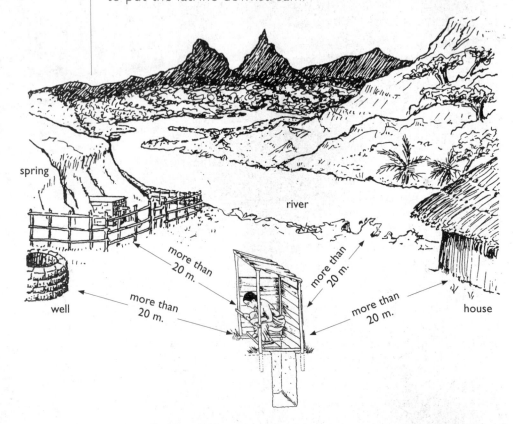

CLEANLINESS IN THE HOME

Since family members are in close contact with each other, it is very easy to spread germs and illness to the whole family. A family will have less illness if they:

- wash cooking and eating pots and utensils with soap (or clean ash) and clean water after using them. If possible, let them dry in the sun.

- clean the living space often. Sweep and wash the floors, walls, and beneath furniture. Fill in cracks and holes in the floor or walls where roaches, bedbugs, and scorpions can hide.

- hang or spread bedding in the sun to kill parasites and bugs.

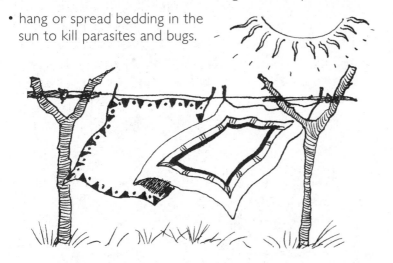

➤ *Sunlight kills many germs that cause illness.*

- do not spit on the floor. When you cough or sneeze, cover your mouth with your arm, or with a cloth or handkerchief. Then, if possible, wash your hands.

- get rid of body wastes in a safe way. Teach children to use a latrine or to bury their stools, or at least to go far away from the house or from where people get drinking water.

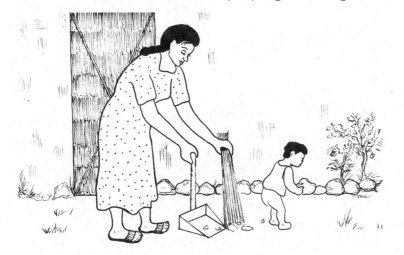

➤ *If children or animals pass stool near the house, clean it up at once.*

caring for yourself during monthly bleeding, 55

infections of the urine system, 365

PERSONAL CLEANLINESS

It is best to wash with soap and clean water every day, if possible. Also:

- wash your hands before eating or preparing food, after passing *urine* or stool, and before and after caring for a baby or someone who is sick.

- wash the *genitals* every day with mild soap and water. **But do not *douche*.** The vagina cleans and protects itself by making a small amount of wetness or discharge. Douching washes away this protection and makes a woman more likely to get a vaginal infection.

- pass urine after having sex. This helps prevent infections of the urine system (but will not prevent pregnancy).

- wipe carefully after passing stool. Always wipe from front to back. Wiping forward can spread germs and worms into the urinary opening and vagina.

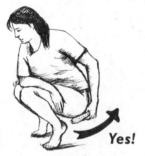
Yes!

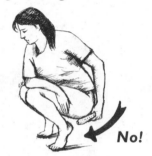
No!

Protect your teeth

Taking good care of the teeth is important because:

- strong, healthy teeth are needed to chew and digest food well.

- painful cavities (holes in the teeth caused by decay) and sore gums can be prevented by good tooth care.

- decayed or rotten teeth caused by lack of cleanliness can lead to serious infections that may affect other parts of the body.

- people who do not care for their teeth are more likely to lose them when they get old.

Teeth should be cleaned carefully twice a day. This removes the germs that cause decay and tooth loss. Clean the surface of all front and back teeth, then clean between the teeth and under the gums. Use a soft brush, tooth stick, or finger wrapped with a piece of rough cloth. Toothpaste is good but not necessary. Salt, charcoal, or even plain, clean water will also work.

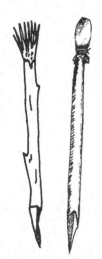

You can make a toothbrush to keep your teeth clean.

CLEAN WATER

Drinking water should be taken from the cleanest possible source. If the water is cloudy, let it settle and pour off the clear water. Then, before drinking, kill the harmful germs as described below. This is called purification.

Store the purified water in clean, covered containers. If the container has been used for storing cooking oil, wash it well with soap and hot water before storing clean water in it. **Never store water in containers that have been used for *chemicals, pesticides,* or fuels.** Wash water containers with soap and clean water at least once a week.

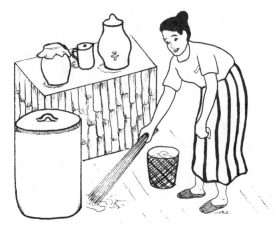

Store water in covered jars and keep your living space clean.

Here are some simple and inexpensive ways to purify your water:

Sunlight. Sunlight kills many harmful germs. To purify water using sunlight, fill clean, clear glass or plastic containers with water, and leave them outside from morning to late afternoon. Be sure to place the containers in an open space where they will be in the sun all day. (If drinking water is needed right away, putting the containers in the sun for 2 hours in the middle of the day should be enough for purification.)

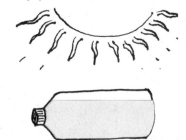

To avoid getting germs in the water, choose a spot away from children, dust, and animals. If you want the water to cool before using, bring the containers inside overnight. Water can be stored for a day or two in the same container. Sunlight purification works best in warm climates.

Lemon juice sometimes kills cholera (but not other germs). Add 2 tablespoons lemon juice to a liter (1 quart) of water and let it sit for 30 minutes.

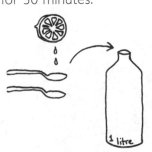

Boiling water for 5-10 minutes will kill most germs. Because boiling water uses so much fuel, use this method only if there is no other way to purify your water. If you want to kill all possible germs, you will have to boil the water for 20 minutes.

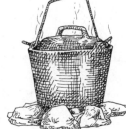

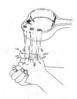

➤ *Washing your hands prevents the spread of disease. Keep a special clean rag for drying your hands. Wash it often and dry it in the sun.*

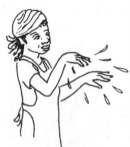

Or dry your hands in the air by shaking the water off.

➤ *In some communities there are special ways to prepare raw meat or fish that make them safe to eat.*

FOOD SAFETY

Many common diseases of the intestines are spread through food. Sometimes people who harvest, handle, or prepare food pass germs from their hands into the food. Sometimes germs and molds in the air begin to grow in the food and it goes bad (spoils). This happens when food is not stored or cooked properly, or when it gets old.

To prevent the spread of germs in food:

- wash your hands with soap and water before preparing food, before eating, and before feeding your children.
- wash or peel all fruits and vegetables that are eaten raw.
- do not let raw meat, poultry, or fish touch other food that is eaten raw. Always wash your hands, knife, and cutting board after cutting these meats.
- avoid coughing, spitting, and chewing things like gum or betel near food so your saliva does not get in the food.
- do not allow animals to lick dishes or utensils clean. If possible, keep animals out of the kitchen.
- throw food out when it spoils.

Here are some of the most common signs of spoiled foods:

- bad smell
- bad taste or a change in taste
- changed color (for example, if raw meat changes from red to brown)
- many bubbles on the top (for example, on the top of old stew or soup) along with a bad smell
- slime on the surface of meat or cooked foods

Cooked food

Cooking food kills germs. All meats, fish, and poultry should be well cooked. Nothing should look raw or have a raw color.

If the food begins to cool, the germs quickly start to grow again. If the food is not eaten within 2 hours, reheat it until it is very hot. Liquids should be bubbling, and solids (like rice) should be steaming.

Food selection. Sometimes food is bad even before it is cooked or stored. Here are some things to look for when selecting food.

Fresh (raw) foods should be:

• fresh and in season.

• whole—not bruised, damaged, or eaten by insects.

• clean (not dirty).

• fresh smelling (especially fish, shellfish, and meat, which should not have a strong smell).

Processed (cooked or packaged) foods should be stored in:

• tins that look new (no rust, bulges, or dents).

• jars that have clean tops.

• bottles that are not chipped.

• packages that are whole, not torn.

Strong-smelling fish and bulging cans are signs that the food has spoiled.

Food storage

Whenever possible, eat freshly prepared food. If you store food, keep it covered to protect it from flies and other insects, and dust.

Food keeps best if it stays cool. The methods described below cool food using evaporation (the way that water disappears into the air). Put the food in shallow pans for more complete cooling.

➤ *Women in the community who know which local foods keep well and good ways to store them can teach others.*

Pottery Cooler. This double-pot cooler is made of a small pot inside a large pot. The space between the pots is filled with water. Use a large pot and lid that have not been glazed (coated with a hard, smooth, baked-on covering) so that the water will evaporate through the pot. The small pot should be glazed on the inside to stop water from seeping into the stored foods.

Cupboard Cooler. Put a wooden crate or box on its side, and then set it on bricks or stones to raise it off the floor. Put a container of water on top of the crate and drape sackcloth or other coarse cloth over the bowl and around the crate. The cloth should not quite reach the floor. Dip the cloth in the water, so that the wetness spreads throughout the cloth. Place the food inside the crate. As the water in the cloth evaporates, it will cool the food. This method works best if you can keep the cloth wet all the time.

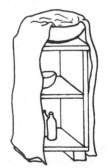

Cover the entire crate when you make a cupboard cooler. The front is open here just so you can see inside.

Special Needs of Women

> work

> ➤ Work with your community to lower women's workload. Stoves that use less fuel (page 395) and village water sources improve everyone's lives.

REST AND EXERCISE

Rest

Most women work very hard cooking, carrying water, and collecting fuel to help their families survive. If a woman also works outside her home, she has a double burden. She may work all day at a factory, in an office, or in the fields, and then return home to her second job—caring for her family. All this hard work can lead to *exhaustion, malnutrition*, and sickness, because she does not have enough time to rest or enough food to give her energy for her tasks.

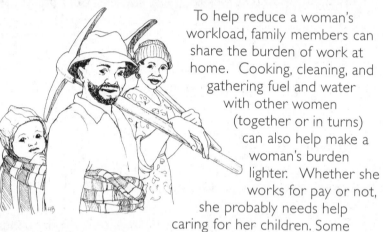

To help reduce a woman's workload, family members can share the burden of work at home. Cooking, cleaning, and gathering fuel and water with other women (together or in turns) can also help make a woman's burden lighter. Whether she works for pay or not, she probably needs help caring for her children. Some women organize child care cooperatives, where one woman cares for young children so that others can work. Each woman pays something to the woman caring for the children or they each take a turn.

If a woman is pregnant, she needs even more rest. She can explain to her family why she needs rest, and ask them for extra help with her workload.

> *I am so tired of sitting! I need to get more exercise. Maybe I should walk home...*

Exercise

> sitting or standing for a long time

Most women get plenty of exercise doing their daily tasks. But if a woman does not move much while she works—for example, if she sits or stands all day in a factory or office—she should try to walk and stretch every day. This will help keep her heart, lungs, and bones strong.

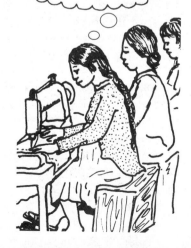

REGULAR HEALTH EXAMS

If possible, a woman should see a trained health worker to check her *reproductive* system (see page 44) every 3 to 5 years, even if she feels fine. This exam should include a pelvic exam, a breast exam, a test for weak blood (*anemia*), and an exam for *sexually transmitted diseases* (STDs) if she is at risk (see page 263). It may also include a *Pap test* (explained below) or other test for cervical cancer. This is especially important for women over 35, because women are more likely to get *cancer* of the cervix (the opening of the womb) as they get older.

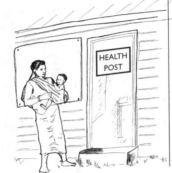

HEALTH POST

➤ *Many STDs and cancers do not show signs until the illness is very serious. By then it may be too late to treat the problem.*

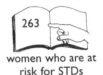

263

women who are at risk for STDs

These are the steps in the pelvic exam:

I am going to use this speculum to look inside your vagina now.

1. The health worker will look at your outer genitals for any swelling, bumps, sores, or changes in color.

2. Usually, the health worker will put a speculum into your vagina. A speculum is a small metal or plastic tool that holds the inside of the vagina open. He or she can then examine the walls of the vagina and the cervix for swelling, bumps, sores, or discharge. You may feel slight pressure or discomfort with the speculum inside, but it should not hurt. The exam is more comfortable if your muscles are relaxed and your *bladder* is empty.

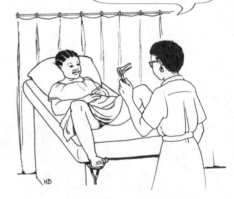

3. If the clinic has *laboratory* services, the health worker will do a Pap test for cancer and, if needed, tests for STDs. To do a Pap test, the health worker scrapes a few *cells* from the cervix. This is not painful. You should only feel a little pressure. The cells are sent to a laboratory where they are checked for signs of cancer. If the cancer is found and treated early, it can almost always be cured (see page 377).

4. After the health worker removes the speculum, she will put on a clean plastic glove and put two fingers of one hand into your vagina. She will press her other hand on your lower belly. In this way she can feel the size, shape, and location of your womb, *tubes*, and *ovaries*. This part of the exam should not be painful. If it is, tell her. It may mean something is wrong.

5. For some problems, the health worker may need to do a rectal exam. One finger is put into your *rectum* and one finger into your vagina. This can give the health worker more information about possible problems of the vagina, and of the womb, tubes, and ovaries.

safer sex, 186

pelvic infection, 272

➤ *AIDS has become a major cause of death among women.*

SAFER SEX

Having unprotected sex or sex with many partners makes a woman more at risk for getting an STD, including *HIV/AIDS*. Untreated STDs can cause *infertility, pregnancies in the tube*, and *miscarriage*. Having many partners also makes a woman more at risk for developing *pelvic inflammatory disease (PID)* and cancer. A woman can help prevent all these problems by practicing safer sex.

197

family planning

FAMILY PLANNING

A young woman should use family planning to delay her first pregnancy until her body is fully grown. Then, after her first baby is born, she should wait 2 or more years between each pregnancy. This method, called child spacing, lets her body get strong again between pregnancies, and her baby can finish breastfeeding. When she has the number of children she wants, she can choose not to have any more.

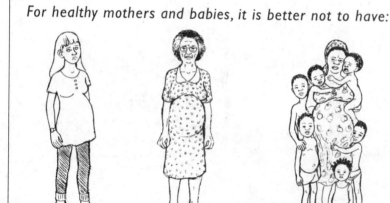

For healthy mothers and babies, it is better not to have:

| babies too early, | babies too late, | too many babies, | babies too close together. |

GOOD CARE DURING PREGNANCY AND BIRTH

Many women do not seek care during their pregnancy because they do not feel sick. But feeling well does not mean there are no problems. Many of the problems of pregnancy and birth, such as high blood pressure or the baby lying the wrong way, do not have any signs. A woman should try to get regular prenatal (before birth) checkups, so that a midwife or health worker trained in giving care during pregnancy can examine her body and see if her pregnancy is going well. Good prenatal care can prevent problems from becoming dangerous.

Family planning and good care during pregnancy and birth can prevent:

Fallen womb (prolapse). If a woman has been pregnant often, had long labors, or pushed too early during labor, the muscles and *ligaments* that hold up her womb may have become weak. When this happens the womb can fall part or all of the way into the vagina. This is called a prolapse.

treatment for
fallen womb

Signs:

- leaking urine
- in severe cases, the cervix can be seen at the opening of the vagina

leaking urine

Prevention:

- Space children at least 2 years apart.
- During labor, push only when the cervix is fully open and there is a strong need to push. Never let anyone push down on your womb to get the baby out quickly.

giving birth

Urine leaking from the vagina (VVF). If a baby's head presses too long against the wall of the vagina during labor, the vaginal *tissue* may be damaged. Urine or stool may leak out of the vagina. For more information, see page 370.

squeezing exercise

Prevention:

- Wait to get pregnant until your body is fully grown.
- Avoid labor that goes on too long.
- Space babies at least 2 years apart so that your muscles can get strong again in between pregnancies.

VACCINATIONS AGAINST TETANUS

Tetanus is an infection that kills. A woman can get tetanus when a germ that lives in the stools of people or animals enters her body through a wound. Although anyone can get tetanus, women and babies are especially at risk during childbirth. Tetanus can enter the body if an instrument that is not properly disinfected is put into the womb or used to cut the baby's cord.

All girls and pregnant women should be *vaccinated* against tetanus. If a woman is pregnant and has not been vaccinated, she should have an *injection* at her first prenatal checkup, and a second injection at least a month later. Then, if possible, she should follow the rest of the schedule.

Tetanus immunization schedule:

No. 1: at first visit

No. 2: at least 1 month after first injection

No. 3: at least 6 months after 2nd injection

No. 4: at least 1 year after 3rd injection

No. 5: at least 1 year after 4th injection

Then get an injection every 10 years.

➤ *A woman should examine her breasts every month, even after her monthly bleeding has stopped forever.*

➤ *If a woman has a disability that makes examining her breasts difficult, she can ask someone she trusts to do it for her.*

REGULAR BREAST EXAMS

Most women have some small lumps in their breasts. These lumps often change in size and shape during her monthly cycle. They can become very tender just before a woman's monthly bleeding. Sometimes—but not very often—a breast lump that does not go away can be a sign of breast cancer.

A woman can usually find breast lumps herself if she learns how to examine her breasts. If she does this once a month, she will become familiar with how her breasts feel, and will be more likely to know when something is wrong.

How to examine your breasts

Look at your breasts in a mirror, if you have one. Raise your arms over your head. Look for any change in the shape of your breasts, or any swelling or changes in the skin or nipple. Then put your arms at your sides and check your breasts again.

Lie down. Keeping your fingers flat, press your breast and feel for any lumps.

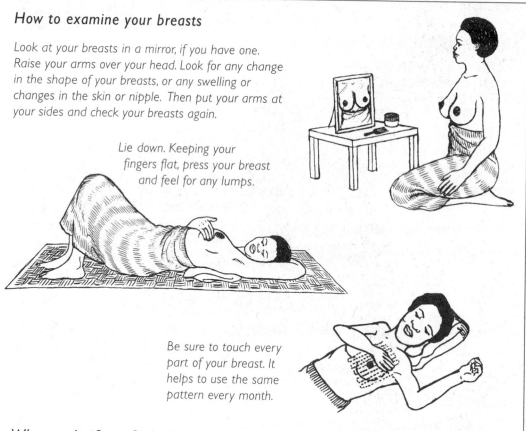

Be sure to touch every part of your breast. It helps to use the same pattern every month.

What to do if you find a lump

If the lump is smooth or rubbery, and moves under the skin when you push it with your fingers, do not worry about it. But if it is hard, has an uneven shape, and is painless, keep watching it—especially if the lump is in only one breast and does not move even when you push it. See a health worker if the lump is still there after your next monthly bleeding. This may be a sign of cancer (see page 382). You should also get medical help if there is a *discharge* that looks like blood or pus.

Things to Avoid to Stay Healthy
Tobacco, alcohol, and other drugs can all be bad for a woman's health. For more information, see page 435.

WORKING TOWARD A BALANCE BETWEEN TREATMENT AND PREVENTION

Working for Change

Health workers, or anyone working to improve the health of women in the community, can play an important role in stopping illnesses before they start. But often a woman's main need is not preventing illness but getting relief from an illness she already has. One of the first concerns of a health worker, then, must be to help with healing.

But treatment can be used as a doorway to prevention. One of the best times to talk to a woman about prevention is when she comes to see you for help. For example, if a woman comes to you with an infection of the urine system, treat the problem first. Then take time to explain how she can prevent these infections in the future.

Work toward a balance between prevention and treatment that is acceptable to the women you see. This balance will depend a lot on how the women already feel about sickness, healing, and health. As daily survival becomes less of a challenge, as their ideas about health change, and more diseases are controlled, you may find that they become more interested in prevention. Then much needless suffering can be avoided, and you can help women work toward more effective self-care.

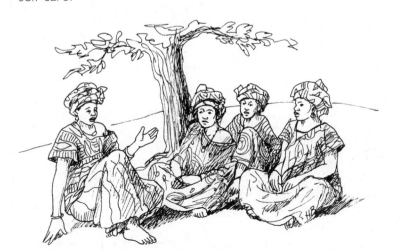

➤ Health workers can play an important role in helping women work together to prevent women's health problems in the community.

Chapter 11

In this chapter:

Eating for Good Health

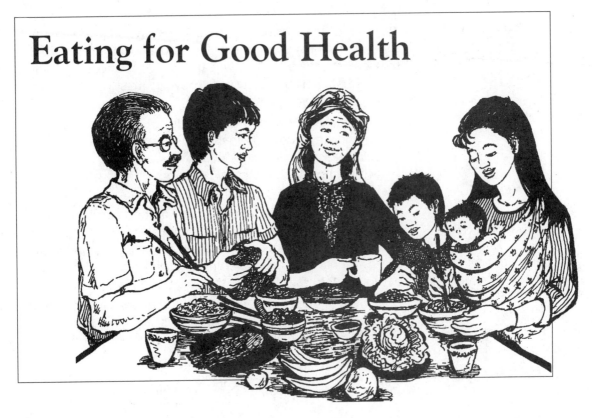

A woman needs good food to do her daily work, to prevent illness, and to have safe and healthy births. And yet, around the world, more women suffer from poor nutrition than any other health problem. This can cause exhaustion, weakness, disability, and general poor health.

There are many reasons for hunger and not eating well. One main reason is poverty. In many parts of the world, a few people own most of the wealth and the land. They may grow crops like coffee or tobacco instead of food, because they can make more money that way. Or poor people may farm small plots of borrowed land, while the owners take a big share of the harvest.

This poverty is hardest on women. This is because in many families women are fed less than men, no matter how little there is to eat. So the problems of hunger and poor nutrition will never be completely solved until land and other resources are shared fairly, and women are treated equally with men.

Still, there are many things people can do now to eat better at low cost. By eating as well as they can, they will gain strength. And when people are not feeling hungry every day, they are more able to think about their families' and communities' needs and to work for change.

> ➤ *Many illnesses could be prevented if people had enough good food to eat.*

Main Foods and Helper Foods

In much of the world, most people eat one main low-cost food with almost every meal. Depending on the region, this may be rice, maize, millet, wheat, cassava, potato, breadfruit, or plantain. This main food usually provides most of the body's daily food needs.

By itself, however, the main food is not enough to keep a person healthy. Other 'helper' foods are needed to provide protein (which helps build the body), vitamins and minerals (which help protect and repair the body), and fats and sugar (which give energy).

The healthiest diets have a variety of foods, including some foods with protein, and fruits and vegetables rich in vitamins and minerals. You need only a small amount of fat and sugar. But if you have problems getting enough food, it is better to eat foods with sugar and fat than to eat too little food.

A woman does not need to eat all the foods listed here to be healthy. She can eat the main foods she is accustomed to, and add as many helper foods as are available in her area.

➤ *Good nutrition means eating enough food and the right kind of food for the body to grow, be healthy, and fight off disease.*

Helper Foods

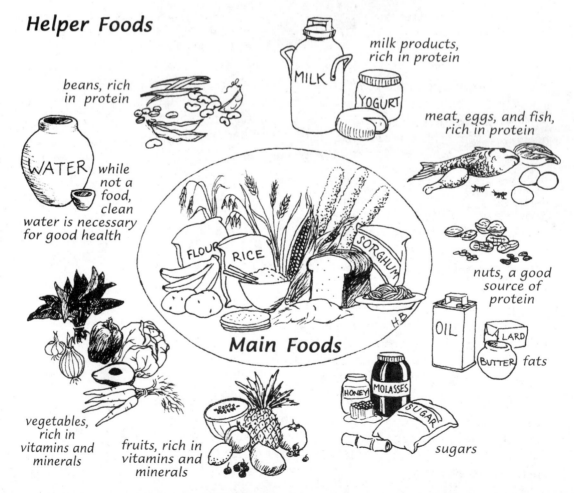

beans, rich in protein

milk products, rich in protein

meat, eggs, and fish, rich in protein

WATER while not a food, clean water is necessary for good health

nuts, a good source of protein

Main Foods

OIL LARD BUTTER fats

vegetables, rich in vitamins and minerals

fruits, rich in vitamins and minerals

sugars

IMPORTANT VITAMINS AND MINERALS

There are 5 important vitamins and minerals that women need, especially women who are pregnant or breastfeeding. The 5 are: iron, folic acid (folate), calcium, iodine, and vitamin A.

Iron

Iron is needed to make blood healthy and to help prevent weak blood *(anemia)*. A woman needs to get a lot of iron throughout her life, especially during the years she has monthly bleeding and during pregnancy.

These foods have a lot of iron:

- meat (especially liver, heart, and kidney)
- blood
- chicken
- eggs
- fish
- beans
- grasshoppers, crickets, termites
- peas

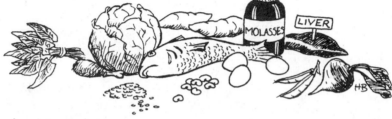

These foods also have some iron:

- cabbage with dark-colored leaves
- potatoes
- cauliflower
- lentils
- brussels sprouts

- turnips
- sunflower, sesame, pumpkin seeds
- strawberries
- dark green leafy vegetables

- pineapples
- yams
- seaweed
- broccoli

- dried fruit (especially dates, apricots, and raisins)
- black-strap molasses

It is possible to get even more iron if you:

- Cook food in iron pots. If you add tomatoes, lime juice, or lemon juice (which are high in vitamin C) to the food while it is cooking, more iron from the pots will go into the food.

- Add a clean piece of iron—like an iron nail or horseshoe—to the cooking pot. These should be made of pure iron, not a mixture of iron and other metals.

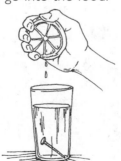

- Put a clean piece of pure iron, like an iron nail, in a little lemon juice for a few hours. Then make lemonade with the juice and drink it.

➤ *It is best to eat iron foods along with citrus fruits or tomatoes. These contain vitamin C, which helps your body use more of the iron in the food.*

Folic acid (folate)

➤ *Avoid cooking food for a long time. This destroys folic acid and other vitamins.*

The body needs folic acid to make healthy red blood cells. Lack of folic acid can lead to anemia in women and severe problems in newborn babies. So getting enough folic acid is especially important during pregnancy.

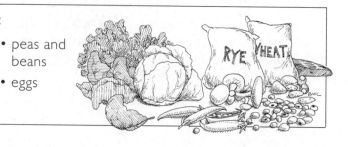

Good sources of folic acid are:

- dark green leafy vegetables
- whole grains
- mushrooms

- liver
- meats
- fish
- nuts

- peas and beans
- eggs

Calcium

Everyone needs calcium to make their bones and teeth strong. In addition, girls and women need extra calcium:

- during childhood. Calcium helps a girl's hips grow wide enough to give birth safely when she is fully grown.
- during pregnancy. A pregnant woman needs enough calcium to help the baby's bones grow, and to keep her own bones and teeth strong.
- during breastfeeding. Calcium is necessary for making breast milk.
- during mid-life and old age. Calcium is needed to prevent weak bones *(osteoporosis)*.

133

weak bones

These foods are rich in calcium:

- milk, curd, yogurt
- cheese
- ground sesame

- bone meal
- green leafy vegetables
- almonds

- beans, especially soy
- shellfish
- lime (carbon ash)

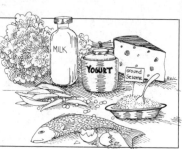

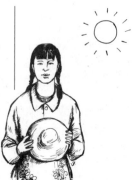

Sunshine will help you use calcium better. Try to be in the sun at least 15 minutes every day. Remember that it is not enough to just be outdoors. The sun's rays must touch the skin.

To increase the amount of calcium you get from food:

- Soak bones or egg shells in vinegar or lemon juice for a few hours, and then use the liquid in soup or other food.
- Add a little lemon juice, vinegar, or tomato when cooking bones for soup.
- Grind up egg shells into a powder and mix with food.
- Soak maize (corn) in lime (carbon ash).

Iodine

Iodine in the diet helps prevent a swelling on the throat called *goiter* and other problems. If a woman does not get enough iodine during pregnancy, her child may be mentally slow. Goiter and mental slowness are most common in areas where there is little natural iodine in the soil, water, or food.

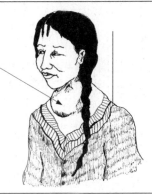

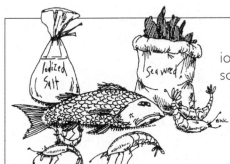

The easiest way to get enough iodine is to use iodized salt instead of regular salt. Or you can eat some of these foods (either fresh or dried):

- shellfish (like shrimp)
- cassava
- fish
- cabbage
- seaweed

If iodized salt or these foods are hard to get, or if there is goiter or mental slowness in your area, check with the local ministry of health to see if they can give iodized oil by mouth or by injection. If not, you can make an iodine solution at home with polyvidone iodine (an antiseptic that is often available at a local pharmacy). It contains 6 ml of iodine per drop. To make an iodine solution to drink:

➤ *The easiest way to get enough iodine is to use iodized salt instead of regular salt.*

1. Pour 4 glasses of clean drinking water into a jug or jar.

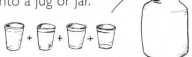

Store iodine at room temperature and in dark containers to protect it from light.

2. Add 1 drop of polyvidone iodine.

Everyone over 7 years old should drink 1 glass of this iodine solution every week of her or his life. This is especially important for pregnant women and children.

Vitamin A

Vitamin A prevents night blindness and helps fight off some infections. Many pregnant women have problems with night blindness, which probably means that their diet lacked vitamin A before they got pregnant. The problem shows up when pregnancy places extra demands on the body.

Dark yellow and green leafy vegetables, and some orange fruits, are rich in vitamin A.

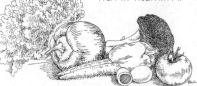

Lack of vitamin A also causes blindness in children. By eating foods rich in vitamin A during pregnancy, a woman can increase the amount of vitamin A her baby will get in breast milk.

Eating Better for Less Money

When money is limited, it is important to use it wisely. Here are some suggestions for getting more vitamins, minerals, and proteins at low cost:

1. **Protein foods.** Beans, peas, lentils, and other similar foods (called legumes) are a good, cheap source of protein. If allowed to sprout before cooking and eating, they have more vitamins. Eggs are one of the cheapest sources of animal protein (see page 168 for ways to use the shells, too). Liver, heart, kidney, blood, and fish are often cheaper than other meats and are just as nutritious.

2. **Grains.** Rice, wheat, and other grains are more nutritious if their outer skins are not removed during milling.

3. **Fruits and vegetables.** The sooner you eat fruits and vegetables after harvesting, the more nutrition they have. When you store them, put them in a cool, dark place to preserve vitamins. Cook vegetables in as small an amount of water as possible, because vitamins from the vegetables go into the water during cooking. Then use the water in soups or drink it.

   The tough outside leaves or tops from vegetables like carrots or cauliflower contain many vitamins and can be used to make healthy soups. For instance, cassava (manioc) leaves contain 7 times as much protein and more vitamins than the root.

   Many wild fruits and berries are rich in vitamin C and natural sugars, and can provide extra vitamins and energy.

4. **Milk and milk products.** These should be kept in a cool, dark place. They are rich in body-building proteins and in calcium.

5. **Avoid spending money on packaged foods or vitamins.** If parents took the money they often use for sweets or sodas (fizzy drinks) and spent it on nutritious foods, their children would be healthier for the same amount of money.

You can buy more nutritious food than packaged food for the same amount of money.

Since most people can get the vitamins they need from food, it is better to spend money on nutritious foods than on pills or *injections*. If you must take vitamins, take pills. They work as well as injections and cost less.

Harmful Ideas About Eating

In many parts of the world, certain traditions and beliefs about women and food are more harmful than helpful. For example:

It is not true that girls need less food than boys. Some people believe that boys need more food. But these people are wrong! Women work just as hard as men in most communities, if not harder, and need to be as healthy. Girls who are healthy and well-fed during childhood grow up into healthy women, and have fewer problems at school and at work.

It is not true that women should avoid foods during pregnancy and breastfeeding. In some communities, people believe that a woman should avoid certain foods—like beans, eggs, chicken, milk products, meat, fish, fruits, or vegetables—at different times in her life. These times may include her monthly bleeding, pregnancy, immediately after childbirth, while breastfeeding, or during *menopause*. But a woman needs all these foods, especially during pregnancy and while breastfeeding. Avoiding them can cause weakness, illness, and even death.

It is not true that a woman should feed her family first. A woman is sometimes taught to feed her family before herself. She eats only what is left and often does not get as much food as the rest of the family. This is never healthy. And when a woman is pregnant, or has just had a baby, it can be very dangerous.

If a family does not help a woman eat well, we encourage her to do what she must to get enough food. She may need to eat while cooking, or hide food and eat it when her husband is out of the house.

It is not true that a sick person needs less food than a healthy person. Good food not only prevents disease but also helps a sick person fight disease and become well again. As a general rule, the same foods that are good for people when they are healthy are good for them when they are sick.

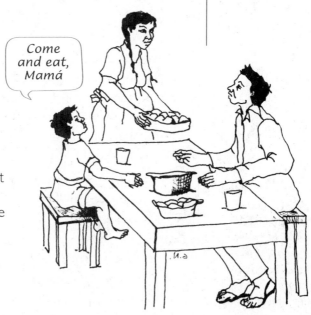

Come and eat, Mamá

Poor Nutrition Can Cause Disease

Because girls and women often get less food—and less nutritious food—than they need, they are more likely to get sick. Here are some common illnesses caused by poor nutrition.

ANEMIA

A person with anemia has weak blood. This happens when red blood cells are lost or destroyed faster than the body can replace them. Because women lose blood during their monthly bleeding, anemia is often found in women who are between *puberty* and *menopause*. About half of the world's pregnant women are anemic, because they need to make extra blood for the growing baby.

Anemia is a serious illness. It makes a woman more likely to get other kinds of diseases, and affects her ability to work and learn. Anemic women are more likely to bleed heavily or even die during childbirth.

Signs:

- pale inner eyelids, tongue, and nails
- weakness and feeling very tired
- *dizziness*, especially when getting up from a sitting or lying position
- fainting (loss of consciousness)
- shortness of breath
- fast heartbeat

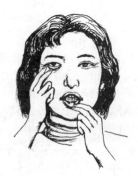

Causes of anemia:

The most common cause of anemia is not eating enough food rich in iron, since iron is needed to make red blood cells. Other causes are:

- *malaria*, which destroys red blood cells
- any kind of blood loss, such as:
  - heavy monthly bleeding (an *intra-uterine device*, or IUD, can make bleeding heavier)
  - childbirth
  - bloody diarrhea (dysentery) from *parasites* and worms
  - bleeding stomach *ulcers*
  - a wound that bleeds a lot

➤ *For more information about malaria, parasites, and worms, see* **Where There Is No Doctor** *or another general medical book.*

Treatment and prevention:

- If malaria, parasites, or worms are causing your anemia, treat these diseases first.
- Eat foods rich in iron (see page 167), along with foods rich in vitamins A and C, which help the body absorb iron. Citrus fruits and tomatoes are rich in vitamin C. Dark yellow and dark green leafy vegetables are rich in vitamin A. If a woman cannot eat enough foods rich in iron, she may need to take iron pills (see page 73).
- Avoid drinking black tea or coffee, or eating bran (the outer layer of grains) with meals. These can prevent the body from absorbing iron from food.
- Drink clean water to prevent infection from parasites.
- Use a *latrine* for passing stool, so that worm eggs will not spread to food and water sources. If hookworms are common in your area, try to wear shoes.
- Space births at least 2 years apart. This will give your body a chance to store some iron between pregnancies.

clean water

cleanliness

BERIBERI

Beriberi is a disease caused by lack of thiamine (one of the B vitamins), which helps the body turn food into energy. Like anemia, beriberi is most often seen in women from puberty to menopause, and in their children.

Beriberi occurs most often when the main food is a grain whose outer skin has been removed (for example, polished rice) or a starchy root, like cassava.

Signs:

- not wanting to eat
- severe weakness, especially in the legs
- the body becomes very swollen or the heart stops working

Treatment and prevention:

Eat foods rich in thiamine, like meat, poultry, fish, liver, whole grain cereals, legumes (peas, beans, clover), milk, and eggs. If this is difficult, a person may need thiamine pills.

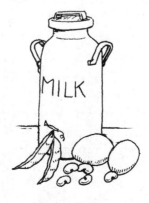

high blood pressure, 130
cancer, 376
arthritis, 133

PROBLEMS FROM EATING TOO MUCH FOOD OR THE WRONG KIND OF FOOD

If a woman weighs too much or eats too much fat, she is more likely to have high *blood pressure*, heart disease, a *stroke*, *gallstones*, diabetes, and some *cancers*. Being overweight can also cause *arthritis* in the legs and feet.

People who weigh too much should lose weight by exercising more, and by replacing fatty and sweet foods in their diet with fruits and vegetables. Here are some suggestions for cutting down the amount of fat in the diet:

- When cooking, try to use as little butter, ghee, lard, or oil as possible. Or cook with broth or water instead.
- Remove fat from meat before cooking. Do not eat the skin of chicken or turkey.
- Avoid processed snack foods that are high in fat, like chips and crackers.

Diabetes

People with diabetes have too much sugar in their blood. This disease is usually more serious if it starts when a person is young (juvenile diabetes). But it is most common in people over age 40 who are overweight.

Early signs:

- always thirsty
- urinates often and a lot
- always tired
- always hungry
- weight loss
- frequent *vaginal* infections

Later, more serious signs:

- itchy skin
- periods of blurry eyesight
- some loss of feeling in the hands or feet
- sores on the feet that do not heal
- loss of consciousness (in extreme cases)

All these signs may be caused by other diseases. To find out whether you have diabetes, you can test your urine yourself. Use special paper strips, like *Uristix,* that change color when dipped in urine that has sugar in it. If the strips are not available, see a health worker to get a simple urine test for sugar.

➤ *Diabetes is more likely to develop during pregnancy than at other times. If you are pregnant and are always thirsty or are losing weight, see a health worker who can test your urine for sugar.*

Treatment:

If you have diabetes and are less than 40 years old, you should be treated by a health worker whenever possible. If you are over 40, you may be able to control diabetes by watching your diet:

- Eat smaller meals more often. This helps keep the same amount of sugar in the blood.
- Avoid eating a lot of sweet foods.
- If you are overweight, try to lose weight.
- Avoid foods high in fat (for example, butter, ghee, lard, and oils), unless you have trouble getting enough food to eat.

If possible, you should also see a health worker regularly to make sure your illness is not getting worse.

To prevent infection and injury to the skin, clean your teeth after eating, keep your skin clean, and always wear shoes to prevent foot injuries. Check your feet and hands once a day to see if you have any sores. If you have a sore and there are any signs of infection (redness, swelling, or heat), see a health worker.

➤ *There may be plants in your area that are helpful for diabetes. Check with a health worker.*

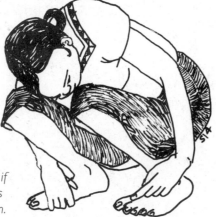

Check your feet once a day to see if you have any sores or signs of infection.

Whenever possible, rest with your feet up. This is especially important if your feet get darker in color and become numb. These signs mean that the blood flow to and from your feet is poor.

Other health problems that can be caused or made worse by poor nutrition:

- high blood pressure (see page 130)
- weak bones (see page 133)
- constipation (see page 70)
- stomach ulcers, acid indigestion, and heartburn

For more information on stomach ulcers, indigestion, and *heartburn*, see **Where There Is No Doctor** or another general medical book.

Ways to Work toward Better Nutrition

There are many different ways to approach the problem of poor nutrition, because many different things help cause the problem. You and your community must consider the possible actions you might take and decide which are most likely to work.

Here are a few examples of ways to improve nutrition. These suggestions can help you grow more food or different kinds of food, or store it better so the food does not spoil. Some of these examples bring quick results. Others work over a longer time.

Some ways people can improve their nutrition

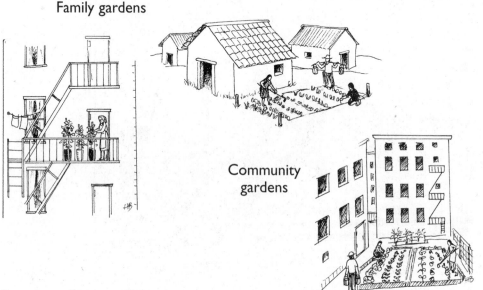

Family gardens

Community gardens

Rotation of crops

Every other planting season, plant a crop that returns strength to the soil—like beans, peas, lentils, alfalfa, peanuts, or some other plant with seeds in pods (legumes or pulses).

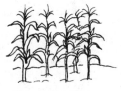

This year **maize**

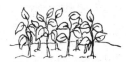

Next year **beans**

Try to grow a variety of foods. That way, even if one crop fails there will still be something to eat.

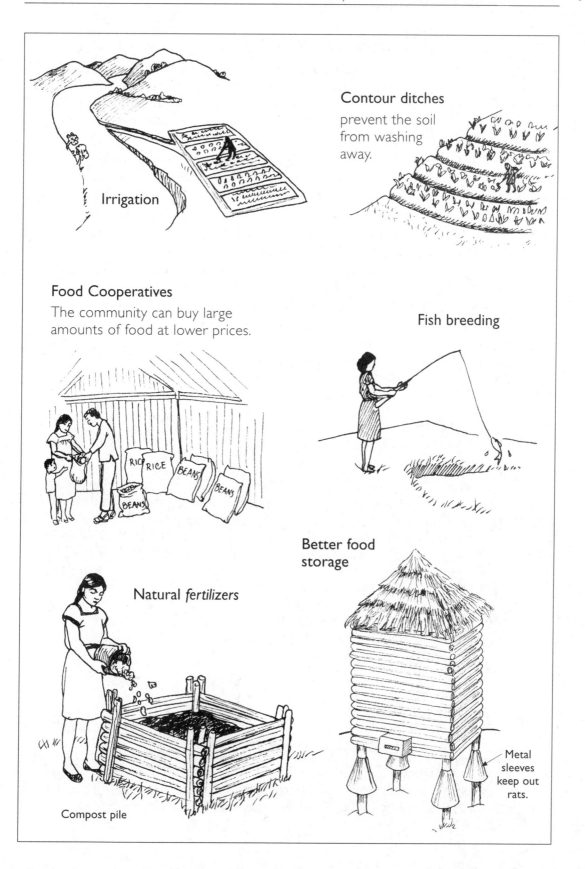

Irrigation

Contour ditches prevent the soil from washing away.

Food Cooperatives
The community can buy large amounts of food at lower prices.

Fish breeding

Natural *fertilizers*

Better food storage

Metal sleeves keep out rats.

Compost pile

TRYING A NEW IDEA

Not all the suggestions in this chapter are likely to work in your area. Perhaps some will work if they are changed for your particular community and the resources at hand. Often you can only know whether something will work or not by trying it—that is, by experiment.

When you try out a new idea, **always start small.** If you start small and the experiment fails, or something has to be done differently, you will not lose much. If it works, people will see that it works and can begin to use it in a bigger way.

Here is an example of experimenting with a new idea:

You learn that a certain kind of bean, such as soya, is an excellent body-building food. But will it grow in your area? And if it grows, will people eat it?

➤ *Do not be discouraged if an experiment does not work. Perhaps you can try again with certain changes. You can learn as much from your failures as from your successes.*

Start by planting a small patch—or 2 or 3 small patches under different kinds of conditions (for example, with different kinds of soil or using different amounts of water). If the beans do well, try cooking them in various ways, and see if people will eat them. If so, try planting more beans using the conditions in which they grew best.

You can also try out even more conditions (for example, adding fertilizer or using different kinds of seed) in more small patches to see if you can get an even better crop. To best understand what helps and what does not, try to change only one condition at a time and keep the rest the same.

Here is an example of adding animal fertilizer (manure) to see if it helps beans grow. This person planted several small bean patches side-by-side, under the same conditions of water and sunlight, and using the same seed. Before planting, each patch of soil was mixed with a different amount of manure, something like this:

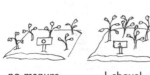

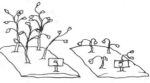

| no manure | 1 shovel manure | 2 shovels manure | 3 shovels manure | 4 shovels manure | 5 shovels manure |

This experiment shows that a certain amount of manure helps, but that too much can harm the plants. This is only an example. Your experiments may give different results. Try for yourself!

Other ideas to experiment with

- To increase the amount of food a piece of land will produce, try planting different kinds of crops together. For example, plants that grow along the ground can be mixed with plants that grow tall. Fruit trees can be planted above both. Or plants that take a shorter time to grow can be mixed with those that take a longer time. Then the first crop can be harvested before the second crop gets too large.

- If you must plant cash crops (non-food crops that you sell), try planting food crops together with the cash crops. For example, plant nut or fruit trees to shade coffee. Or plant cassava with cotton.

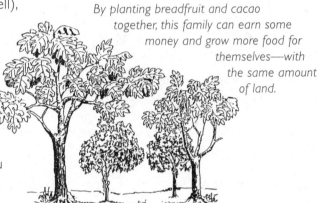

By planting breadfruit and cacao together, this family can earn some money and grow more food for themselves—with the same amount of land.

- Try to find nutritious plants that grow well in local conditions, so that you will need less water and fertilizer for good results.

WORKING TOWARD A BALANCE BETWEEN PEOPLE AND LAND

Most food comes from the land. Land that is used well can produce more food. But even the best used piece of land can only feed a certain number of people. And today, many of the people who farm do not have enough land to meet their needs or to stay healthy.

For this reason, some people argue that 'the small family lives better'. For many poor families, however, having many children is an economic necessity. Because of the work they do to help the family, children of poor families often produce more than they cost by the time they are 10 or 12 years old. Having a lot of children also makes it more likely the parents will have someone to give the help and care they need in old age.

So lack of social and economic security creates the need for parents to have many children. Therefore, the answer to gaining a balance between people and land does not come from telling poor people to have smaller families. It comes from sharing the land more fairly, paying fair wages, and taking other steps to overcome poverty. Only then can people afford small families. Then we can hope to achieve a lasting balance between people and land.

Chapter 12

In this chapter:

Sexual Health

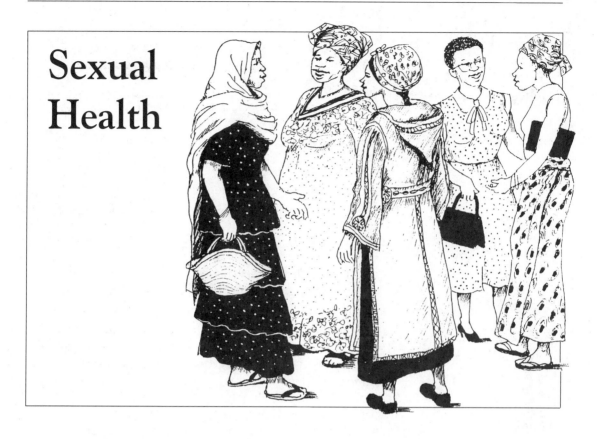

Sex is a natural part of life. For many women, it is a way to feel pleasure, express love or sexual desire for their partners, or to become pregnant with the children they hope for.

But sex can also lead to serious problems, such as pregnancies that are unwanted or that threaten a woman's health, *sexually transmitted diseases* (STDs), or physical and emotional harm from forced sex.

To be free from these problems, a woman must have control over her sexual life. This control should include:

- choosing her sexual partner.
- negotiating when and how to have sex.
- choosing if and when she becomes pregnant.
- preventing STDs, including *HIV/AIDS*.
- being free from sexual violence, including forced sex.

When a woman has this control, we say she has good sexual heath. But in many communities, harmful beliefs about what it means to be a woman make it hard for women to have good sexual health. This chapter gives information and suggestions about how women can overcome these beliefs and gain control over their sexual lives.

> *We have been ignorant for so long, and full of fear about our bodies.*
> — *Oaxaca, Mexico*

Sex and Gender Roles

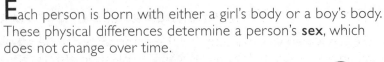

Each person is born with either a girl's body or a boy's body. These physical differences determine a person's **sex**, which does not change over time.

A person's **gender role** refers to the way a community defines what it is to be a woman or a man. Each community expects women and men to think, feel, and act in certain ways, simply because they are women or men. In most communities, for example, women are expected to prepare food, gather water and fuel, and care for their children and partner. Men, however, are often expected to work outside the home to provide for their families and parents in old age, and to defend their families from harm.

Unlike the physical differences between men and women, gender roles and the activities associated with them are created by the community. Some activities, like preparing food and caring for children, are considered 'women's activities' in many communities. But others vary from place to place—depending on a community's traditions, laws, and religions. Gender roles can even vary within communities, based on how much education a person has, her race, or her age. For example, in some communities women of a certain race are expected to do domestic work, while other women have more choice about the jobs they hold.

HOW GENDER ROLES ARE LEARNED

Gender roles are passed down from parents to children. From the time children are very young, parents treat girls and boys differently—sometimes without realizing they do so. Children watch their parents closely, noticing how they behave, how they treat each other, and what their roles are in the community.

As children grow up, they accept these roles because they want to please their parents and because parents have more authority. These roles also help children know who they are and what is expected of them. So in the same way that children learn their own names, they also learn about their gender—that is, what it means to be a woman or a man.

As the world changes, gender roles also change. Many young people want to live differently from their parents. But they sometimes find it difficult to change, because the family and community expect them to continue following old 'rules'. As women struggle to gain the freedom to redefine their gender roles, they can also gain more control over the things that determine sexual health.

WHEN GENDER ROLES CAUSE HARM

Fulfilling the roles expected by the community can be satisfying and can give a woman a sense of belonging. But these roles can also limit a woman's activities and choices, and make her feel less valued than a man. When this happens, everyone—the woman herself, her family, and her community—suffers.

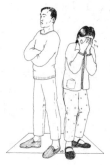

In most communities, women are expected to be wives and mothers. Many women like this role because it can be very satisfying and it gives them *status* in the community. Other women would prefer to follow their own interests—or they want to have only a few children—but their families and communities do not give them this choice. If she is expected to have many children, a woman may have less chance to learn new skills or go to school. Most of her time and energy will be spent taking care of others' needs. Or, if a woman is unable to have children, her community may value her less than other women.

Most communities value men's work more than women's work. For example, this woman has worked all day—and then cooks, cleans, and cares for her children at night. But because her husband's work is considered more important, she is concerned about his rest—not her own. Her children will grow up thinking men's work is more important, and value women less.

Don't bother your father. He works hard and needs his rest.

Women are often considered more emotional than men, and they are free to express these emotions with others. Men, however, are often taught that showing emotions like sadness or tenderness is 'unmanly', so they hide their feelings. Or they express their feelings in angry or violent ways that are more acceptable for men. When men are unable to show their feelings, children may feel more distant from their fathers, and men are less able to get support from others for their problems.

Women are often discouraged from speaking—or forbidden to attend or speak—at community meetings. This means the community only hears about what men think—for example, how they view a problem and their solutions for it. Since women have much knowledge and experience, the whole community suffers when they cannot discuss problems and offer suggestions for change.

Women and men who have sexual relations with people of the same sex (homosexuals) are sometimes made to feel like outcasts in their own communities. Even if they are community leaders in other ways, they may be forced to live and love in secrecy and shame. In some communities, fear or lack of understanding of people in same sex relationships may even lead to physical violence against them. Any time a person is made to feel afraid or ashamed about who he or she is, it harms the person's mental and sexual health.

How Gender Roles Affect Sexual Health

HARMFUL BELIEFS ABOUT WOMEN'S SEXUALITY

What it means to be a woman or a man in a particular community includes beliefs about men's and women's sexuality—that is, about sexual behavior, and how people feel about their own bodies.

A few harmful beliefs about women's sexuality that are common in many communities are described below. These beliefs and other harmful effects of gender roles—the lack of opportunity and choice for women, and the lack of value they feel—prevent women from having control over their sexual lives. This puts them at great risk for sexual health problems.

Harmful belief: Women's bodies are shameful

Mothers and fathers begin to teach their children about their bodies as soon as they are born. Parents do not do this directly. But a baby learns it by the way the parents hold her, and the tone of their voices.

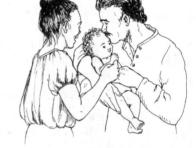

As a little girl grows, she becomes curious about her body. She wants to know what the different parts are called and why her *genitals* are different from a boy's. But unlike little boys, she is often scolded for being curious, and is told that 'nice girls' do not ask such things. If she touches her genitals, she is taught that it is dirty or shameful—and that she should keep her sexual parts hidden.

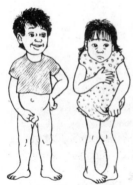

Parents act differently when little boys and little girls touch their bodies.

Her parents' reactions teach a little girl that her body is shameful. As a result, she will find it difficult to ask questions about changes in her body as she enters *puberty*, and about her *monthly bleeding*, or about sex. She may be too embarrassed to talk to a health worker, because she does not know what parts of her body are called or what questions to ask. When she starts having sex, she is less likely to understand how her body feels sexual pleasure, or to know how to protect herself from unwanted pregnancy or sexually transmitted diseases (STDs).

➤ *A woman's body is NOT shameful. Her body is something to discover, love, and value.*

Our bodies are not causes for shame. Our bodies allow us to touch and care for others, and to feel sexual pleasure. Our bodies are something to discover, love, and value.

Harmful belief: Women's bodies belong to men

In many communities, a woman is treated like the property of her father or husband. As a child, she belongs to her father, and he can arrange to have her marry whomever he chooses. Sometimes she will be sold—like property—to her husband or to an employer. Her future husband wants his property to be 'pure' and unspoiled by other men, so he expects her to be a *virgin*. After marriage, he feels he has the right to use her body for his pleasure whenever he wants. He may have sex with other women, but she is to be his alone.

These beliefs can cause great harm. A girl learns that other people make the important decisions about her life—it does not matter what she wants or what skills she could contribute to the community. Because virginity is valued so highly, she may be forced to marry at a young age. Or she may try to remain 'virgin' by using unsafe sexual practices. For example, she may have sex in the anus (so that her *hymen* will not be torn), which puts her at great risk for STDs, including HIV/AIDS. When she starts having sex, she may have little power to discuss *family planning methods* with her partner or to protect herself from STDs.

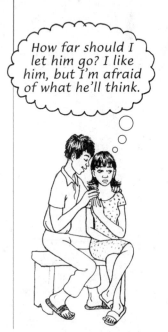

Some girls are married as children to make sure they will be virgins. This can cause serious health problems for a girl and her babies (see page 59).

But men do not own women's bodies! A woman's body is hers alone, and she should be able to decide how, when, and with whom to share it.

Harmful belief: Women have less sexual desire

A woman is often taught that it is part of her duty as a wife to meet her husband's sexual demands. But if she is a 'good' woman, she will endure sex, not want it.

Again, these beliefs harm a woman's sexual health. First, a woman who believes she should not think about sex will be unprepared to have sex safely. She is less likely to learn about family planning or about how to get and use condoms. Even if she has the information, it will be hard for her to discuss these things with her partner beforehand. If she can discuss sex, her partner may think she is sexually experienced, and therefore 'bad'.

How far should I let him go? I like him, but I'm afraid of what he'll think.

Once she is in a sexual relationship, she is likely to let her partner control the kind of relationship they have. This includes when and how they have sex, whether they try to prevent pregnancy or STDs, and whether he has sex with other women. This puts her at great risk for getting STDs.

But sexual desire is a natural part of life, and a woman can feel as much sexual desire and pleasure as a man.

Gaining More Control over Your Sexual Health

➤ *It is best for family planning and STD services to be included in the other health services women already use.*

STDs, 261
HIV/AIDS, 283

➤ *Safer sex can save your life.*

Improving sexual health means:

• **reducing the risk of unwanted pregnancy and STDs.** This means women must have *access* to information about family planning methods and ways to prevent STDs, including HIV/AIDS (safer sex methods and practices). Women also need control over when to use these methods. For information about family planning and choosing a method that works best for you, see the chapter on "Family Planning." For information about safer sex, see the next section below.

• **feeling more pleasure from sex**. What brings pleasure to one person should not be harmful to another. See page 192 for more information about sexual pleasure.

• **changing harmful gender roles, including harmful beliefs about women's sexuality.** This kind of change takes time, because it means women and men must develop different ways of relating to each other. See page 194 for suggestions about how you and your community can work to change these roles.

SAFER SEX FOR SEXUAL HEALTH

In the past, the main danger from sex was unwanted pregnancy. Now STDs, including HIV/AIDS, have become a serious sexual health problem.

STDs are caused by *germs* that are passed from one person to another during sex. Some STDs, like genital warts and herpes, are spread by germs on the outer genitals of an infected person. Other STDs are passed by contact with germs in a man's *semen*, the liquid in a woman's *vagina*, or blood. *Infection* can happen when the germs pass through the *cervix* into the *womb*, or through breaks in the skin—especially in the vagina, *anus*, tip of the *penis*, or mouth.

Because STDs are spread through sexual contact, avoiding direct contact with an infected man's genitals, semen and blood is the best way to avoid getting an STD. This is called 'safer sex'.

When should a woman practice safer sex?

Everyone should always have sex safely. Women have many different kinds of sexual relationships. Some have one faithful sex partner their entire lives. Others have one sex partner at a time but several partners over the course of their lives. And others have multiple partners (or their partners have multiple partners) at one time. This means different women have different risks of getting STDs.

Many women think they are not at risk for an STD if they have just one sex partner. This is true ONLY if you and your partner know for sure that neither of you already has an STD, and that both of you have sex only with each other.

Most women cannot be sure of this because:

- it is possible to have an STD and not know it. If a woman's past partners—or her partner's past partners—had an STD, she or her partner could have one, too.

- they do not know for sure that their partner does not have other sex partners now. If someone your partner has sex with has an STD, you can get it too.

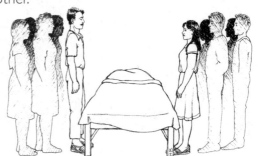

You can be infected by past partners—and your partner's past partners.

Fátima's story: Every woman should protect herself

Fátima lives in a rural town called Belem—and she is dying of AIDS. When she was 17, she married a man named Wilson. He was killed a few years later in an accident at the cooperative where he worked. Fátima had to leave her baby with Wilson's parents and go to the city to find work. When she had extra money, she sent it back home. The work was hard, and she was very lonely.

When she learned that the government was building a highway near Belem, Fátima got a job cooking for the road construction workers so that she could stay at home. It was there that she met Emanuel. He was handsome, had cash in his pockets, and charmed her little girl when he came around after work. When the work crew had to move on, he promised to return.

Emanuel did come back, but he never stayed long. He got a new job driving trucks that kept him on the road most of the time. Fátima thought he probably had other women, but he always told her she was his only one. They had a baby boy, but he was small and sickly and died after a year. Soon Fátima began to feel sick, too. The nurse at the health post gave her different medicines, but nothing helped. Finally she went to the hospital in the city. They did some tests, and later told her she had AIDS. When she asked how she could have got AIDS, the doctor replied, "You shouldn't have slept with so many men." Fátima did not think she was at risk for HIV/AIDS—she had only had sex with 2 men in her life! She thought that only prostitutes and homosexuals in the cities got AIDS.

Practicing safer sex means using barriers that keep germs from being passed between you and your partner during sex (**safer sex methods**), and having sex in ways that make infection with an STD less likely (**safer sex practices**).

Safer sex methods

Using *condoms* for either men or women can protect you from STDs, including HIV/AIDS. If they are used correctly, they keep a man's genitals and semen from touching your genitals. Condoms can also prevent unwanted pregnancy. For more information about how to use condoms, see page 202.

➤ *The more often you use a condom, or avoid sex in the vagina or anus without one, the less likely you will be to get AIDS.*

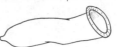
latex condom for men

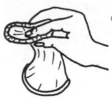
condom for women

Note: Spermicides—chemicals that kill sperm—used alone or with a diaphragm, also provide some protection against the germs that cause gonorrhea and chlamydia.

To encourage your partner to use condoms:

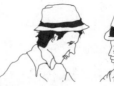

If he says. . .   *try saying. . .*

It will not feel as good.	*It may feel different, but it will still feel good. Here, let me show you.* *You can last even longer and then we will both feel good!*
I do not have any diseases.	*I do not think I have any, either. But one of us could and not know it.*
You are already using family planning.	*I would like to use it anyway. One of us might have an infection from before that we did not know about.*
Just this once without a condom.	*It only takes one time without protection to get an STD or HIV/AIDS. And I am also not ready to be pregnant.*
Condoms are for prostitutes. Why do you want to use one?	*Condoms are for everyone who wants to protect themselves.* *NO CONDOM, NO SEX!*

Do what you can to make sure that you both enjoy having sex with a condom. That way, it may be easier to get him to use one the next time.

Safer sex practices

Sexual practices in which there is less contact with a man's semen are also less likely to spread STD germs, including HIV. The box below shows which kinds of practices are safer than others. Sex with the penis in the vagina (vaginal sex) is the most common kind of sexual practice for many men and women. But other couples give and receive sexual pleasure by using many different kinds of talk and touch. If your partner does not want to use condoms, try to get him to have other kinds of sex with you. These other practices may feel just as good to him—and mean less risk for you.

➤ *Make sex safer:*
• *Use a latex condom every time.*
• *Replace risky practices with touching and kissing.*
• *If you cannot use a condom, it is better to use spermicide alone or with a diaphragm.*

Some kinds of sex are safer than others

Kissing. Kissing mouth-to-mouth is safe, even if your mouths are open or your tongues touch.
But if you or your partner has a sore in the mouth, you should wait until the sore has healed.

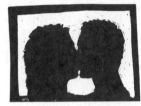
Safe

Touching. Touching is always safe, as long as neither person has blood, discharge, or sores on the genitals or hands.

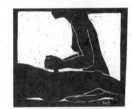
Safe

Oral sex. *Oral sex* is much safer than vaginal or anal sex. But the less time you have semen in your mouth, the better. So, if the man *ejaculates* into your mouth, you should swallow or spit right away, and rinse your mouth afterward. If you get a sore throat a couple of days after having oral sex, be sure to have it checked by a health worker. You can get gonorrhea in your throat and herpes sores in your mouth. The safest way to have oral sex is if the man's penis is covered with a condom before you take it into your mouth.

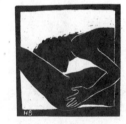
Safer with a condom

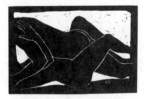
Safer with a condom

Vaginal sex. Vaginal sex is less safe than oral sex, but safer than anal sex. Always use a condom to keep the semen from touching your vagina. If you cannot, try to have the man withdraw his penis before he ejaculates. You can still get HIV and you can still get pregnant, but it is safer because less semen gets into your body.

Anal sex. Sex in the anus is very dangerous because the skin there tears even more easily than the skin in the vagina. If you and your partner have anal sex, it is important that you use condoms and make the anus wet first. Never have sex in the vagina **after** having sex in the anus without the man washing his penis first, or you could get an infection.

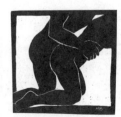
Safer with a condom

Avoid 'dry sex'. In some places people prefer to have sex when the vagina is very dry, so some women put herbs or powders in their vaginas or *douche* before sex. But if the vagina (or anus) is dry or irritated, it will tear easily during sex and make infection more likely. You can make the vagina less dry by not using powders, herbs, or douches, and by taking more time with sex to allow the body to make more of its own wetness. Or use saliva, spermicide, or *lubricant* to make the vagina slippery so the skin will not tear. **Do not use oil or petroleum gel**, which can make a condom break.

MAKING CHANGES FOR SAFER SEX

Everyone needs to think about ways to make sex safer, even if you do not think you are at risk. How you make these changes will depend on whether you expect your partner to support your wish to have safer sex.

If your partner is supportive, it is best to talk together about the health risks of STDs. But this is not always easy! Most women are taught that it is not 'proper' to talk about sex—especially with their partners or other men—so they lack practice. A man may talk with other men about sex, but is often uncomfortable talking with his partner. Here are some suggestions:

I want to talk about these things, but I'm not sure how.

I really want to talk about these things, but I am afraid of what he will think.

Practice talking with a friend first. Ask a friend to pretend to be your partner and then practice what you want to say. Try to think of the different things he might say and practice for each possibility. Remember that he will probably feel nervous about talking too, so try to put him at ease.

Talk with your partner. Do not wait until you are about to have sex. Choose a time when you are feeling good about each other and when you are not likely to be interrupted. If you have stopped having sex because you have a new baby, try to talk with him before you have sex again. If you and your partner live far apart or must travel often, talk ahead of time about what having other partners would mean for your sexual health.

➤ *Work with your community to educate women and men about condoms and how to use them. This will help make condoms more acceptable.*

Learn as much as you can about the risks of unsafe sex, and about safer sex methods and practices. If your partner does not know much about STDs and how they are spread, or about their lasting health effects, he may not understand the real risks involved in unsafe sex. If you give him this information, or encourage him to talk to a health worker about it, you can help convince him of the need to practice safer sex.

If you think your partner will not want to practice safer sex, you will need to be more creative to get what you want:

Bargaining for safer sex

Think about how you bargain for the other things you need. In these situations, you must know what you want and then talk to the other person in such a way that you get it. Start by asking yourself: Exactly what changes do I want my partner to make? Is there something I can offer him that will make him more likely to agree? What am I willing to offer?

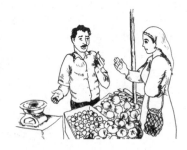

Focus on safety. When you talk about safer sex, your partner may say that you do not trust him. Tell him the issue is safety, not trust. Since a person may have an STD without knowing it, or may get HIV/AIDS from something other than sex, it is difficult for a person to be sure he or she is not infected. Safer sex is a good idea for every couple, even if they only have sex with each other.

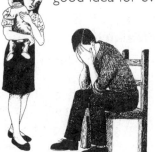

But if you or your partner has had or now has another sexual partner, it may be hard to talk about. If your partner is having sex with others now, do not use this discussion to punish him. Try to talk honestly about why you are scared and how each of you will behave in the future. If he is not willing to stop having sex with others, ask him to use condoms every time he has sex with you and with anyone else.

Use other people as examples. Sometimes learning that others are practicing safer sex can help influence your partner to do so, too.

My brother told me he always uses condoms now.

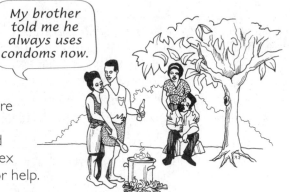

Ask for help if you need it. If you are afraid your partner will get angry or violent when you talk, you may need someone to help you discuss safer sex with him. Ask someone you trust for help.

If your partner does not want to change

If your partner does not want to change his sexual habits, you must decide what to do. You may be able to choose not to have sex, to find protection you can control—like the female condom, or the diaphragm with spermicides (see pages 204 to 206)—or think about ending the relationship.

Getting AIDS

He stays. You get AIDS.

He Leaves

He leaves. You do not get AIDS.

What you must weigh if your partner is unwilling to stop unsafe sexual practices.

FEELING MORE PLEASURE FROM SEX

➤ *Both men and women are capable of feeling—and controlling—their desires.*

It is natural for women and men to want to share sexual pleasure with their partners. When each partner knows the kind of sexual talk and touch that the other likes, they can both enjoy sex more.

If a woman does not feel pleasure with sex, there may be many reasons. Her partner may not realize that her body responds differently to sexual touch than a man's body does. Or she may have been taught that women should enjoy sex less than men, or that she should not tell her partner what she likes. Understanding that women are capable of enjoying sex just as much as men, and that it is OK to do so, may help her like sex more. But she should remember that these kinds of changes often take time.

➤ *What brings pleasure to one person should not be harmful to another.*

How the body responds to sexual pleasure

Both women and men feel sexual desire but their bodies respond differently to sexual thoughts and touch. When men and women have sexual thoughts or are touched in a sexual way, they feel excited. More thought and touch makes the body more excited. It is easy to see sexual excitement in a man, because his penis gets hard. When a man reaches his peak of pleasure, his penis releases fluid with his sperm (ejaculation). This is called *orgasm*, or *climax*. After orgasm, the penis becomes soft again.

The woman's body also gets excited, but it is harder to see. The *clitoris* gets hard and may swell, and the *labia* and walls of the vagina become sensitive to touch. If sexual touch and thought continue, sexual tension builds up until she reaches her peak of pleasure and has an orgasm. Touching the clitoris is the most common way this happens. It often takes longer for a woman to reach orgasm than a man. But when orgasm happens, the energy and tension in her body releases, and she feels relaxed and full of pleasure.

It is possible for almost all women to have orgasms, but many women have them only once in a while, or never. If she wants, a woman may be able to learn how to have an orgasm, either by touching herself (see the next page), or by letting her partner know what feels good. It may make him feel good too, to know that he pleases her.

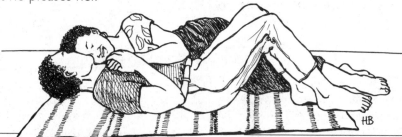

Touching oneself for pleasure (masturbation)

A woman can touch herself in a way that gives sexual pleasure. This is a good way for her to learn about her body and what kinds of sexual touch feel best. Many communities have beliefs that touching oneself is wrong, so sometimes people feel shame about doing it. But touching oneself does not cause harm or use up sexual desire.

Lack of desire

Many things—including everyday life events—can affect how much sexual desire a woman or man feels. For example, when life seems exciting—such as when starting a new relationship or a new job—a woman or man may feel more sexual desire. But you may feel less desire when:

- you feel stress from hard work, not enough food, illness, or a new baby.
- you have a partner you do not like.
- you fear that others will see or hear you having sex.
- you are afraid of becoming pregnant or getting an STD.

When a woman lacks desire, her body makes less of its natural wetness, and she may need to use lubrication, like saliva, so that sex is not painful. When a man lacks desire, it is more difficult for his penis to get hard (impotence). He may feel ashamed, and this may make it more difficult for him to get hard the next time.

If you or your partner is having less desire, try to forgive each other and to talk about it. Plan time for sex when you both want it, and try to do things that awaken sexual thoughts and feelings for both of you.

> ➤ *If a woman has been raped or forced to have sex, she may need time—or to talk with someone she trusts or a trained mental health worker— before she wants to have sex again.*

If sex is painful

Sex should not be painful. Pain during sex is usually a sign that something is wrong. A woman may feel pain with sex when:
- her partner enters her too soon, before she is relaxed or wet enough.
- she feels guilt or shame, or does not want to have sex.
- she has an infection or growth in her vagina or lower belly (see page 356).
- she has been *circumcised* (see page 463).

IMPORTANT *Pain with sex after recent childbirth, miscarriage, or abortion can be a sign of serious infection. See a health worker right away.*

Working for Change

CHANGING HARMFUL GENDER ROLES

Changing harmful gender roles takes time, because ideas about gender are some of the most deeply-held beliefs a community has. But over time, women and men can learn to take on new roles, especially if they understand how these roles will help girls and women live healthier, more productive lives.

To begin changing these gender roles, you will need to find ways to help your community. Here are some suggestions:

- Develop an awareness of what gender roles are, and how they are passed on by parents, community traditions, and the media (the radio, television and newspapers).
- Examine different gender roles to see which are harmful and need changing.
- Make plans for change.

Here are some suggestions for fun activities that have been used in some communities to help women and men think about gender roles and how they affect sexual health:

Using sexual language

Understanding that men and women see each others' sexuality differently can help people think about how gender roles affect their beliefs about sexuality. This activity can help women and men learn how to talk openly about sex without shame, and to begin to think about the different ways that men and women view sexuality.

1. *Write down (or draw) several sexual terms, each at the top of a separate piece of paper: for example 'male genital organ', 'female genital organ', 'sex', 'condoms', etc.*

2. *Divide into groups of 2 or 3 people. Give each small group one of the pieces of paper. Let each group have a few minutes to think of every polite, rude, medical, and common way to say the words on their paper, and call them out. Then pass the papers to a different group until each group has had a chance to add to each list.*

3. *Discuss the words with the whole group.*

   What does each word make people feel? Do they make the women in the group feel differently than the men? What words are used more by men? Which are used more by women? If a woman uses these words, what do people think of her? What do they think of a man who uses the same words? Why? What words are the best to use in different situations? Why?

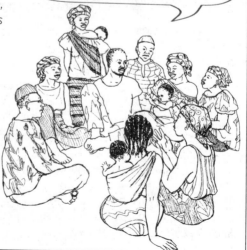

If a woman says 'rubber', 'gumboot', or even 'condom', people will think she's a bad woman. But it's ok for a man to say it if he's talking with his buddies...

Gender messages in the media

If people understand how harmful ideas about women's sexuality and gender roles are learned, they can begin to think about how to change those ideas. This activity will help people think about how radio, movies, popular songs, and advertising communicate ideas about gender roles.

1. Listen to some popular songs on the radio (record them ahead of time if you have a tape recorder) or have members of the group sing (or act out) the songs. Listen carefully to what the words of the songs are saying about women and men. How are the women and men being described? Are these songs passing on ideas about women's roles and sexuality? Note each 'gender' message the group identifies in the songs, and decide whether it is harmful or helpful to women.

2. Divide into small groups. Give each group an advertisement cut out of a magazine or newspaper, or copied from a billboard (pick advertisements that have women in them). Ask each group to identify what the advertisements say about women's roles and sexuality. Then, bring everyone together again to say what messages are being passed on in each advertisement. Then decide as a group whether the messages are harmful or helpful to women.

3. Discuss how messages about women are passed on by radio, songs, and advertisements. How do these ideas influence us, our husbands, our children? Do these ideas lead to practices and beliefs which are harmful to women?

4. Identify ideas about women's roles and sexuality **that are important and helpful** to pass on. How can these ideas be communicated in advertisements, songs, and movies? Ask small groups to draw an advertisement, or prepare a song or a skit that teaches helpful and healthy ideas about women. Have each group present their work to the others.

IMPROVING SEXUAL HEALTH IN YOUR COMMUNITY

Gender roles are different in each community, and so are the difficulties women and men face when trying to improve their sexual health. Here is a way to begin a discussion about why it may be hard for women to practice safer sex in your community.

➤ To work for change in your community, it is important to identify the barriers to practicing safer sex.

1. Begin by telling a story, like "Fátima's story" (page 187). Talk about Fátima and Emanuel as if they lived in your community.

2. After telling the story, start a discussion with questions like, "Why didn't Fátima protect herself from AIDS?" "Do you think she realized that she could get AIDS?" "If no, why not?"

3. Once the group has talked about the importance of understanding risk, you can talk about other barriers to safer sex. For example: What are the difficulties that women like Fátima face if they try to practice safer sex? Why do women find it hard to talk with their partners about safer sex? What can women do to convince their partners to practice safer sex?

4. Talk about what can be done in your community to help women like Fátima. Discuss how you can help to overcome barriers to safer sex in your community. (For ideas about ways to work for safer sex in your community, see page 280.) End the discussion by making a plan to improve sexual health in your community.

Chapter 13

In this chapter:

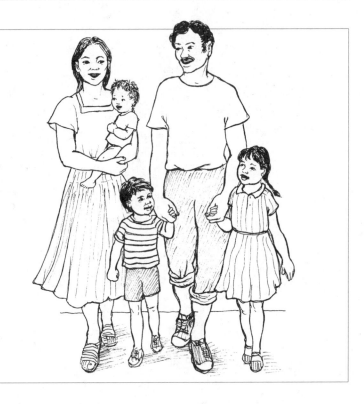

Family Planning

Having the number of children you want, when you want them, is called family planning. If you decide to wait to have children, you can choose one of several methods to prevent pregnancy. These methods are called family planning methods, child spacing methods, or contraception.

➤ *Family planning saves lives.*

Every year, half a million women die of problems from pregnancy, childbirth, and unsafe *abortion*. Most of these deaths could be prevented by family planning. For example, family planning can prevent dangers from pregnancies that are:

- **too soon.** Women under the age of 17 are more likely to die in childbirth because their bodies are not fully grown. Their babies have a greater chance of dying in the first year.
- **too late.** Older women face more danger in child bearing, especially if they have other health problems or have had many children.
- **too close.** A woman's body needs time to recover between pregnancies.
- **too many.** A woman with more than 4 children has a greater risk of death after childbirth from bleeding and other causes.

Benefits of Family Planning

➤ *In poor countries about half of all deaths in women of child-bearing age are caused by problems of pregnancy and childbirth. Family planning prevents these pregnancies and deaths.*

As well as saving lives, family planning has other benefits

Mothers and babies will be healthier, because risky pregnancies are avoided.

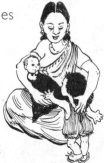

Fewer children means more food for each child.

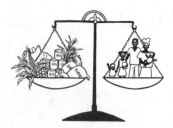

Waiting to have children can allow young women and men time to complete their education.

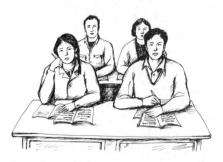

Fewer children can mean more time for yourselves and your children.

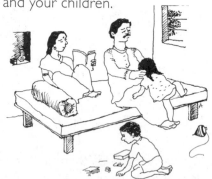

Family planning can also help you and your partner enjoy sex more, because you are not afraid of unwanted pregnancy. And some methods have other health benefits. For example, *condoms* and *spermicides* can help protect against the spread of *sexually transmitted diseases (STDs)*, including *HIV/AIDs*. *Hormonal methods* can help with irregular bleeding and pain during a woman's *monthly bleeding*.

Is Family Planning Safe?

All of the family planning methods found in this chapter are used safely by millions of women. In fact, these methods are much safer than pregnancy and childbirth:

Of 15,000 women who become pregnant, 500 are likely to die from problems of pregnancy or childbirth.

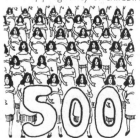

Of 15,000 women who use family planning methods, only one is likely to die from using these methods.

Some women want a lot of children—especially in communities where poor people are denied a fair share of land, resources, and social benefits. This is because children help with work and provide care for their parents in old age. In these places, having just a few children may be a privilege only wealthier people can afford.

Other women may want to limit the number of children they have. This often happens where women have opportunities to study and earn income, and where they can negotiate with men in a more equal way.

No matter where a woman lives, she will be healthier if she has control over how many children she has, and when she will have them. Still, deciding to use—or not to use—family planning should always be a woman's choice.

Choosing to Use Family Planning

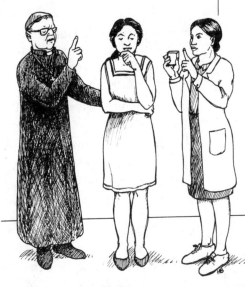

You have a right to make your own decisions about family planning.

Talking with your husband or partner about family planning

It is best if you can talk together with your husband or partner about choosing to use family planning and what method you will use.

Some men do not want their wives to use family planning, often because they do not know very much about how different methods work. A man may worry about his wife's health, because he has heard stories about the dangers of family planning. He may fear that if a woman uses family planning, she will have sex with another man. Or he may also think it is 'manly' to have lots of children.

Try sharing the information in this chapter with your partner. It may help him understand that:

• family planning will allow him to take better care of you and your children.

• child spacing is safer for you and your children.

• family planning can make sex with him more pleasant, because neither of you will have to worry about an unplanned pregnancy. Being protected against unwanted pregnancy will not make you want to have sex with other men.

If your husband still does not want you to use family planning even after learning about its benefits, you must decide whether you will use family planning anyway. If you do, you may need to choose a method that can be used without your partner knowing about it.

Choosing a Family Planning Method

Once you have decided to use family planning, you must choose a method. To make a good decision you must first learn about the different methods, and their advantages and disadvantages.

There are 5 main types of family planning methods:

- **Barrier methods**, which prevent pregnancy by keeping the *sperm* from reaching the egg.
- **Hormonal methods**, which prevent the woman's *ovary* from releasing an egg, make it harder for the sperm to reach the egg, and keep the lining of the *womb* from supporting a pregnancy.
- **IUDs**, which prevent the man's sperm from *fertilizing* the woman's egg.
- **Natural methods**, which help a woman know when she is *fertile*, so that she can avoid having sex at that time.
- **Permanent methods**. These are operations which make it impossible for a man or a woman to have any children.

These methods of family planning are described on the following pages. As you read about each method, here are some questions you may want to consider:

- How well does it prevent pregnancy (its effectiveness)?
- How well does it protect against STDs, if at all?
- How safe is it? If you have any of the health problems mentioned in this chapter, you may need to avoid some types of family planning methods.
- How easy is it to use?

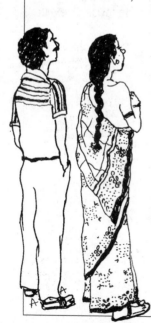

  - Is your partner willing to use family planning?
  - What are your personal needs and concerns? For example, do you have all the children you want, or are you breastfeeding your baby?
  - How much does the method cost?
  - Is it easy to get? Will you need to visit a health center often?
  - Will the side effects (the problems the method may cause) create difficulties for you?

After reading about these methods, you can get more help with choosing one on page 226. It may also help to talk with your partner, other women, or a health worker about different methods.

Only you can decide which family planning method is right for you.

How well each method works

Here is some basic information about the effectiveness of the different methods, their usefulness in protecting against STDs as well as pregnancy, and whether you can use them while breastfeeding.

For every 100 women who use this method for one year...	This many women will become pregnant:	Protection against STDs
Condom	12	good
Condom for Women	20	good
Diaphragm	18	some
Spermicide	20	some
Pill (the combined pill)	3	none
Progestin Only Pill	5	none
Implants	Less than 1	none
Injections	Less than 1	none
IUD	1	none
Breastfeeding (1st 6 mo.)	2	none
Natural Family Planning	20	none
Sterilization	Less than 1	none
No Method	85	none

All of these methods can be used safely while breastfeeding except the combined pill, and injections that have estrogen.

Barrier Methods of Family Planning

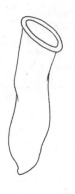

Barrier methods prevent pregnancy by blocking the sperm from reaching the egg. They do not change the way the woman's or man's body works, and they cause very few side effects. Barrier methods are safe if a woman is breastfeeding. Most of these methods also protect against STDs, including HIV/AIDs. When a woman wants to become pregnant, she simply stops using the barrier method.

The most common barrier methods are the condom, condoms for women, the diaphragm, and spermicides.

THE CONDOM

The condom is a narrow bag of thin rubber that the man wears on his *penis* during sex. Because the man's semen stays in the bag, the sperm cannot enter the woman's body.

Condoms work best when they are used with spermicide (see page 206). Condoms made of *latex* are the best protection against STDs and HIV/AIDS, and can be used alone or along with any other family planning method.

Condoms can be bought at many pharmacies and markets, and are also available at health posts and through AIDS prevention programs. They can help some men last longer during sex.

➤ *Condoms can help some men last longer during sex.*

Be careful not to tear the condom as you open the package. Do not use a new condom if the package is torn or dried out, or if the condom is stiff or sticky. The condom will not work. Do not unroll the condom before putting it on.

How to use a condom:

1. *If the man is not circumcised, pull the foreskin back. Squeeze the tip of the condom and put it on the end of the hard penis.*

2. *Keep squeezing the tip while unrolling the condom, until it covers all of the penis. The loose part at the end will hold the man's sperm. If you do not leave space for the sperm when it comes out, the condom is more likely to break.*

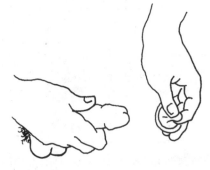
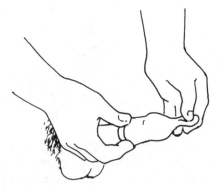

The condom must be put on the man's penis when it is hard, but before it touches the woman's *genitals*. If his penis touches the woman's genitals or goes into her *vagina*, he can make the woman pregnant or can give her an STD, even if he does not spill his sperm (ejaculate).

Remember:

- Use a condom every time you have sex.
- If possible, always use condoms made of latex. They give the best protection against HIV. Condoms made of sheepskin will not protect against HIV.
- Keep condoms in a cool, dry place away from sunlight. Condoms that are from old or torn packages are more likely to break.
- Use a condom only once. A condom that has been used before is more likely to break.

Use *lubricants* to keep condoms from breaking. Lubricants should be water based, such as spit (saliva), spermicide, or K-Y Jelly. Rub the lubricant on the sides of the condom after it is on the hard penis. Do not use cooking oils, baby oil, mineral oil, petroleum gel, skin lotion, or butter. They can make the condom break.

A man may not want to use a condom at first, but often a woman can convince her partner to use condoms by explaining the advantages of family planning and the importance of protection against HIV/AIDs and STDs.

➤ *If the condom tears or slips off, the woman should immediately put spermicide into her vagina. If possible, use an emergency method of family planning (see page 224).*

➤ *Since condoms are the best protection against STDs and HIV/AIDS, they should be used with other family planning methods when a woman needs protection from both pregnancy and STDs.*

188

encouraging your partner to use condoms

---

3. *After the man ejaculates, he should hold on to the rim of the condom and withdraw from the vagina while his penis is still hard.*

4. *Take off the condom. Do not let sperm spill or leak.*

5. *Tie the condom shut and dispose by burning or burying it away from children and animals.*

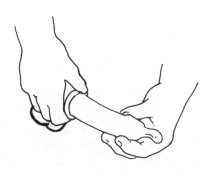

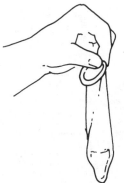

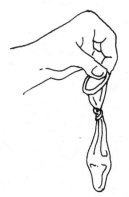

CONDOMS FOR WOMEN (female condoms)

A female condom, which fits into the vagina and covers the outer lips of the *vulva*, can be put in the vagina any time before sex. It should be used only once, because it may break if it is washed and reused. But reusing a female condom is better than no condom.

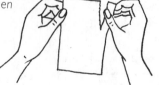

The female condom is the most effective of the methods controlled by women in protecting against both pregnancy and STDs, including HIV/AIDS. It is available only in a few places now. But if enough people demand this method, more programs will make them available.

➤ *Female condoms are larger than condoms made for men and are less likely to break.*

The female condom should not be used with a male condom.

How to use the female condom:

1. Carefully open the packet.

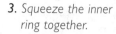

2. Find the inner ring, which is at the closed end of the condom.

Outer ring →

Inner ring →

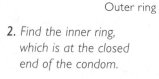

3. Squeeze the inner ring together.

4. Put the inner ring in the vagina.

5. Push the inner ring up into your vagina with your finger. The outer ring stays outside the vagina.

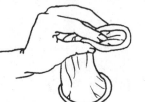

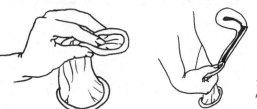

6. When you have sex, guide the penis through the outer ring.

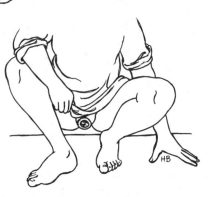

7. Remove the female condom immediately after sex, before you stand up. Squeeze and twist the outer ring to keep the man's sperm inside the pouch. Pull the pouch out gently, and then burn or bury it. Do not flush it down the toilet.

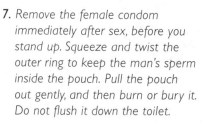

THE DIAPHRAGM

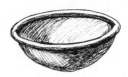

The diaphragm is a shallow cup made of soft rubber that a woman wears in her vagina during sex. The diaphragm works by covering the opening to the womb (cervix), preventing the sperm from entering it. The spermicide jelly used with the diaphragm helps kill the sperm, and also protects against gonorrhea and chlamydia (2 common STDs).

Diaphragms come in different sizes, and are available at some health posts and family planning clinics. A health worker who has been trained to do *pelvic exams* can examine you and find the right size diaphragm.

Diaphragms can get holes, particularly after being used for more than a year. It is a good idea to check your diaphragm often. Replace it when the rubber gets dry or hard, or when there is a hole in it.

When you use a diaphragm with spermicide, it can be put in just before you have sex, or up to 6 hours before.

➤ *New research shows that using a diaphragm without spermicide can also help prevent pregnancy. You can leave the diaphragm in all the time, except during monthly bleeding.* **Remove it once a day for cleaning.**

How to use a diaphragm:

1. If you have spermicide, squeeze it into the center. Then spread a little bit around the edge with your finger.

2. Squeeze the diaphragm in half.

3. Open the lips of your vagina with your other hand. Push the diaphragm into your vagina. It works best if you push it toward your back.

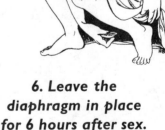

4. Check the position of your diaphragm by putting one of your fingers inside of your vagina and feeling for your cervix through the rubber of the diaphragm. The cervix feels firm, like the end of your nose. The diaphragm must cover your cervix.

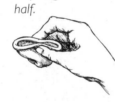

5. If the diaphragm is in the right place, you will not be able to feel it inside you.

6. Leave the diaphragm in place for 6 hours after sex.

To remove the diaphragm:

Put your finger inside your vagina. Reach behind the front rim of the diaphragm and pull it down and out. It sometimes helps to push your muscles down at the same time, as if you were passing stool. Wash your diaphragm with soap and water, and dry it. Check the diaphragm for holes by holding it up to the light. If there is even a tiny hole, get a new one. Store the diaphragm in a clean, dry place.

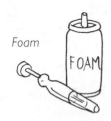

Foam

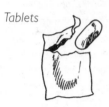

Tablets

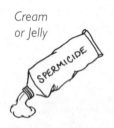

Cream or Jelly

SPERMICIDE
(contraceptive foam, tablets, jelly, or cream)

Spermicide comes in many forms—foam, tablets, and cream or jelly—and is put into the vagina just before having sex. Spermicide kills the man's sperm before it can get into the womb. Spermicide made with nonoxynol-9 also provides some protection from gonorrhea and chlamydia, which are 2 common STDs.

If used alone, spermicide is less effective than some other methods. But it is helpful when used as extra protection along with another method, like the diaphragm or condom.

Spermicides can be bought in many pharmacies and markets. Some women find that some types of spermicides cause itching or irritation inside the vagina (see page 520).

When to insert spermicide:

Tablets or suppositories should be put in the vagina 10 to 15 minutes before having sex. Foam, jelly, or cream work best if they are put in the vagina just before having sex.

If more than one hour passes before having sex, add more spermicide. Add a new tablet, suppository, or applicator of foam, jelly, or cream each time you have sex.

How to insert spermicide:

1. Wash your hands with soap and water.
2. **To use foam**, shake the foam container rapidly, about 20 times. Then press the nozzle to fill the applicator.

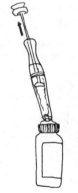

To use jelly or cream, screw the spermicide tube onto the applicator. Fill the applicator by squeezing the spermicide tube.

To use vaginal tablets, remove the wrapping and wet them with water or spit on them. (DO NOT put the tablet in your mouth.)

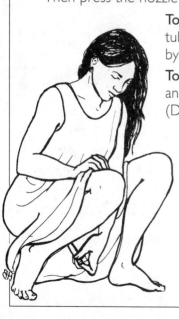

3. Gently put the applicator or vaginal tablet into your vagina, as far back as it will go.
4. If you are using an applicator, press in the plunger all the way and then take out the empty applicator.
5. Rinse the applicator with clean water and soap.

Leave the spermicide in place for at least 6 hours after sex. Do not douche or wash the spermicide out. If cream drips out of your vagina, wear a pad, cotton or clean cloth to protect your clothes.

Those methods contain *hormones,* called estrogen and *progestin,* that are similar to the estrogen and progesterone a woman makes in her own body.

Hormonal methods include:

- birth control pills, which a woman takes every day.

- injections, which are given every few months.

- implants, which are put into a woman's arm and last for several years.

Hormonal Methods of Family Planning

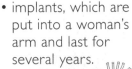

47
hormones

Hormonal methods work by preventing the woman's ovaries from releasing an egg. The hormones also make the mucus at the opening of the womb very thick, which helps stop the sperm from getting inside the womb.

Most birth control pills and some injections contain both estrogen and progestin. These are called 'combination' pills or injections. The two hormones work together to give excellent protection against pregnancy. However, some women should not use pills or injections with estrogen for health reasons, or because they are breastfeeding.

'Progestin-only' pills (also called mini-pills), implants, and some injections contain only one hormone—progestin. These methods are safer than combined pills or injections for women who should not use estrogen, or are breastfeeding.

These women should avoid ANY kind of hormonal method:

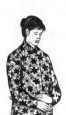

- Women who have breast *cancer,* or a hard lump in the breast (see page 382). Hormonal methods do not cause cancer. But if a woman already has breast cancer, these methods can make it worse.

- Women who might be pregnant or whose monthly bleeding is late (see page 67).

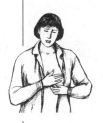

- Women who have *abnormal bleeding* from the vagina during the 3 months before starting hormonal methods (see page 360). They should see a health worker to find out if there is a serious problem.

Some hormonal methods are harmful for women with other health problems. Be sure to check each method to see if it is safe for you. If you have any of the health problems mentioned and still wish to use a method, talk to a health worker who has been trained in hormonal methods of family planning.

IMPORTANT

Hormonal methods do not protect against STDs, or HIV/AIDS.

➤ *A woman controls hormonal methods and they can be used without a man knowing.*

➤ *Some medicines for seizures (fits) or for tuberculosis (TB) make hormonal methods less effective. A woman taking these medicines should use other family planning methods.*

Side effects of hormonal methods

Because hormonal methods contain the same *chemicals* that a woman's body makes when she is pregnant, these things may happen during the first few months:

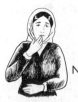

Nausea

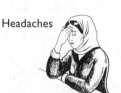

Headaches

Swelling of the breasts

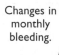

Changes in monthly bleeding.

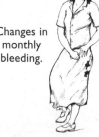

Side effects often get better after the first 2 or 3 months. If they do not, and they are annoying or worrying you, see a health worker. She may be able to help you change the amount of the hormones in your method or to change methods. For more information about the specific side effects that are common with each hormonal method, see pages 209 to 215.

➤ *Some women find that taking the pill helps their monthly bleeding to be more regular, with less bleeding and less pain.*

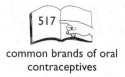

common brands of oral contraceptives

➤ *If you must change to a lower dose pill, use a barrier method of family planning or do not have sex during the first month.*

THE PILL

Birth control pills that contain estrogen and progestin

If you take birth control pills every day, they will protect you from pregnancy for your entire *monthly cycle*. These pills are usually available at family planning clinics, health posts, pharmacies, and through health workers.

There are many different brands of pills. The pill you get should be what is called a 'low-dose' pill. This means it has 35 micrograms (mcg) or less of estrogen, and 1 milligram (mg) or less of progestin. (Mini-pills and low-dose pills are different—low-dose pills have both estrogen and progestin, while the mini pill has only progestin.) Never use a method with more than 50 mcg of estrogen.

Once you start taking pills, you should try to stick with one brand (and if you can, buy several packets at once). If you must change brands, try to get another with the same hormone names and strength. You will have fewer side effects and better protection.

Who should not take combined pills:

Some women have health problems that make it dangerous for them to use the pill. **NEVER take the pill if you have any of the conditions listed on page 207, or if you:**

- have *hepatitis*, or yellow skin and eyes.
- have ever had signs of a *stroke*, *paralysis*, or heart disease.
- have ever had a *blood clot* in the *veins* of your legs or in your brain. *Varicose veins* are usually not a problem, unless the veins are red and sore.

If you have any of the following health problems, try to use a method other than combined birth control pills. But if you cannot, it is still better to take the combined pill than to become pregnant. **Try not to take combined pills if you:**

- **smoke and are over 35 years old**. You have a greater chance of having a stroke or heart attack if you take combined pills.

- **have diabetes or epilepsy**. If you are taking medicine for fits *(seizures)* you will need to take a stronger (50 mcg estrogen) birth control pill. Get medical advice from a health worker or doctor.

- **have high blood pressure** (more than 140/90). If you have ever been told you have high blood pressure or think you might have it, have your *blood pressure* checked by a health worker. If you weigh too much, have frequent headaches, get out of breath easily, feel weak or *dizzy* often, or feel pain in the left shoulder or chest, you should be tested for high blood pressure.

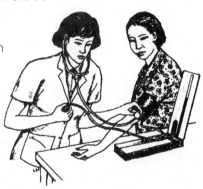

➤ *If you are breastfeeding you should also **try not to take the combined pills**. The estrogen in combined pills will reduce your milk supply. This could affect your baby's health.*

Common side effects of combined pills:

- **Irregular bleeding or spotting** (bleeding at other times than your normal monthly bleeding). Combined pills often make your monthly bleeding shorter and lighter. It is also normal to sometimes skip your monthly bleeding. This is the most common side effect of combined birth control pills. To reduce spotting, be extra careful to take the pill at the same time every day. If the spotting continues, talk with a health worker to see if changing doses of progestin or estrogen will help.

- **Nausea.** Nausea, the feeling that you want to throw up, usually goes away after 1 or 2 months. If it bothers you, try taking the pills with food or at another time of day. Some women find that taking the pill just before going to sleep at night helps.

- **Headaches.** Mild headaches in the first few months are common. A mild pain medicine should help. If the headache is severe or comes with *blurred eyesight*, this could be a serious warning sign, see page 210.

➤ *If your monthly bleeding does not come at the normal time **and** you have missed some pills, continue to take your pills but see a health worker to find out if you are pregnant.*

Warning signs for problems with combined pills:

STOP taking the pill and see a health worker if you:

➤ *If you are given a new medicine while on the pill, ask your health worker if you should use a barrier method or not have sex while taking the medicine. Antibiotics and some other medicines make the pill less effective.*

- have severe headaches with blurred vision *(migraines)* that begin after you start taking the pill.
- feel weakness or numbness in your arms or legs.
- feel severe pain in your chest and shortness of breath.
- have severe pain in one leg.

If you have any of these problems, pregnancy can also be dangerous, so use another type of family planning such as condoms until you can see a health worker trained in hormonal family planning methods.

How to take combined birth control pills:

The pill comes in packets of 21 or 28 tablets. If you have a 28-day packet, take one pill every day of the month. As soon as you have finished one packet, begin taking pills from another packet.

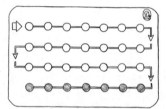

28-Day Pill Packet

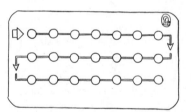

21-Day Pill Packet

If you have a 21-day packet, take a pill every day for 21 days, then wait 7 days before beginning a new packet. Your monthly bleeding will usually happen during the days you are not taking pills. But begin a new packet even if your monthly bleeding has not come.

With both 21-day and 28-day packets, take the first pill on the first day of your monthly bleeding. This way you will be protected right away. If it is after the first day, you can start taking a pill on any of the first 7 days of your monthly cycle. But you will not be protected right away, so for the first 2 weeks you are taking the pill you should also use another family planning method or not have sex.

You must take one pill every day, even if you do not have sex. Try to take your pill at the same time every day. It may help to remember that you will always start a new packet on the same day of the week.

Forgetting to take pills:

If you miss pills you could get pregnant.

If you forget one pill, take it as soon as you remember. Then take the next pill at the regular time. This may mean that you take 2 pills in one day.

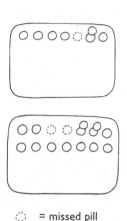

If you forget to take 2 pills in a row, start taking them again immediately. Take 2 pills for 2 days and then continue taking 1 pill each day until you finish the packet. Use condoms (or do not have sex) until you have taken a pill for 7 days in a row. If you forget to take 3 or more pills, stop taking the pills and wait for your next monthly bleeding. Use condoms (or do not have sex) for the rest of your cycle. Then start a new packet.

    Late or missed pills will cause some bleeding, like a very light monthly bleeding.

🔘 = missed pill
x = take 2 pills

    If you have trouble remembering to take pills, try taking a pill when you do a daily task, like preparing the evening meal. Or take the pill when you see the sun go down or before you

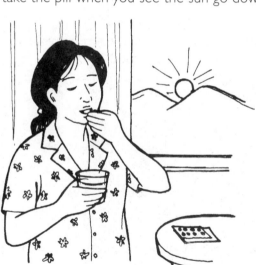

sleep. Keep the packet where you can see it every day. If you still forget to take your pills often (more than once a month), think about changing to a different method of birth control.

    If you vomit within 3 hours after taking your pill or have severe diarrhea, your birth control pill will not stay in your body long enough to work well. Use condoms, or do not have sex, until you are well and have taken a pill each day for 7 days.

Stopping the pill:

    If you want to change methods or get pregnant, stop taking the pills when you finish a packet. You can get pregnant right after you stop. Most women who stop taking pills because they want to get pregnant will get pregnant sometime within the first year.

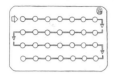

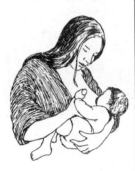

The Mini Pill or Progestin-only Pills

Because this pill does not contain estrogen, it is safer for women who should avoid combined birth control pills (see pages 208 and 209) and for women who have side effects from combined pills. But this pill is less effective than combined birth control pills.

The mini pill is also a better choice for women who are breastfeeding because it does not cause a decrease in the milk supply. The mini pill is very effective for most breastfeeding mothers. Like the combined pill, it is usually available at family planning clinics, health posts, pharmacies, and through health workers. See page 518 for brand names.

Women with any of the conditions on page 207 and women who are taking medicine for seizures should not take the mini pill. The medicine makes the mini pill less effective.

Common side effects of the mini pill:

- **irregular bleeding or spotting.** This is the most common side effect. If it becomes a problem, taking ibuprofen may help stop spotting.

- **no monthly bleeding**. This is fairly common, but if you go more than 45 days without bleeding you may be pregnant. Keep taking your pills until you can see a health worker to find out if you are pregnant.

- **occasional headaches.**

➤ *If you forget a pill, use a barrier method (or do not have sex) for 7 days, AND keep taking your pills.*

How to take the mini pill:

- Take your first pill on the first day of your monthly bleeding.

- **Take one pill at the same time each day, even if you do not have sex**.
  If you take a pill even a few hours late or forget only one day's pill, you can become pregnant.

- When you finish a packet, start your new packet the next day, even if you have not had any bleeding. Do not skip a day.

If you are breastfeeding and have not started your monthly bleeding, you can start taking the pills any day. You may not begin bleeding. This is normal.

What to do if you miss a mini pill:

Take it as soon as you remember. Take the next pill at the regular time, even if it means taking 2 pills in one day. You may have bleeding if you take your pill at a later time than usual.

Stopping the mini pill:

You can stop taking the pill any time. You can get pregnant the day after you stop, so be sure to use another family planning method right away if you do not want to become pregnant.

IMPLANTS

Implants are 6 small, soft tubes that are placed under the skin on the inside of a woman's arm. These tubes contain the hormone progestin and work like mini pills. They prevent pregnancy for 5 years. The only brand available when this book was written is called *Norplant*.

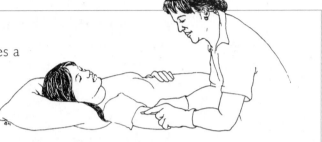

How to use implants:

A trained health worker makes a small cut in the skin to insert and remove the implants. This is usually done at a clinic or family planning center.

IMPORTANT *Before trying implants, be sure a health worker near you is trained and willing to remove the implants, in case you want them removed. It is harder to take implants out than it is to put them in.*

Implants can be used by women who are breastfeeding and others who have problems with estrogen. Women should not use implants if they have any of the conditions described on page 207, if they have heart disease, or if they want to become pregnant in the next few years. If you are taking medicines for seizures, you will need to use a backup method, like a condom or a diaphragm, as well as the implants.

contraceptive implant

Common side effects of implants:

During the first months, the implants may cause irregular bleeding (in the middle of your monthly cycle) or more days of monthly bleeding. Or you may have no bleeding at all. This does not mean that you are pregnant or that something is wrong. These changes will go away as your body becomes used to having more progestin. If this irregular bleeding causes problems for you, a health worker may have you take low-dose combined birth control pills along with the implants for a few months.

➤ *Ibuprofen or aspirin will also help control irregular bleeding.*

You may also have occasional headaches and the same side effects common with progestin-only injections (see page 214).

To stop using implants:

Although *Norplant* implants last for 5 years, they can be removed at any time—though it can be hard to find a health worker who knows how to remove them. After removal, you can get pregnant right away, so use another family planning method if you do not want to become pregnant.

➤ *Many women want their implants removed early because they do not like the side effects. The most common concern is irregular bleeding.*

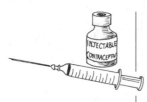

BIRTH CONTROL INJECTIONS

In this family planning method, a woman is given injections of hormones every 1 to 3 months, usually at a health center or family planning clinic, by someone who knows how. The protection lasts until you need a new injection, and can be used without others knowing.

Progestin-only injections

Progestin-only injections, such as *Depo Provera* and *Noristerat*, contain only the hormone progestin. These are especially good for women who are breastfeeding and women who should not use estrogen (see pages 208 and 209). They are given every 2 to 3 months.

Women should not begin progestin-only injections if they have any of the conditions listed on page 207, if they are unable to get regular injections, or if they want to become pregnant within the next year.

➤ *Progestin-only injections almost always cause changes in the monthly bleeding. You may have light bleeding every day or every once in a while. You will probably stop having monthly bleeding by the end of the first year. These changes are normal.*

Common side effects of progestin-only injections:

Because of the large doses of progestin given with each injection, women experience more changes in their monthly bleeding during the first few months than with other hormonal methods.

Other common side effects are:

- **irregular bleeding or heavy spotting**. If this is a problem, a health worker can give 2 cycles of a combined low-dose birth control pill to take along with the injections to stop the spotting. Most irregular bleeding will stop after a few months.
- **no monthly bleeding**.
- **weight gain**.

Combined injections

Other injections, such as *Cyclofem* and *Mesigyna*, contain both estrogen and progestin. This type of injection is good for women who want to have regular monthly bleeding. Combined injections are given every month, are more expensive than progestin-only injections, and are harder to find.

Women who should not take combined birth control pills or progestin-only injections should not take combined injections either. Do not begin combined injections while breastfeeding.

Common side effects of combined injections:

Because the injection contains the same hormones as combined birth control pills, the same side effects are common (see page 209).

How to use birth control injections:

It is best to get your first injection during your monthly bleeding. This way you know that you are not pregnant. You can start the injections anytime if you are breastfeeding and have not started your monthly bleeding.

The injection protects you against pregnancy immediately if it is given within 5 days after your monthly bleeding begins. If the injection was given 6 or more days after the beginning of your monthly bleeding, you should use condoms or not have sex for the next 2 weeks.

You must have an injection every 1, 2, or 3 months, depending on the kind of injection:

• *Depo Provera:* every 3 months

• *Noristerat:* every 2 months

• *Cyclofem* and *Mesigyna:* every month

Try not to be late getting injections. The injection becomes less effective the longer you wait.

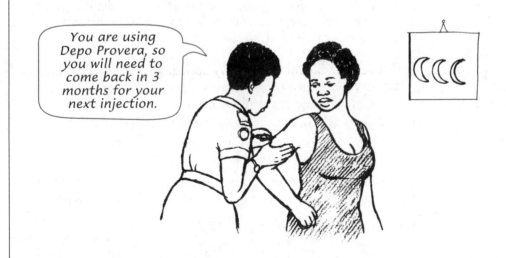

To stop using injections:

You can stop having birth control injections any time you want. But after you stop, it can take a year or more to become pregnant and for your monthly bleeding to return to normal. But it also may come back sooner. So if you do not want to become pregnant right away, you must use another family planning method during this time.

injectable contraceptives

Intra-Uterine Devices

(Devices that go into the womb)

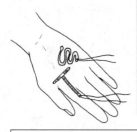

THE IUD (IUCD, Copper-T, The Loop)

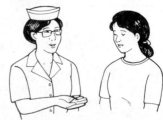

The IUD is a small object or device that is inserted into the womb by a specially trained health worker or midwife. Once in the womb, the IUD prevents the man's sperm from fertilizing the woman's egg. The IUD can stay in the womb for up to 10 years (depending on the kind of IUD it is) before it must be removed and replaced. An IUD can be used without the man knowing you are using it (although sometimes a man can feel the strings).

The most common IUDs are made of plastic, or plastic and copper.

Progestin IUD

This kind of IUD also contains the hormone progestin and is available in some countries. Progestin decreases the pain and bleeding that some women have with the IUD. It protects against pregnancy for 5 years.

261

STDs

➤ *IUDs can be used safely by women who are breastfeeding.*

➤ *Do not use an IUD if you are unable to get to a health center or clinic where you can have the IUD removed if necessary.*

IMPORTANT *IUDs do not protect against STDs, including HIV/AIDS. Not only that, but if a woman has an STD, the IUD can lead to more serious complications, such as* **pelvic inflammatory disease (PID)**. *PID can lead to infertility.*

Who should not use an IUD:

Do not use an IUD if you:

- are pregnant or might be pregnant.
- are in danger of getting an STD. (This includes any woman who has more than one partner, or whose partner may have other sex partners.)
- have ever had an *infection* in your tubes or womb, or an infection after giving birth or after having an abortion.
- have had a pregnancy in your tubes.
- have a lot of bleeding and pain during your monthly bleeding.
- are very *anemic*.
- have never been pregnant.

Common side effects:

You may have some light bleeding during the first week after getting an IUD. Some women also have longer, heavier, and more painful monthly bleeding, but this usually stops after the first 3 months.

How to use the IUD:

An IUD must be inserted by a specially trained health worker after doing a pelvic exam. The best time to have the IUD put in is during your monthly bleeding. After childbirth, it is best to wait 6 weeks for the womb to return to its normal size and shape before getting an IUD.

Occasionally an IUD will slip out of place. If this happens, it will not be effective in preventing pregnancy, so it is important to learn to check your IUD to make sure it is still in place. Most IUDs have 2 thread-like strings attached which hang down into the vagina. You should check the strings after each monthly bleeding to make sure the IUD is in place.

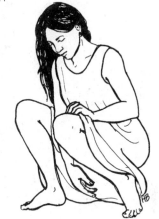

How to check the IUD strings:

1. Wash your hands.

2. Squat down and reach as far as you can into your vagina with your 2 fingers. Feel for the IUD strings, but **do not pull them**.

3. Take out your fingers and wash your hands again.

Warning signs for problems with an IUD:

Pelvic inflammatory disease is the most serious problem that can result from having an IUD. Most infections happen in the first 3 months, usually because the woman already had an infection when the IUD was put in. Or it may happen because the health worker did not put in the IUD under clean conditions.

If you have any of the following signs, you should see a health worker trained to insert IUDs and to treat complications, or go to a hospital immediately:

- Your monthly bleeding is late.
- You have pain in your lower belly or pain during sex.
- You have a heavy or bad-smelling discharge from the vagina.
- You do not feel well, or have fever or chills.
- Your IUD string is missing, or is shorter or longer than usual.
- Your partner can feel the IUD (not just the strings) during sex.

To stop using an IUD:

When you want to stop using an IUD, it must be removed by a trained health worker. Never try to remove an IUD yourself.

You can become pregnant as soon as it has been removed.

Natural Methods of Family Planning

There are also 3 methods to avoid pregnancy that do not require any devices or chemicals (as with barrier methods) or medicines (as with hormonal methods). The methods are:

- breastfeeding for the first 6 months
- the mucus method
- the rhythm method

IMPORTANT *Natural methods of family planning do not protect against STDs, including HIV/AIDS. If you use any of the natural methods listed in these pages, you still need to think about ways to protect yourself from these diseases.*

BREASTFEEDING FOR THE FIRST 6 MONTHS (LACTATIONAL AMENORRHEA METHOD, LAM)

Breastfeeding under certain conditions can prevent the ovaries from releasing an egg. This method does not cost anything, but it is most effective for only the first 6 months after childbirth.

How to use breastfeeding to prevent pregnancy:

Breastfeeding is not an effective method of family planning unless these 3 conditions are true:

1. Your baby is less than 6 months old.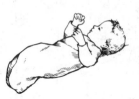

2. You have not had your monthly bleeding since giving birth.

3. You are giving your baby only breast milk, and feeding it whenever it is hungry—with no more than 6 hours between feedings—day and night. Your baby does not sleep through the night without feeding.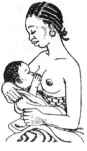

Use another method of family planning that is safe with breastfeeding as soon as any of the following things happen:

- Your baby is more than 6 months old, **or**
- Your monthly bleeding starts, **or**
- Your baby starts taking other kinds of milk or other foods, or starts sleeping for more than 6 hours during the night, **or**
- You must be away from the baby for more than 6 hours and cannot remove milk from your breasts during that time.

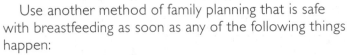

THE MUCUS METHOD AND THE RHYTHM METHOD

To use either of these methods, you must understand when you are fertile during your monthly cycle. This is sometimes called 'fertility awareness'. Then, to avoid pregnancy, you and your partner must not have sex, or must use a barrier method of family planning, during your fertile days.

Because there are no costs or side effects, these methods can be used by women who cannot or do not want to use other methods, or when other methods are not available.

To practice fertility awareness more effectively, both you and your partner should visit a specially trained health worker to learn about your bodies and about fertility. It usually takes about 3 to 6 months of practice to learn how to use these methods.

➤ *All these methods require the man's cooperation or they will not be effective.*

barrier methods

Natural family planning methods do not work as well if:

- you have little control over when you will have sex. During your fertile times, your partner must be willing to wait and not have sex or to use condoms or some other barrier method.

- your fertility signs change from month to month. You will not be able to know when you are fertile.

- you have just had a baby or miscarriage. It is hard to know when you are fertile at these times.

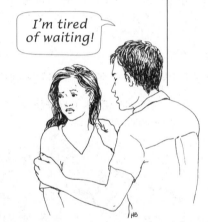

I'm tired of waiting!

What you should know about a woman's cycle of fertility:

- A woman produces one egg each month.
- The egg is released from the ovary about 14 days before the next monthly bleeding.
- The egg lives for about 24 hours (1 day and 1 night) after it has been released from the ovary.
- The man's sperm (seed) can live up to 2 days inside the woman's body.

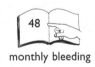

monthly bleeding

To make all natural family planning methods more effective:
- Have sex only on the days between the end of the fertile time and your next monthly bleeding.
- Use both the mucus method and the rhythm method at the same time.
- Use condoms whenever you are not sure if you are fertile, or do not have sex.

Mucus Method

To use the mucus method, you must pay careful attention to the mucus (wetness) in your vagina. Your body produces wet mucus during your fertile time to help the sperm get into the womb. So if you check your mucus every day, you will know when you are becoming fertile. Then you can avoid sex during this time.

How to tell when you are fertile:

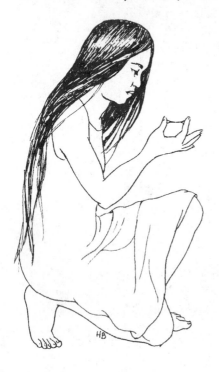

1. Wipe the outside of your vagina with your finger or a piece of paper or cloth.

2. If there is mucus there, take some between your fingers. How does it feel? Wet and slippery? Dry and sticky?

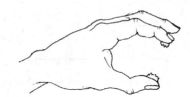

clear, wet, slippery mucus = fertile

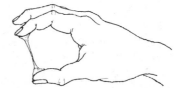

white, dry, sticky mucus = not fertile

How to use the mucus method:

• Do not have sex on any day you see or feel wetness or mucus. Or, if you want to have sex on those days, use a condom or a diaphragm **without** spermicide (these are the only methods that do not change the mucus).

• Do not have sex until 4 days after the last day of clear, slippery mucus.

• Do not have sex during your monthly bleeding. There is a small possibility you could be fertile and not be able to tell.

• Do not douche or wash out your vagina at any time.

• If you are having trouble knowing when you are fertile, or if you have a vaginal infection, you should use another method.

Rhythm Method

The rhythm method teaches you to find your fertile time by counting the days in your monthly cycle. You can NOT rely on the rhythm method if:

- you are breastfeeding and your monthly bleeding has not returned.
- you have recently been pregnant and your monthly bleeding is not yet regular.

How to use the rhythm method:

- Count the number of days in each of your monthly cycles for 6 months, from the first day of one monthly bleeding until the first day of the next.
- Pick out the longest and the shortest cycles.
- Take away or subtract 20 days from your shortest cycle and 10 days from your longest cycle. The time between these 2 days is your fertile time.
- Although you can have sex any time before or after your fertile time, the safest time is between the end of your fertile time and the beginning of your next monthly bleeding.

For example: Julia kept track of her monthly bleeding for 6 months. Her shortest cycle was 26 days and her longest cycle was 34 days:

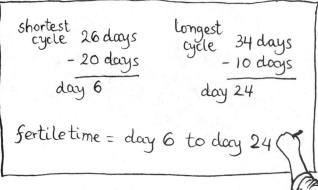

shortest
cycle 26 days
− 20 days
day 6

longest
cycle 34 days
− 10 days
day 24

fertile time = day 6 to day 24

To avoid pregnancy, Julia should not have sex, or she should use another family planning method, from day 6 after her monthly bleeding starts until day 24.

   You must use another method of family planning while you are counting your 6 monthly cycles. But you should not use the pill, implants, or injections during the time you are counting, because these methods change the time when your monthly bleeding starts.

Traditional and Home Methods to Prevent Pregnancy

Every community has traditional methods to prevent or stop pregnancy. Many of these can be very useful in limiting the number of children a couple has, although they are usually not as effective as modern methods. But some traditional methods are not effective at all, and some can even be very harmful.

TRADITIONAL METHODS THAT WORK

Withdrawal or pulling out (coitus interruptus). With this method, a man pulls his penis out of the woman and away from her genitals before he ejaculates. This method is better than no method, but it does not always work. Sometimes a man is not able to pull out before he ejaculates. Even if the man pulls out in time, some liquid that contains sperm can leak out of his penis before ejaculation and cause pregnancy.

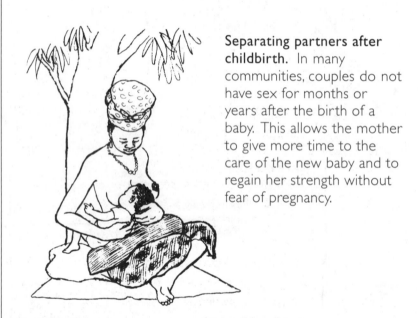

Separating partners after childbirth. In many communities, couples do not have sex for months or years after the birth of a baby. This allows the mother to give more time to the care of the new baby and to regain her strength without fear of pregnancy.

TRADITIONAL METHODS THAT DO NOT WORK OR THAT CAN BE HARMFUL

- Omens and magic do not prevent pregnancy.
- Putting grasses, leaves, pods, and dung in the vagina can cause infection and irritation.
- Washing out the vagina (douching) with herbs or powders does not prevent pregnancy. Sperm move very fast and some will reach the inside of the womb before they can be washed out.
- Urinating after sex does not prevent pregnancy. (But it can help to prevent infections of the *urine* system.)

STERILIZATION
(the operation for no more children)

There are operations that make it almost impossible for a man or a woman to have any children. Since these operations are permanent, they are only good for those women or men who are certain that they do not want any more children.

To have one of these operations, you must go to a health center or hospital. The surgery is fast and safe, and does not cause side effects.

The operation for the man (Vasectomy)

A vasectomy is a simple operation in which the tubes that carry the sperm from the *testicles* to the penis are cut. The man's testicles are not cut. This operation can be done in any health center where there is a trained health worker. It takes only a few minutes to do.

The man's tubes are cut here and here.

HB

The operation does not change a man's ability to have sex or to feel sexual pleasure. He still ejaculates semen but there are no sperm in the semen. He must ejaculate 20 times after the operation before all the sperm are gone. During this time, keep using your regular method of family planning.

The operation for the woman (Tubal Ligation)

A tubal ligation is a slightly more difficult operation than a vasectomy, but it is still very safe. It takes about 30 minutes.

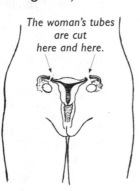

The woman's tubes are cut here and here.

A trained health worker makes 1 or 2 small cuts in the woman's belly, and then cuts or ties the tubes that carry the egg to the womb. **It does not change a woman's ability to have sex or to have sexual pleasure.**

IMPORTANT   *Sterilization does not protect against STDs, including HIV/AIDS. So you will still need to think about ways to protect yourself from these diseases.*

Permanent
Methods

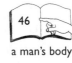
46

a man's body

Emergency Methods of Family Planning

Emergency methods are ways for women to avoid pregnancy after having unprotected sex. These methods prevent a fertilized egg from attaching to the womb wall. They are only effective if used soon after having sex.

Emergency methods are safe and effective. But they are not as effective as consistent use of the other family planning methods discussed in this chapter and they can cause unpleasant side effects.

EMERGENCY PILLS

The pills used for emergency family planning are the same combined birth control pills that some women take each day. But in emergencies, you take a much higher dose for a short time. You must take the pills within 3 days (72 hours) of having unprotected sex. **The pills will not work if you are pregnant from having sex more than 3 days earlier.**

➤ *Emergency family planning methods should not be used instead of other methods.*

How to take Emergency Pills:

Low dose pills. Take 4 low-dose birth control pills, which contain 35 mcg of the estrogen called ethinyl estradiol. Then take 4 more tablets 12 hours after the first dose. Some common brands are *Brevicon 1+35, Lo-Femenal, Lo-Ovral, Microgynon 30, Microvlar, Neocon, Nordette, Ortho-Novum1/35, 1/50*.

OR

High dose pills. Take 2 high-dose birth control pills, which contain 50 mcg of the estrogen called ethinyl estradiol. Then take 2 more tablets 12 hours after the first dose. Some common brands are *Ovral, Femenal, Primovlar, Norlestrin, Ovcon 50, Nordiol, Eugynon,* and *Neogynon*.

Emergency pills can make you have headaches or feel nauseous. Try eating something at the same time you take the pills and, if possible, take a medicine that will keep you from vomiting. If you vomit within 3 hours of taking the pills, you should take them again. For more information, see page 519.

Until your next monthly bleeding, you should use a barrier method of family planning, like condoms, or not have sex. After your monthly bleeding, you can use any family planning method you choose.

Your next monthly bleeding should begin in about 2 weeks. If it does not, you may have become pregnant despite the emergency family planning. You should continue to use a barrier method of family planning until you know for sure.

OTHER EMERGENCY METHODS

Mini pills (progestin only pills). These pills contain no estrogen, so they cause less nausea than combined birth control pills. They only work if taken within 2 days (48 hours) of having unprotected sex.

- Take 20 mini pills followed by 20 more pills 12 hours after the first dose.

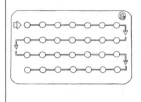

Mifepristone, also known as RU 486 or the 'French Pill', causes less nausea and vomiting than the other emergency pills.

- Take 600 mg within 3 days of having unprotected sex. Take this amount only once.

mifepristone

IUD (Intra Uterine Device): An IUD can also keep the egg from attaching to the womb wall.

- The IUD must be inserted by a specially trained health worker within 5 days after having unprotected sex. The IUD can be kept in and continue to protect you from pregnancy for up to 10 years. Do not have an IUD inserted if you are at risk of having an STD.

IUD

how to know if you are at risk for an STD

New methods of family planning

The following new methods of family planning are available or are being developed. They may only be available in some places and may be expensive. We include them here because the more women know about new methods and ask for them, the more likely it is that the methods will become available for everyone and perhaps be less costly. The more methods there are, the more likely it is that every woman who wants to prevent pregnancy will be able to find a method that suits her needs.

1. **Plastic condoms** are made from very fine polyurethane. They are thinner than latex condoms and allow for more feeling. They are less likely to be damaged by heat or oils.

2. **Once-a-week birth control pills** work by changing a woman's natural balance of estrogen, which prevents a fertilized egg from attaching to the womb wall. The once-a-week pill is less effective than regular daily birth control pills at preventing pregnancy. Little is known about its side effects.

3. **Vaginal rings** slowly release progestin into a woman's vagina. Vaginal rings come in only one size and a woman can put one in herself. They last from 3 months to a year. After taking the ring out, fertility returns within 24 hours.

If you are offered a new method of family planning, be sure to discuss any concerns you have before choosing that method (see page 200). Make sure you have all the information you need to make a good choice, and that you are not being pressured into using a method that is not right for you.

Choosing the Best Method

After reading this chapter, if you still have questions about which family planning method is best for you, the chart below may help. It is important to choose a method that meets your needs, because then you will be likely to use it regularly and it will be more effective.

Personal Needs	You Might Prefer	You Should Probably Avoid
Your partner is not willing to take an active role in family planning.	Hormonal methods, diaphragm, female condom, IUD	Male condoms, natural methods
Other bleeding, besides your normal monthly bleeding, worries you or creates difficulties for you.	Barrier methods, IUD	Hormonal methods
You do not want any more children.	Sterilization, implants, IUD, injections	Natural methods, barrier methods
No matter what you say, your partner does not want you to use family planning.	Injections, inserts, IUDs	Barrier methods, pills, natural methods
You feel embarrassed to touch your vagina.	Hormonal methods, male condoms	Diaphragm, female condoms
You do not feel comfortable asking your partner to avoid or to interrupt sex.	IUD, hormonal methods	Barrier methods, natural methods
Your are concerned that your partner has had sex with others and may infect you with STDs	Male or female condom, or other methods combined with condoms	IUD, hormonal methods
You have more than one sex partner or have had STDs.	Male or female condom	IUD
You think you will want to have a child within a year.	Male or female condom, diaphragm, natural methods, combined or progestin-only pills	IUD, injections, implants
You are breastfeeding.	IUD, male or female condoms, diaphragm with spermicide, mini pill, progestin-only injections	Combined birth control pills, injections with estrogen
You have not had a child.	Hormonal methods, barrier methods	IUD
You do not want to have to remember to do anything.	IUD, implants, injections	Birth control pills, natural methods

After you choose a new method

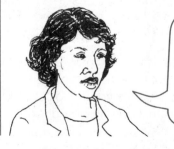

It is very important to understand the instructions for using your method and to follow those instructions. If you have questions, read the instructions again or ask a health worker to explain them.

Sometimes a woman would like to space her children or limit the number she has, but cannot use family planning. This can happen because:

- she cannot get the information about different methods.
- some family planning methods are not easily available or cost too much for the family to afford.
- there are no women's health or family planning services nearby, or the local health worker is not trained to provide family planning services.
- religious beliefs forbid the use of family planning.
- a woman's husband does not agree to use family planning.

Working for Change

Here are some things that groups of people can do to make family planning services more available to all women in the community, and to encourage the use of family planning:

- **Provide education.** Make information about family planning available to everyone—boys and girls as well as women and men. Education programs can show the benefits of family planning and help couples choose the best methods for them. Perhaps you can lead discussions with women or couples about their concerns and experiences related to family planning. Include information about preventing STDs and HIV/AIDS when you talk about family planning.
- **Make family planning methods accessible at a low cost.** Have a local health worker trained to provide family planning services start a women's health center or include family planning services at your local clinic.
- **Train male outreach workers** to educate men about the importance and benefits of family planning. Help men understand their role in reproduction so they can see that they should share the responsibility for family planning. Try to change attitudes about what is 'manly' so that men will support and participate in family planning with their partners.
- **Address local religious concerns** about family planning. If a family planning method can be explained in a way that respects religious beliefs, it will help create more acceptance of it.

As you talk about family planning in your community, it helps to remember and remind others that family planning is important to improve not just women's health and well being, but the health and quality of life of **everyone** in your community.

Chapter 14

In this chapter:

Infertility (When You Are Not Able to Have a Baby)

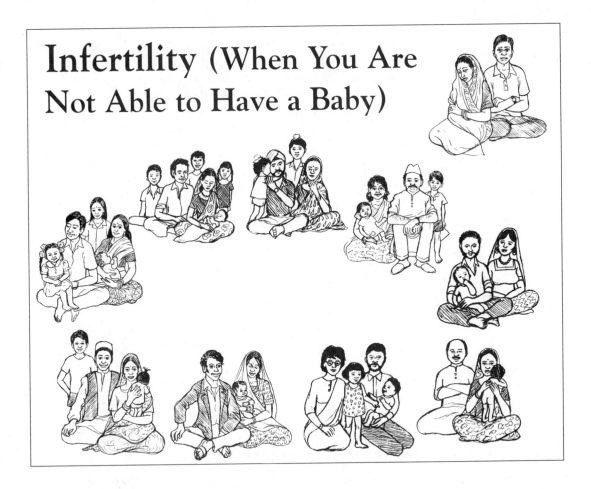

Most men and women assume they will be able to have children. The truth is that **about 1 out of every 10 couples has trouble getting pregnant.** Some men and women do not want to have children. But for couples who look forward to having children, infertility can bring sorrow, anger, and disappointment.

Often it is the woman who is blamed if a couple does not have children. But about half the time, it is the man who is infertile. Sometimes a man will not believe it is his problem, or that it may be a shared problem. He may refuse to go for an *examination*, or he may react with anger. Most often this is because infertility causes shame in communities where a man is expected to produce children as a sign of his manhood.

Infertility has many causes. Some of them can be treated and some cannot. This chapter will help you understand infertility and what you can do about it.

➤ *When a couple cannot have a baby, it may be because the man, the woman, or both have a fertility problem. It is a problem that few people talk about.*

What Is Infertility?

We say a couple is infertile if they cannot get pregnant after having sex together a few times a month for a year, without using a family planning method. A couple may also have a fertility problem if they have had 3 or more miscarriages (lost pregnancies) in a row.

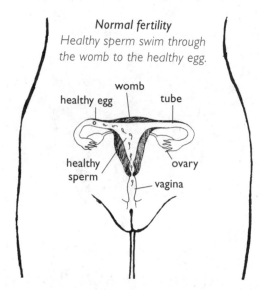

Normal fertility
Healthy sperm swim through the womb to the healthy egg.

womb

healthy egg

tube

healthy sperm

ovary

vagina

A man or woman who has already had a child can also become infertile. A problem can develop in the years after the last child was born.

Sometimes the problem is not the man's or the woman's alone but a combination of the two. And sometimes both partners seem to be healthy and no doctor or test can find out what is causing the problem.

Habits such as drinking too much alcohol, smoking or chewing tobacco, and using drugs can all affect a man's or a woman's fertility.

What Causes Infertility?

INFERTILITY IN A MAN

The main causes of infertility in a man are:

1. **He does not produce enough sperm**. Or his *sperm* may not be able to swim to the woman's tubes or to *fertilize* the eggs.

2. **He had *mumps* after *puberty*** that harmed his *testicles*. When this happens, the man can still climax *(ejaculate)*, but the liquid that comes out has no sperm in it.

3. **His sperm cannot leave his penis** because he has scars in his tubes from a past or present *sexually transmitted disease (STD)*.

4. **He has a swelling** of the veins in his *scrotum* (varicocele).

5. **He may have problems during sex because:**
   • his *penis* does not get hard.
   • his penis gets hard but does not stay hard during sex.
   • he has a *climax* too quickly, before his penis is deep in the woman's *vagina*.

6. **Illnesses** such as *diabetes*, *tuberculosis*, and *malaria* can all hurt a man's fertility.

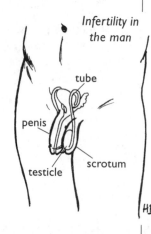

Infertility in the man

tube

penis

testicle

scrotum

HB

INFERTILITY IN A WOMAN

The main causes of infertility in a woman are:

1. **She has scarring in her tubes or inside her womb.** Scarring in the *tube* can prevent the egg from moving through the tube, or the sperm from swimming to the egg. Scarring in the *womb* can prevent the fertilized egg from attaching to the wall of the womb. Sometimes a woman gets scarring but does not know it because she does not feel ill. But years later she learns she is infertile.

   Scarring can be caused by:

   • an infection from an untreated STD that goes up into the womb or tubes (pelvic inflammatory disease or PID).

   • unsafe *abortion* or problems in childbirth that caused damage or *infection* in the womb.

   • unclean conditions when an IUD is put in that caused an infection.

   • problems from an operation of the vagina, womb, tubes, or *ovaries*.

2. **She does not produce an egg** (no ovulation). This can be because the body does not make enough of the needed *hormones* at the right time. If her monthly bleedings are less than 25 days apart, or more than 35 days apart, she may have a problem with ovulation.

   Sometimes a woman does not produce eggs if she loses weight very quickly, or if she is too fat.

3. **She has growths in her womb** (fibroids). Fibroids can prevent *conception* or make it difficult to carry the pregnancy.

4. **Illnesses** such as diabetes, tuberculosis, and malaria can also hurt a woman's fertility.

➤ *Infertility caused by infection can be prevented. For more information, see page 272 and 279.*

Infertility in the woman

1. blocked tube

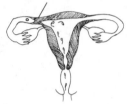

2. ovary does not produce an egg

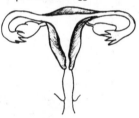

3. fibroids

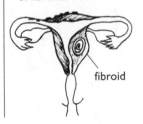

fibroid

Family Planning Is Safe

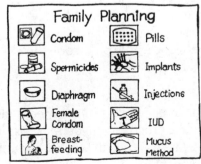

Family Planning
- Condom
- Pills
- Spermicides
- Implants
- Diaphragm
- Injections
- Female Condom
- IUD
- Breastfeeding
- Mucus Method

Family planning methods are often blamed for infertility. But family planning methods (other than sterilization) do not cause infertility except in some cases when an IUD has not been put in correctly and causes an infection in the womb or tubes. For more information, see the chapter on "Family Planning," page 197.

Dangers at Work or Home That Can Hurt Fertility

These dangers can hurt fertility in many ways—from the making of sperm and eggs to the birth of a healthy baby:

- **Contaminated air, food, or water caused** by dangerous *pesticides* or *toxic chemicals* used in factories and farms.

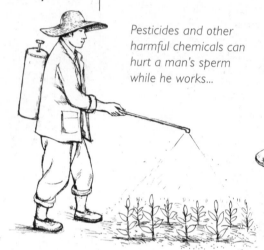

Pesticides and other harmful chemicals can hurt a man's sperm while he works...

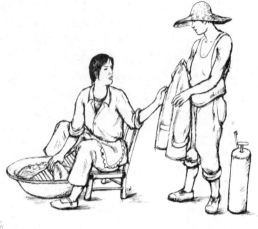

...and if the woman washes his clothes, the harmful chemicals are passed to her.

- **Smoking or chewing tobacco, or drinking alcohol or strong coffee.** Women who smoke or chew tobacco, or who drink a lot of alcohol or strong coffee take longer to become pregnant and have more miscarriages. Men who smoke or drink a lot have fewer sperm, and these are often damaged or weak.

- **High temperatures.** A man's sperm need to stay cool. That is why the testicles hang in the scrotum outside a man's body. When the testicles get too warm they can stop making healthy sperm. For example, this can happen if a man wears tight clothes that press his testicles up inside his body, or if he takes a hot bath, or works near hot things such as boilers, furnaces, or the hot engine of a long-distance truck—especially if he drives for many hours without a break. Once the testicles become cool, they start making healthy sperm again.

Working in hot places, like sitting near the hot engine of a truck for many hours, can kill sperm and cause a man to be infertile.

- **Medicines.** Some medicines can hurt fertility. The best choice is for you and your partner not to use any medicines while you are trying to become pregnant. If you must use medicines because of illness, talk to a health worker and tell her you are trying to get pregnant.

If you or your partner think you have a fertility problem:

1. **Try to have sex during your fertile time.** Although a man makes millions of sperm every day, a healthy woman releases only one egg a month. This is called her fertile time—the only time during the month when she can get pregnant. For most women their fertile time starts about 10 days after the first day of the *monthly bleeding* and lasts about 6 days.

   The body has several signs that tell you when you are in a fertile time. The easiest signs to check are the changes in the *mucus* in your vagina.

What to Do for Infertility

Checking your mucus

During your fertile time, your *cervix* makes mucus that helps sperm get into the womb. This mucus looks clear and wet, like raw egg white, and can be stretched between your fingers. Later in your monthly cycle, you may see sticky or dry mucus. This kind of mucus stops the man's sperm from getting into the womb.

B = monthly bleeding
W = wet days (fertile)
D = dry days (not fertile)

B	B	B	B	B	D
D	D	D	D	W	W	W
W	W	W	D	D	D	D
D	D	D	D	D	D	D
B	B	B	B	B	

See page 220 to learn how to check your mucus. Write down the changes every day on a chart. During the week that you see wet, shiny, clear mucus, try to have sex every day.

When you have sex, the best positions for getting the sperm close to the opening of your womb are:

- to lie on your back with the man on top.
- to lie on your side.

   Then, after having sex, lie flat on your back for about 20 minutes. This will help the sperm swim into your womb and find the egg.

Avoiding these things can also help:

- Do not use oils or creams during sex. They can kill the sperm or stop it from reaching the egg.
- Do not *douche* or wash inside your vagina. Douching before or after sex can change the wetness inside your vagina, making it harder for the sperm to live.
- Your partner should not have a hot bath before having sex. Heat on the testicles kills sperm.

➤ *Try not to worry if you do not get pregnant right away. Many couples get pregnant within a year if they continue to have sex during the woman's fertile days.*

261

STDs

2. Treat any health problems.
Both you and your partner
should have medical exams
and be checked for STDs. If
either of you has an STD,
both of you must be treated.
Be sure to finish all the
medicines you are given.

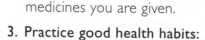

3. Practice good health habits:

- Eat good, healthy food. If you do not have
regular monthly bleeding and you are very
thin or very fat, try to gain or lose weight.
- Avoid smoking or chewing tobacco, using drugs,
or drinking alcohol.
- Avoid *caffeine* in drinks like coffee, black tea, and
cola drinks.
- Get plenty of rest and regular exercise.

staying healthy, 149
eating for good
health, 165

**4. Try to see a health worker if you are not pregnant after
one year.** There are some simple tests that do not cost
much that may be able to tell you what the problem is. For
example, the health worker may look at your partner's
sperm under a *microscope* to see if they are healthy. She
may give you a *pelvic exam* to check your vagina, womb, and
tubes for infection or growths. Or she may teach you to tell
if your ovaries are releasing an egg by taking your
temperature every morning.

It is important to remember that these tests only tell you
what the problem is—they will not solve it. Even the most
expensive medicines and operations often cannot cure
infertility.

Losing a Pregnancy (Miscarriage)

For many couples, the problem is not getting pregnant but
staying pregnant. Losing 1 or even 2 pregnancies is common.
It can be the body's way of ending a pregnancy that is too weak
to survive.

But if you have lost 3 or more pregnancies, there may be
another problem, such as:

- unhealthy eggs or sperm.
- a problem with the shape of the womb.
- growths (fibroids) in the womb.
- the wrong balance of *hormones* in your body.
- infection in the womb or vagina.
- an illness, such as malaria.

272

infection in the womb

The warning signs of miscarriage are:

- small amounts of brown, red, or pink blood from your vagina.
- pains or *cramping*, no matter how small.

What to do when signs start:

Once a miscarriage starts there is usually not much that can be done to stop it. If you are bleeding slightly, without pain:

- lie down and rest for 2 or 3 days.
- do not have sex.

If bleeding continues or becomes heavy, or if you are more than 4 months pregnant, go to a hospital and tell them you are pregnant.

IMPORTANT *If you are in the first 3 months of pregnancy and you have severe pain, feel faint, and have some bleeding, you could have a pregnancy in the tube.* Go to a hospital immediately. *Be sure to tell them you are pregnant.*

Before you try to get pregnant again:

- Follow the guidelines on page 234 about treating health problems and practicing good health habits. It is especially important to avoid caffeine, to stop smoking or chewing tobacco, and to stop drinking alcohol or using drugs. These things can all help cause miscarriage.

- If your miscarriages always happen after you have been pregnant for 3 months, it may be that the opening to your womb is weak. This can sometimes be treated by having a doctor put a small tie around the *cervix* to keep it closed. Make sure that the doctor has experience giving this treatment. When it is time to give birth, the tie has to be removed.

If you do become pregnant:

- try not to lift heavy things.
- try not to have sex for the first 6 to 8 weeks of your pregnancy.
- rest when you can.

Losing a pregnancy is common. If it happens to you, it does not mean you cannot have a healthy pregnancy the next time.

➤ *Miscarriage often happens no matter how careful you are. Do not blame yourself.*

67

pregnancy

Living with Infertility

helping relationships,
support groups

Infertility can make a woman or man feel sad, nervous, alone, frustrated, or angry.

When this happens, it is important to know you are not alone. Try to talk with people who love and care about you. You may also be able to find other couples with the same problem and learn to help each other.

The stories below describe some ways that people have coped with infertility:

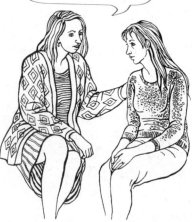

I understand how you feel. I also have been unable to have a child.

Adopting a child: Lina's story

Lina was 25 years old and had been married 3 times. She was very unhappy because each of her husbands divorced her when she did not become pregnant. In the village, people spoke about her and blamed her, saying that she must have used some magic to avoid pregnancy before she was married, and that it must have been so strong it had made her infertile.

Her sisters all had children, and sometimes Lina cared for them. Her older sister had *tuberculosis (TB)* and she was very ill when she gave birth to twins. Lina asked if she might adopt one of the twins and her sister agreed. Lina went to the health center and asked the health worker to help her find a way to feed the baby. The health worker taught Lina how to feed the baby from a cup and spoon and arranged to have the baby breastfed during the day by a healthy woman in the village with another baby. At night Lina fed her baby from a cup, with breast milk that another sister gave her each evening.

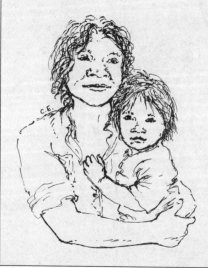

Lina's friends and neighbors were not sure that her baby would be healthy. But when they saw the baby grow strong, they were pleased and proud of Lina. In fact, Lina came to be seen as an expert in raising adopted babies. When a village mother died in childbirth, her baby was given to Lina to care for.

The twins have grown up now, and people often say that the one Lina adopted is taller and stronger than the other. They credit this to Lina's loving care.

— *Bundoora, Australia*

Building a life without children: Sara and Tito's story

Sara and Tito tried for many years to have children, but they were not able to. At first they were sad, because in their community, couples were expected to have as many children together as they could. But then they decided to stop thinking that their lives were not complete without children and to plan a future for themselves.

They decided to start a business and to travel from town to town, market to market, selling pots and pans and other goods. With children, it would have been very difficult for them to travel in this way.

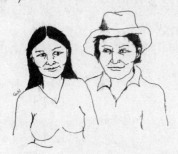

Now that Sara and Tito are older, people say they look alike in their faces and attitudes. They care for each other, share many laughs and many friends. They are not grandparents like their neighbors, but they have many interesting stories to tell. They are respected by everyone in the community.

— *Lima, Peru*

To help others with infertility problems:

- be kind and sympathetic. It is a difficult time, and they need support and understanding. Do not blame couples who cannot get pregnant.
- teach couples to value and respect each other as companions.
- help a couple who cannot have children to look for other ways to be with children or to make peace with their lives.

Health workers can also:

- provide information on ways to adopt children.
- teach young people about STDs and how to prevent them.
- make sure your local health center is prepared to diagnose and treat STDs and to take women's complaints about *pelvic* pain seriously. Too often women are sent home without treatment after being told there is nothing wrong with them.
- teach women the signs of pelvic infection and the importance of getting immediate and complete treatment.
- teach men and women the signs of STDs, the importance of getting treated right away, and the importance of treating all partners.

Working for Change

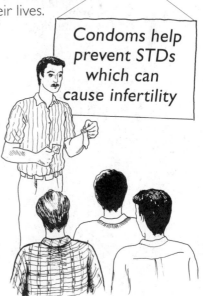

Condoms help prevent STDs which can cause infertility

There are many causes of infertility, but STDs are the easiest to prevent.

Chapter 15

In this chapter:

Abortion and Complications from Abortion

If family planning methods fail, safe and legal abortion is a woman's safety net.

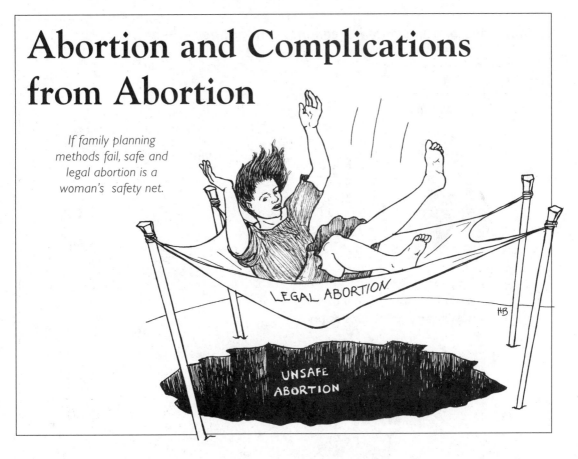

When a woman does something to end a pregnancy, this is called an 'abortion'. We use the word abortion in this book only to describe an action that is planned. The unplanned, natural loss of a pregnancy we call a 'miscarriage'.

➤ Lack of family planning services and lack of information about sex lead to unwanted pregnancy and abortion.

Deciding to have an abortion is always hard. A woman may seek abortion because:

- she already has all the children she can care for.
- a pregnancy is a danger to her health or her life.
- she has no partner to help support the child.
- she wants to finish school.
- she does not want to have children.
- she got pregnant after being forced to have sex.
- someone is forcing her to have an abortion.
- the child will be born with serious problems (*birth defects*).

Why Do Some Women Have Abortions?

Unplanned and unwanted pregnancy can happen when. . .

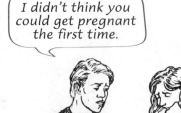

...the woman and her partner do not know how pregnancy happens.

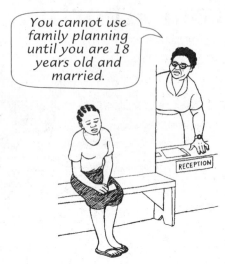

. . . health workers think some women are too young to get family planning.

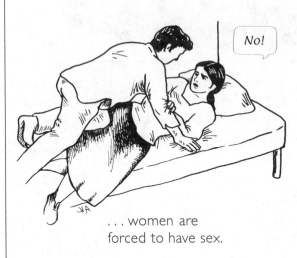

...women are forced to have sex.

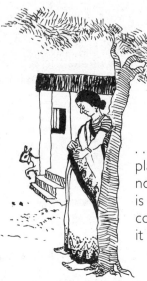

. . . family planning is not available, is not used correctly, or it fails.

Emergency Family Planning Methods

A woman who has had unprotected sex within the last 3 days may be able to prevent pregnancy if she acts quickly (see page 224).

Safe and Unsafe Abortion

A safe abortion is less likely to cause harm than having a baby.

Abortion is very safe when it is done:

- by a trained and experienced health worker.
- with the proper instruments.
- under clean conditions. Anything that goes into the *vagina* and *womb* must be sterile (without any germs).
- up to 3 months (12 weeks) after the last *monthly bleeding*.

Abortion is unsafe when it is done:

- by someone who has not been trained to do it.
- with the wrong instruments or medicines.
- under unclean conditions.
- after 3 months (12 weeks) of pregnancy, unless it is done in a health center or hospital that has special equipment.

DEATH FROM UNSAFE ABORTION

Around the world, 55 million abortions are done every year. Women survive most of them, even if they are not legal. But unsafe abortions can cause death, or complications like *infection*, lasting pain, and *infertility*.

Women have always tried to find ways to end pregnancy when they are desperate. **Stay away from the following methods. They are very dangerous.**

- **Do not** put sharp objects like sticks, wire, or plastic tubing into the vagina and womb. These can tear the womb and cause dangerous bleeding and infection.
- **Do not** put herbs or plants in the vagina or womb. These can burn or irritate badly, causing damage, infection, and bleeding.
- **Do not** put substances such as bleach, lye, ashes, soap, or kerosene in the vagina or womb. Also, do not drink them.
- **Do not** take medicines or traditional remedies in large amounts to cause abortion (either by mouth or in the vagina). For example, taking too much of the medicines for *malaria* (chloroquine) or to stop bleeding after childbirth (ergometrine, oxytocin) can kill you before they cause abortion.
- **Do not** hit your abdomen or throw yourself down stairs. This can cause injury and bleeding inside your body, but may not cause abortion.

IMPORTANT *Never put anything inside the womb yourself or allow an untrained person to do so. This can kill you.*

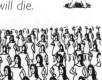

*Out of 100,000 women getting a **safe abortion**, only 1 will die.*

*But out of 100,000 women having **unsafe abortions**, between 100 and 1000 will die.*

➤ *Avoid unsafe abortion. Try to prevent unwanted pregnancy before it happens.*

ACCESS TO SAFE ABORTION

When a woman is faced with an unwanted pregnancy, she should be able to get a safe and legal abortion. But laws about abortion differ from one country to another.

Legal abortion. If abortion is legal a woman can walk into a health center or hospital, pay a fee, and have a safe abortion. In countries where this happens, almost no women get sick or die from complications of abortion.

Legal abortion in some cases. In some countries an abortion is only legal for certain reasons, such as:

• if a woman becomes pregnant from *rape* or incest (sex with a close family member).

• if a doctor says pregnancy would be a danger to a woman's health.

But abortion is often difficult to get, even for those reasons. Doctors and health workers may not be sure what the law really says. They may be unwilling to do abortions openly, or they may charge a lot of money. Women may not know if abortion is legal or available in their country.

Illegal abortion. If abortion is not legal, both the women who get abortions and those who perform them can be arrested. **In most places this does not happen.** But where abortion is against the law, more women die from unsafe abortion and unsafe pregnancies. Money that could be spent on women's health services is spent instead on treating *complications* of unsafe abortion.

Never assume abortion is illegal. Try to find out about the laws in your own country. It may be easier to work around the laws than to try and change them. Even if abortion is illegal, there may be people providing safe abortions. Finding a safe abortion may mean the difference between staying alive and dying.

➤ *Even if abortion is illegal, a woman should be able to get medical help for complications after an abortion. It is often difficult to tell the difference between abortion and miscarriage, unless something from the abortion has been left in the womb.*

If you don't have any money, we can't help you.

But please, I MUST have an abortion!

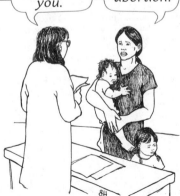

Other barriers to finding a safe abortion

Legal or not, it can be hard to get a safe abortion because it is too costly, too far away, or because there are confusing rules, or papers to fill out.

These reasons often make it especially difficult for women who are poor, or who are not familiar with the medical system, to get safe abortions. Unfortunately, in many places, the only women who can easily get a safe abortion are women who can afford to pay a private doctor.

Deciding about an Abortion

Your decision to have an abortion will often depend on whether safe abortion is available where you live. It also depends on how an abortion or a baby would affect your life.

It may help to think about these questions:

- Will you be able to care for a baby? Do you have enough money to raise a child?
- Is pregnancy a danger to your health?
- Do you have a partner or husband who will help support a child? Can you talk with him about this decision?
- Is your religion or family against abortion? If yes, how will you feel if you have one?
- How will the abortion be done? (See page 248.)
- For how long have you been pregnant?
- Could you have a sexually transmitted disease (STD)? You may be at more risk of having an STD if you are young, single, and have a new partner, or if you have signs of an STD. If you feel that you are at risk, see page 263 in the STD chapter. You may need treatment before the abortion.
- What complications (problems) can be caused by the abortion? (See pages 251 to 258.)
- Where can you go for emergency care if you have complications? How will you get there?

The information on the next 4 pages may help you decide whether safe methods of abortion are available in your community.

➤ *If safe abortion is not available, you might consider giving the baby up for adoption, if this is acceptable to you and your community.*

261 | STDs

I will be your friend no matter what you decide to do.

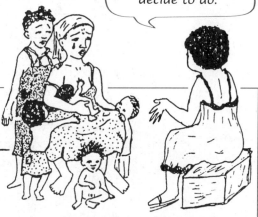

If you are helping someone decide about an abortion:

She needs respectful advice and friendly support. Do not tell anyone else about her decision unless she wants others to know.

Safe Methods of Abortion

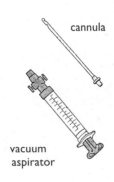

cannula

vacuum aspirator

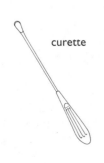

curette

➤ *As time goes on, medicines for abortion may be used in more places and be more available to women who need them.*

A pregnancy can be removed from the womb by a trained health worker in the following ways:

Abortion by suction (vacuum aspiration, MVA)

The pregnancy is removed by suction using a special tube (cannula) that is put into the womb through the vagina and *cervix*. This can be done without putting the woman to sleep, though sometimes medicine is injected into the *cervix* to help with the pain. When vacuum aspiration is done by hand (manual vacuum aspiration or MVA), the pregnancy is removed using a special *syringe*. Otherwise, a small electric machine is used.

Vacuum aspiration is simple and safe, and takes only about 5 to 10 minutes. It is usually done in a clinic or health post, or doctor's office. This kind of abortion is easiest to do during the third month of pregnancy, but is sometimes done a bit later. Vacuum aspiration causes fewer complications than dilation and curettage (described below).

In some places MVA is used to bring on late monthly bleeding. The woman may not even know if she is pregnant— just that her monthly bleeding has not come. This is called menstrual regulation.

Abortion by scraping (dilation and curettage, or D and C)

The pregnancy is scraped out with a curette, a small spoon-shaped instrument that is made especially to go into the womb. A curette is larger than a cannula and because it is sharp, the cervix must first be stretched open. This stretching can cause some pain.

The D and C takes more time to do (about 15 to 20 minutes), is more painful, and costs more than vacuum aspiration. It is usually done in an operating room, and the woman is often given medicine to make her sleep.

Abortion by medicine (medical abortion)

Certain medicines are now being used by doctors and health workers to cause abortion. These medicines work by causing the womb to contract and squeeze out the pregnancy. Some medicines are put into the vagina (NOT in the womb), some are swallowed, and some are injected. If the right medicine to cause abortion is used, it may be safer than putting something inside the womb, which may cause severe injury or infection.

If you use medicines for abortion

- Never use a medicine you are not sure of.
- Medicines to cause abortion should only be used if there is a health clinic or hospital close by, so you can get there soon after bleeding starts. The clinic or hospital should have trained health workers who can empty a womb in case the abortion medicines do not work.
- Go to the clinic or hospital when bleeding starts so your womb can be checked to see if it has emptied completely. If it has not, you must have the rest of the pregnancy removed by suction or scraping. If you do not, you could suffer dangerous complications. (If you go on to give birth, the baby may be born with severe birth defects.)

Some medicines used for abortion

1. **Mifepristone** (RU-486, the 'French Pill') is available in some countries to cause abortion in women who are up to 9 weeks pregnant. It is given only in special programs in clinics and hospitals where the woman can be watched for complications and treated if needed. Two days later a second medicine, such as misoprostol, is given. This usually causes complete abortion.

2. **Misoprostol** is a medicine used to treat stomach *ulcers*, and is used with mifepristone or other medicines to cause abortion. It can also be used by itself to start abortion, but usually the abortion will not finish, so a woman must get medical care after bleeding starts. Misoprostol can be used during the first 3 months (12 weeks) of pregnancy, and works better close to 12 weeks. The tablets are put into the vagina, not swallowed.

3. **Methotrexate** is an anti-*cancer* medicine which has been used together with misoprostol to cause abortion. It has dangerous side effects for the woman, and if it fails to cause abortion, it can cause severe birth defects in the baby. Not enough is known yet about how to use methotrexate safely, especially in places without modern hospital equipment.

IMPORTANT

Follow the instructions for misoprostol very carefully. If you do not, the womb can split open (rupture) and cause death.

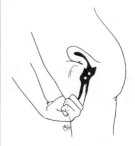

➤ *For more information about these medicines, see page 508.*

Incomplete abortion

An incomplete abortion is when part of the pregnancy remains in the womb after an abortion. The signs are heavy bleeding for more than one day after the abortion, *cramping* pains, and passing *tissue* and clots or lumps of blood from the vagina. If this happens, go to a hospital right away to have the pregnancy completely removed. If not, you could have serious complications and even die. See page 249 for danger signs after abortion.

How to tell if an abortion will be safe

It is not always easy to tell if an abortion will be safe. Try to go to the place where the abortion will be done, or ask someone who has been there these questions:

- **Have you heard of women getting sick or dying from having an abortion here?** If so, go somewhere else.

- **Who will do the abortion and how were they trained?** Doctors, nurses, health workers, and traditional birth attendants can all do abortions. However, abortions done by someone who is not trained in safe abortion methods and how to prevent infection can be very dangerous.

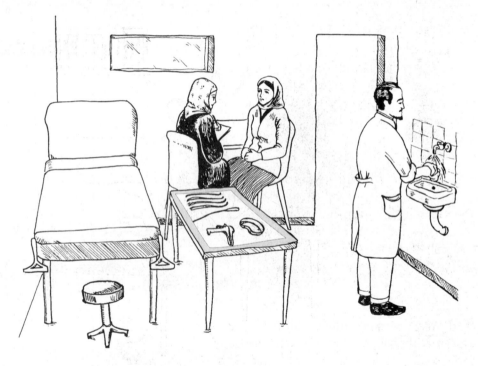

This room looks safe.

- **Is the room where the abortion will be done clean and neat?** If it is dirty and messy, probably the abortion will be also.

- **Is there a place for washing hands?** A health worker who has no place to wash his or her hands cannot do a clean, safe abortion.

- **Do the instruments look like the ones in this chapter on page 244, or do they look like something found or made at home?** Instruments made at home can cause injury and infection.

- **How are the instruments cleaned and made free of germs?** Instruments should be soaked in strong disinfectant or boiled in water to kill germs that cause infection.

- **Does the cost seem fair?** If the cost is very high, sometimes it means the health worker cares only about money, not your health.
- **Are other health-care services also provided along with abortions?** A good health center will also try to provide other services that women need, like family planning, treatment for STDs, and *AIDS* prevention.
- **Where will you be taken if something goes wrong during or after the abortion?** There should always be a plan to get you to a hospital in case of emergency.

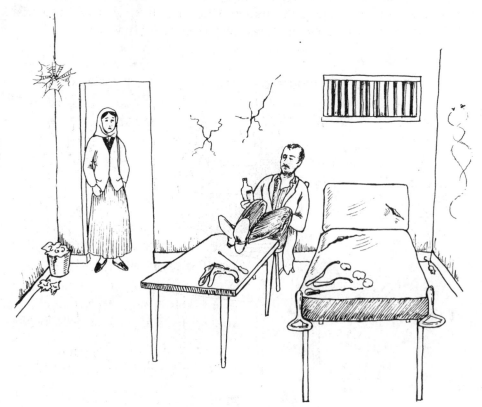

This room does not look safe.

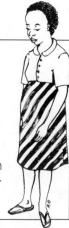

IMPORTANT

An abortion is more dangerous if:

- your last monthly bleeding was more than 3 months ago.
- your pregnancy is starting to show.

The longer you have been pregnant, the greater the chance of complications after abortion. For your safety, an abortion after more than 3 months of pregnancy must be done with special equipment in a clinic or hospital.

What to Expect during a Safe Abortion

➤ *Drink plenty of liquids the day before you have an abortion. This will help you recover more quickly.*

Safe abortions, especially abortions by suction (MVA), are done in both health centers and hospitals. An abortion by scraping (D and C) is usually done in a hospital. An abortion by medicine should be done at a health center or hospital that also has equipment to do MVAs and D and Cs, and health workers trained to do them. For more information about how these abortions are done, see page 244.

When you go to a health center or hospital for an abortion, you should be welcomed and treated with respect. A counselor should talk with you about your decision and explain how the abortion will be done and what the risks are.

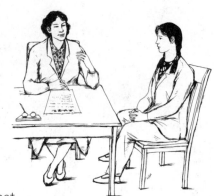

The information below tells what to expect from a safe abortion. An abortion that is very different from this could be dangerous.

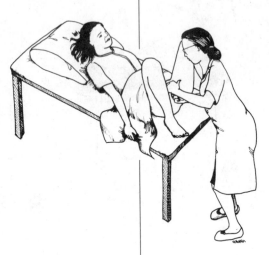

- You should be asked about the time of your last monthly bleeding and whether you might have an STD (see page 263).

- A health worker should do a medical exam. This includes feeling carefully in your vagina and on your belly for the size of your womb.

- During both abortion by suction and by scraping you will feel strong pains in the lower belly. But soon after the abortion is over, the pains will become less strong.

- After the abortion, your genitals should be cleaned, and then you should be taken to rest. A health worker should be there to check you for about an hour.

- Someone should tell you what to do after the abortion, the danger signs to watch for, and who to contact if you have a complication.

In addition, someone should discuss family planning methods with you. You can start using a method the day of the abortion. You should be given an appointment to come back for a check-up in 1 or 2 weeks.

After an abortion, signs of pregnancy, like *nausea* and sore breasts, should disappear within a day. If they do not, you could still be pregnant, either in your womb or in one of your tubes (ectopic pregnancy). **This is an emergency. See a health worker right away.**

You may feel a little tired and have some cramps or pains for a day after the abortion. You will have some bleeding from the vagina for as long as 2 weeks. But after the first day it should be no more than a light monthly bleeding. Your next normal monthly bleeding should start about 4 to 6 weeks after an abortion. It might take longer if you were more than 5 to 6 months pregnant.

If you had no one to talk to before the abortion, it may help to talk to someone now. Talking about your feelings with someone you trust can make you feel better.

How to care for yourself after an abortion:

- To prevent infection, take 100 mg of doxycycline twice a day for 5 days starting the day of the abortion. (**But if you are breastfeeding**, take 500 mg of amoxicillin 3 times a day for 5 days instead.)

- Do not have sex or put anything into your vagina for at least 2 days after bleeding stops.

- If you have cramps or pains, rest and use a hot water bottle on your *abdomen*. Or take paracetamol or ibuprofen (see page 482).

- To lessen pain and bleeding, rub or *massage* your lower abdomen often. This helps the womb to squeeze down to normal size and lessen bleeding.

- Drink plenty of liquids to help you recover faster.

- You can go back to your usual activities as soon as you feel well, usually within a day.

What to Expect after an Abortion

➤ *Normal monthly bleeding should start about 4 to 6 weeks after an abortion. But you can become pregnant again after 11 days.*

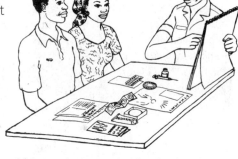

After an abortion, start family planning right away. You can get pregnant again before your next monthly bleeding.

Danger signs

If you have any of these signs, get medical help fast:

- Heavy bleeding from the vagina (see page 251)
- High fever (see 'Infection', page 255)
- Severe pain in the abdomen (see 'Internal Injury' , page 258, and 'Infection', page 255)
- Fainting and confusion (see 'Shock', page 254)
- Bad-smelling *discharge* from the vagina (see 'Infection', page 255)

Family Planning after an Abortion

After an abortion you can get pregnant again right away—in as soon as 2 weeks. Many methods of family planning take time to start working, so talk with someone about family planning and start using one of these methods as soon as possible:

- **The Pill:** You can start taking pills on the same day as the abortion. Do not wait more than one week.

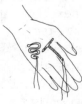

- **Intra-Uterine Device (IUD):** If there is no risk of infection, a trained health worker can put in an IUD right after the abortion.

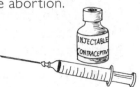

- **Injections:** The first injection should be given on the day of the abortion, or up to one week after.

- **Implants:** Implants can be put in just before or just after the abortion, or up to one week later.

- **Female sterilization:** If your pregnancy was less than 3 months, you can be sterilized during the abortion or right after it. It is very important that you make this decision carefully. **Sterilization is permanent.**

- **Male sterilization:** Sterilization for a man can be done any time and is permanent. This decision must be made carefully.

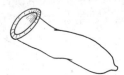

- **Condoms:** You and your partner can use condoms as soon as you have sex again. Condoms also protect against STDs, including HIV.

- **Spermicide:** You can use spermicide as soon as you have sex again. Spermicides made with nonoxynol-9 also give some protection against gonorrhea and chlamydia, 2 common STDs.

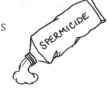

- **Diaphragm:** If there was no infection or injury, you can be fitted with a diaphragm before or after the abortion. Diaphragms with spermicide give some protection against gonorrhea and chlamydia.

- **Natural methods (mucus and rhythm):** These methods do not work until your normal monthly bleeding returns.

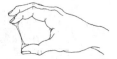

➤ *A woman who has just had an abortion most likely did not want to become pregnant. This is a good time to offer her information about family planning methods and how to get them.*

➤ *For more information on all these methods, see the chapter on "Family Planning."*

A woman with any of the danger signs after abortion (see page 249) **needs medical help fast!** She should go **immediately** to a health center or hospital where she can get the care she needs. Most of the time the womb must be emptied completely using vacuum aspiration or a D and C. In the meantime, the information on the next 8 pages may help if transport is not available immediately or if medical care is very far away.

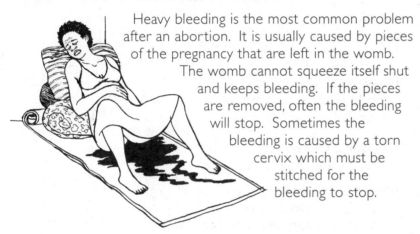

HEAVY BLEEDING FROM THE VAGINA

Heavy bleeding is the most common problem after an abortion. It is usually caused by pieces of the pregnancy that are left in the womb. The womb cannot squeeze itself shut and keeps bleeding. If the pieces are removed, often the bleeding will stop. Sometimes the bleeding is caused by a torn cervix which must be stitched for the bleeding to stop.

A woman is bleeding too much if she soaks a pad, towel, or clothing with bright red blood in less than 30 minutes. A slow, steady trickle of bright red blood is also dangerous. When this happens, a woman may quickly lose a dangerous amount of blood. If it is not possible to get medical help immediately, try to stop the bleeding.

To stop the bleeding

A woman who is bleeding too much may be able to help her womb squeeze shut with massage. She can do this herself or have someone else do it. Rub or massage the lower belly very hard while lying down or squatting.

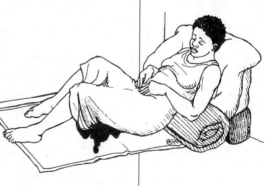

If there are pieces of tissue stuck in the womb or cervix, she may be able to push them out herself by squatting and bearing down as if passing stool or giving birth.

Even if these treatments seem to work, **get medical help as soon as possible**. The woman will need *antibiotics* and may still need to have her womb emptied completely.

> ➤ *Early treatment of abortion complications prevents illness, infertility, and death. Seek help quickly if you have problems after an abortion.* **DO NOT WAIT!**

EMERGENCY HELP FOR TOO MUCH BLEEDING

Health workers and others trained in giving a woman a *pelvic* exam may be able to follow these steps to try and stop the bleeding until the womb can be emptied.

IMPORTANT *Because the entrance to the woman's womb is open, putting anything inside her vagina is very dangerous. She can get a serious infection. Only do this if the bleeding is so heavy the woman's life is in danger. See the previous page for how much bleeding is too much.*

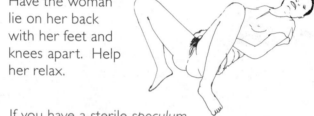

1. Wash your hands and the woman's *genitals* with soap and clean water.

2. Put a clean *latex* or plastic glove or a very clean plastic bag on one hand. **The gloved hand should not touch anything before it goes into the woman's vagina.**

3. Have the woman lie on her back with her feet and knees apart. Help her relax.

4. If you have a sterile *speculum* (you can get the right instruments from an IUD kit if you have one), put it into the vagina so you can see the opening of the womb. If you can see tissue or clots or lumps of blood there, try to get hold of them with sterile forceps or clamps and gently remove them.

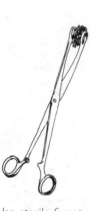

Use sterile forceps to remove any tissue you see at the opening of the womb.

5. If you do not have a speculum, reach inside the woman's vagina with your gloved hand, first with 1 finger, and then with 2 fingers.

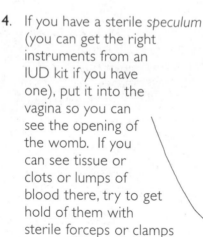

the cervix, opening of the womb

6. Feel for the cervix. It will feel more firm and smooth than the skin around it. It looks like this and is about this size.

7. Move your finger across the opening and feel for bits of the pregnancy that may be sticking out of the opening. They will feel like soft meat. Gently try to remove them. If the pieces are too slippery, take your hand out and wrap 2 fingers with sterile *gauze*, or a clean cloth that has been boiled in water, and try again to remove them.

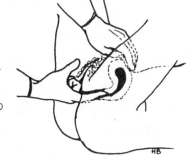

8. After you have removed the pieces, put your gloved hand into the woman's vagina with two fingers under the womb. With your other hand, rub or massage her belly to help stop the bleeding. Her womb should be between your 2 hands.

9. Give the woman an injection of ergometrine (0.2 mg) in a large muscle, such as her *buttock* or thigh. Then give her one 0.2 mg pill of ergometrine, or a 0.1 mg injection, every 4 hours for 24 hours.

how to give an injection

10. Give antibiotics for mild infection immediately (see page 255) to prevent infection. She is at high risk of infection because the womb is open to germs.

11. If she is awake, give her fluids to drink. If she is *unconscious*, see the next page.

12. Take her to a hospital right away, even if you think you have removed the tissue and the bleeding has stopped. She still needs to have her womb emptied completely. If the bleeding does not stop, continue to rub or massage her lower belly while taking her to the hospital.

TRANSPORT!

When there is no health worker to help

If you are bleeding too much after an abortion, and you have tried the steps on page 251, you can also try to remove tissue stuck in your cervix by yourself.

First wash your hands and genitals well with soap and clean water. Then squat and bear down, as in childbirth or passing stool, and follow the instructions above in steps 6 and 7. After you have removed any pieces, massage your lower belly (see page 251). You should still get medical help, even if the bleeding becomes less.

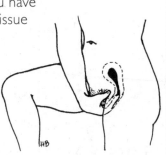

Shock

Shock is a life-threatening condition that can result from heavy bleeding. Bleeding inside the body can also cause shock.

Signs:

- very fast heart rate, more than 110 beats a minute
- pale, cold, damp skin
- pale inner eyelids, mouth, and palms
- fast breathing, more than 30 breaths a minute
- confusion or unconsciousness (fainting)

Treatment if she is conscious:

- Lay the woman down with her feet higher than her head.
- Cover her with a blanket or clothes.
- If she can drink, give her sips of water or rehydration drink.
- Help her to stay calm.
- If you know how, start a fast *intravenous drip (IV)* with a wide needle, or start rectal fluids.

Treatment if she is unconscious:

- Lay her on her side with her head low, tilted back and to one side, and her feet high.

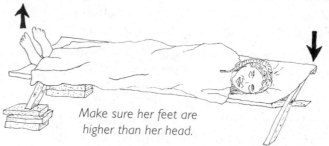

Make sure her feet are higher than her head.

- If she seems to be choking, pull her tongue forward with your finger.
- **If she has *vomited*, clean out her mouth immediately.** Be sure her head is low, tilted back and to one side, so she does not breathe vomit into her lungs.
- Do not give her anything by mouth until she has been awake for one hour.
- If you know how, start a fast IV drip with a wide needle. If you do not, start rectal fluids (see page 537).

Do not wait for a health worker. Take the woman for medical help or to a hospital <u>right away</u>. She needs medical help fast!

DANGER! Heavy bleeding can cause SHOCK, which can kill. Transport immediately.

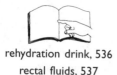

rehydration drink, 536

rectal fluids, 537

TRANSPORT!

INFECTION

If there is infection, it is more likely to be a **mild infection** if the abortion was done sooner than 3 months (12 weeks) after the last monthly bleeding.

Serious infection is an infection that has spread into the blood (sepsis). A woman is more likely to have a serious infection if the abortion was done later than 3 or 4 months from the last monthly bleeding, or if there was an injury to the womb during the abortion. Sepsis is very dangerous and can also cause shock.

Infection can happen because:

* an unclean hand or object was put inside the womb.
* pieces of the pregnancy were left inside the womb and they have become infected.
* the woman already had an infection when she had the abortion.
* a hole was made in the wall of the womb.

Signs of mild infection:

* slight *fever*
* mild pain in the abdomen

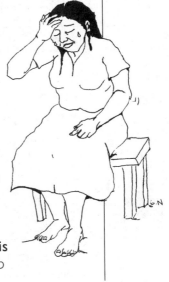

Treatment for mild infection:

To keep mild infection from becoming serious, treat it immediately with the medicines listed below. A woman needs more than one medicine because infections after abortion are caused by several different kinds of germs. If the medicines listed below are not available, see the "Green Pages" for others that will work. **A woman who is breastfeeding** should use the treatment for womb infection after childbirth, see page 97.

Medicines for mild infection after abortion

Medicine	How much to take	When and how to take
Take both medicines:		
amoxicillin	3 grams	all at once, 1 time only, by mouth
and		
doxycycline	100 mg	2 times a day for 10 days, by mouth

IMPORTANT *If the fever is not completely gone in 48 hours (2 days after starting these medicines), the woman should go to a health center.*

Signs of serious infection:

- chills and high fever
- muscle aches, weakness, and tiredness
- swollen, hard, and painful belly
- bad-smelling discharge from the vagina

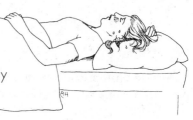

TRANSPORT!

Treatment for serious infection:

- **Take the woman to a health center or hospital immediately.**
- Start the following medicines right away, even if you are already on your way to the hospital. If she can swallow, give her these medicines, with plenty of water:

Medicines for serious infection after abortion

Medicine	How much to take	When and how to take
Take all 3 medicines:		
amoxicillin	3 grams	all at once, 1 time only, by mouth
and		
doxycycline	100 mg	2 times a day by mouth until you reach a hospital
and		
metronidazole	500 mg	3 times a day by mouth until you reach a hospital

If the woman cannot swallow medicines and you know how to give *injections* or IV medicines, start giving the medicines listed on the next page. **But do not delay. Take the woman for medical help or to a hospital right away. She needs medical help fast.**

TETANUS

A woman with an infection or bleeding from an injury after abortion can get a tetanus infection, especially if a dirty object or instrument was put into her womb. She needs a tetanus toxoid vaccination immediately (see page 515).

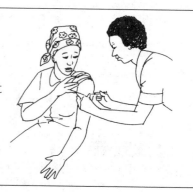

Injectable medicines for serious infection after abortion

IMPORTANT *Medicines in the vein (IV) or in the muscle (IM) should be given until the woman has been completely without fever for 48 hours.*
* *Choose one box and give ALL the medicines in that box.*
* *If the woman still has fever after 24 hours, change to another group of medicines.*
* *After 48 hours without fever, she can change to medicine by mouth (see the box at the bottom of this page).*
For complete information on these medicines, see the "Green Pages."

Best treatment: Give all 3 medicines

Medicine:	How much to give:	When and how to give:
benzylpenicillin	5 Million Units	4 times a day, IV
gentamicin	80 mg first dose, then 60 mg each dose	3 times a day, IM
metronidazole	I gram	2 times a day, by mouth or IV

Second best treatment: Give both medicines

Medicine:	How much to give:	When and how to give:
doxycycline	100 mg	2 times a day, by mouth or IV
metronidazole	I gram	2 times a day, IV or by mouth

Third best treatment: Give both medicines

Medicine:	How much to give:	When and how to give:
benzylpenicillin	5 Million Units	4 times a day, IV
chloramphenicol	I gram	4 times a day, IV

After 48 hours without fever, give this medicine by mouth:

Medicine:	How much to give:	When and how to give:
doxycycline	100 mg	2 times a day, by mouth, for 10 days

If a woman is breastfeeding, give amoxicillin instead, 500 mg 3 times a day for 10 days.

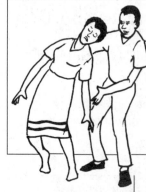

Fainting or loss of consciousness

Fainting can be a sign of shock after abortion, either from heavy bleeding, severe injury to the internal organs, or infection. For signs and treatment of shock, see page 254. If a woman faints but wakes up very soon afterward and does not have signs of shock, give her plenty of liquids to drink and watch her carefully.

Injury inside the body (internal injury)

An internal injury from an abortion is most often caused by a sharp object that makes a hole in the womb. The object may also cause damage to other internal organs, such as the *tubes*, *ovaries*, *intestines*, and *bladder*.

When a woman has internal injuries she may have severe bleeding inside her abdomen but almost no bleeding from her vagina.

Signs (she will have some or all of these):

- her abdomen feels stiff and hard with no sounds or gurgles inside
- very bad pain or cramps in the abdomen
- fever
- nausea and vomiting
- pain in one or both shoulders

Listen for gurgles for 2 minutes.

Treatment:

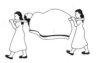

TRANSPORT!

- Immediately take the woman to a hospital or clinic where she can have surgery. An injury inside the body must be repaired right away by a surgeon or it can lead to infection, shock, and death.
- Do not give her anything by mouth—no food, no drink, not even water—unless it will take more than 12 hours to get to a health center. Then give water only in small sips. Or let her suck on a piece of cloth soaked in water.
- If she has signs of shock, treat her for shock (see page 254). Make sure nothing is blocking her mouth and that she can breathe.
- Give her the medicines for severe infection (see page 257), but only by injection or IV. If possible, give her a tetanus toxoid vaccination (see page 515).

Preventing Unsafe Abortion

Here are some things any woman or group of women can do in a community to help prevent illness and death from abortion:

- Educate men, women, and the community about how family planning can help prevent the need for abortion. Get training to provide family planning services to women in your community.

- Educate women and girls in your community about the dangers of unsafe abortion.

- Visit the people in your community who do abortions to make sure they are doing them safely.

- Learn about the complications of abortion and what to do for them. Find out where to take a woman in your community for emergency treatment of complications.

- Find out who could transport a woman who needs emergency care. If there is no emergency medical transport, is there someone in the community with a car or truck? Store extra containers of fuel (gas or petrol) for emergencies.

- Keep some of the medicines from page 484 in a village pharmacy or clinic to treat emergency abortion problems.

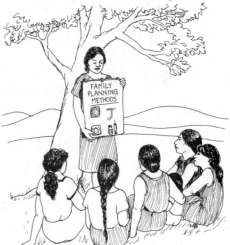

Family planning education can prevent the need for abortion.

If you are a health worker, here are some more suggestions:

- Try to get trained to do MVA, so you can treat women with abortion complications. Perhaps someone can train health workers at your local hospital. Do not do abortions unless you have been trained and have the instruments to do them safely.

- Organize health workers in your community to talk with health authorities about the risks of unsafe abortion. Even where abortion is not legal, treatment for abortion complications should be available to save women's lives.

➤ *Encourage women who are sick to seek help after an abortion, not to hide from it.*

Treat women who need your help with kindness

Many women who seek help after abortion are refused treatment or treated very badly. Some are made to feel ashamed or are given no care as 'punishment' for what they have done. Whatever your own beliefs, try not to judge women who have had an abortion, but rather care for them with compassion. Many of us could have an unwanted pregnancy at some time in our lives. Treat others as you would want yourself or your daughter to be treated.

Chapter 16

In this chapter:

How to use this chapter:

Many STDs have no signs in men or women. This chapter can help you learn when you are at risk for getting STDs and how to treat them. The chapter will also help you treat some problems of the genitals that are not sexually transmitted.

If you have signs: Look up the sign that is bothering you most. You may have to look in more than one place. For example, if you have a discharge but you also feel itchy, look first in the section called 'Abnormal Discharge'. If your problem is not there, look in the section called 'Itching of the Genitals'.

If you do not have signs: Read page 263 to learn when you are at risk for getting an STD.

This chapter suggests many different medicines that treat different STDs. Before you take any medicine, read about how to use medicines safely in the chapter called "Use of Medicines in Women's Health" (see page 469). There is also information you should know about each medicine listed in the "Green Pages," (see page 485).

Sexually Transmitted Diseases and Other Infections of the Genitals

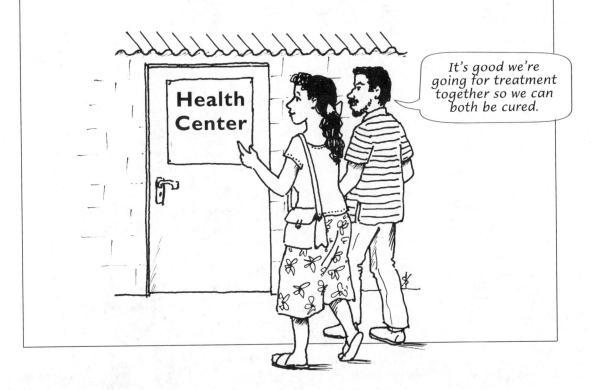

It's good we're going for treatment together so we can both be cured.

Sexually Transmitted Diseases, or STDs, are *infections* passed from one person to another during sex. Any type of sex can cause an STD. It can be *penis* to *vagina* sex, or penis to *anus* sex, or *oral sex* (mouth to penis, mouth to vagina). Sometimes STDs can happen from just rubbing an infected penis or vagina against another person's *genitals*. STDs can be passed from a pregnant woman to her baby before it is born, or during childbirth.

Unless they are treated early, STDs can cause:

- *infertility* in both men and women.
- babies born too early, too small, or blind.
- pregnancy in the tube (outside the womb).
- death from severe infection or *AIDS*.
- lasting pain in the lower *abdomen*.
- *cancer* of the *cervix*.

➤ *Early treatment of STDs in both partners can prevent many serious problems.*

➤ *This chapter will also help you treat some problems of the genitals that are not sexually transmitted.*

Why STDs Are a Serious Problem for Women

➤ *More than half of all women who are infected with an STD do not have any signs.*

➤ *If low-cost, accurate testing for STDs were available, women could avoid taking medicines that they do not need, may not be able to afford, or that cause side effects.*

181

sexual health

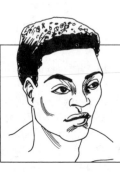

Men and women can both get STDs. **But a woman gets infected from a man more easily than a man gets infected from a woman.** This is because a man's penis goes into some part of a woman's body—such as her vagina, mouth, or anus—during sex. Without a condom, the man's *semen*, which may carry infection, stays inside her body. This gives her a greater chance of getting an infection in the *womb*, *tubes*, and *ovaries*.

Because most STDs are inside a woman's body, the signs of an STD in a woman are harder to see than in a man. So it is often hard to tell if a woman has an infection in her genitals—much less what kind of infection she has.

There are tests that can show if a woman has a particular STD. But these tests are not available in many places, and sometimes they do not give accurate results or do not find all possible STDs. Tests can also be expensive.

Since many women are not able to be tested accurately for STDs, **if you are at risk for being infected** (see the next page), it is usually better for you to take medicine to treat all the STDs you may have—just in case.

Why so many women get STDs

It can be hard for a woman to protect herself from an STD. Often, she must have sex when her partner demands it. She may not know if her partner has sex with other partners, or if he is infected with an STD. If he has another partner who is infected, he may infect his wife.

A woman may not be able to persuade her partner to use condoms. Latex condoms are the best way to protect both partners, but the man has to be willing to use them (see page 188).

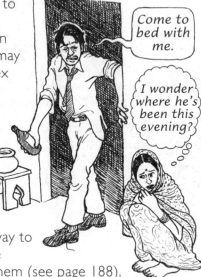

Come to bed with me.

I wonder where he's been this evening?

STDs hurt men, too

When they are not treated, STDs can cause a man to:
- become infertile.
- have lasting pain.
- die of AIDS or other serious infections.

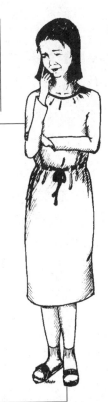

You may have an STD if you have one or more of the following signs:

- unusual *discharge* from the vagina
- pain in your lower abdomen
- a rash, bump, or sore on your genitals

HOW TO KNOW IF YOU ARE AT RISK FOR AN STD

Even if you do not have any signs, you may be at risk (more likely to have an STD) if:

- your partner has signs of an STD. He has probably passed the STD to you, even if you have no signs.
- you have more than one partner. The more partners you have, the greater the chance that one of them has passed an STD to you.
- you have had a new partner in the last 3 months. He may have had another partner just before you who had an STD.
- your partner lives away from home, or you believe your partner has other partners. This means he is more likely to become infected with an STD and infect you.

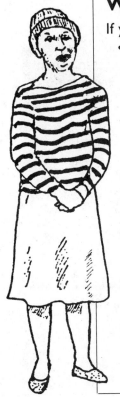

WHAT TO DO IF YOU HAVE AN STD

If you already have an STD or think you are at risk to get one:

- **treat it early.** If you have signs described in this chapter, follow the treatments given. Remember that it is very common to have more than one disease at the same time. If you have no signs but are at risk, take the medicines for discharge (page 266).
- **do not wait until you are very ill.** Early treatment will protect you from more serious problems later on, and will prevent the spread of infection to others.
- **help your partner to get treated at the same time you do.** If he does not, he will infect you again if you have sex. Urge him to take the proper medicine, or to see a health worker.
- **make sure you take *all* the medicine, even if your signs start to go away. Do not buy only part of the medicine.**
  You will not be cured until all the required medicine is gone.
- **practice *safer sex.*** You can always get another STD or HIV/AIDS if you do not protect yourself (see page 186).
- **try to get tested for syphilis.** If you have one STD, you could be infected with another and have no signs. Also consider being tested for *HIV* (see page 288).

Abnormal Discharge

It is normal to have a small amount of discharge, or wetness, that comes from the vagina. This is the way the vagina cleans itself. The amount of discharge changes during the days of your monthly cycle. During your fertile time, your discharge is more wet and slippery, and clear in color. If you are pregnant, you may have more discharge.

A change in the amount, color, or smell of the discharge from your vagina sometimes means you have an infection, but **it can be difficult to tell from your discharge what kind of infection you have.** Infections are often passed during sex (sexually transmitted), but not always. To decide if you are at risk for an STD, see page 263.

If your discharge continues even after taking medicines, see a health worker to have an *exam* and if possible get tested to see what infection you may have. The discharge could also be caused by another problem like *cancer.*

IMPORTANT *If you have discharge from the vagina with pain in the lower abdomen, you could have a serious pelvic infection. Get treatment immediately! See page 272.*

COMMON CAUSES OF ABNORMAL DISCHARGE

Abnormal discharge may be caused by several different types of infections. Below is a list of them and their most common signs.

Yeast (candida, white discharge, thrush)

Yeast is **not sexually transmitted.** It does not cause complications. You are most likely to have a yeast infection when you are pregnant, taking *antibiotics*, or have some other illness like *diabetes* or HIV/AIDS.

Signs:
- white, lumpy discharge, like milk curd or yogurt
- bright red skin outside and inside your vagina that sometimes bleeds
- you feel very itchy inside or outside your vagina
- a burning feeling when you pass urine
- a smell like mold or baking bread

Bacterial vaginosis

Bacterial vaginosis is **not sexually transmitted.** If you are pregnant, it can cause your baby to be born too soon.

Signs:
- more discharge than usual
- a fishy smell, especially after sex
- mild itching

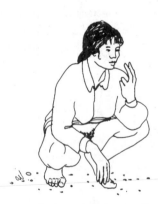

A change in the smell or color of your discharge can mean you have an infection

Trichomonas

Trichomonas is not a dangerous infection, but the itching can make you miserable. A man usually does not have any signs, but he can still carry the disease in his penis and give it to others during sex.

Signs:

- gray or yellow, bubbly discharge
- bad-smelling discharge
- red and itchy genital area and vagina
- pain or burning when you pass *urine*

Gonorrhea (clap, gono, VD) and chlamydia

Gonorrhea and chlamydia are both serious illnesses. But they are easy to cure if they are treated early. If not, they can cause severe infection and infertility in both women and men.

In a man, the signs usually begin 2 to 5 days after he had sex with an infected person. **But a man can have no signs and still be infected.** In a woman, the signs may not begin for weeks or even months. **Even if you do not have any signs, you can still give both gonorrhea and chlamydia to another person.**

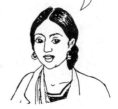

Remember that you can have any of these infections without any signs.

➤ *Gonorrhea and chlamydia have the same signs, so it is best, if possible, to get treated for both.*

Signs in a woman:

- yellow or green discharge from the vagina or *anus*
- pain or burning when passing urine
- *fever*
- pain in the lower belly
- pain or bleeding during sex
- or no signs at all

Signs in a man:

- discharge from his penis
- pain or burning when he passes urine
- pain or swelling of the *testicles*
- or no signs at all

Itching of the Genitals

Itching of the genitals can have many causes. Itching around the opening of the vagina could be yeast or trichomonas.

Itching in the hair of the genitals or close to the genitals, could be caused by *scabies* or *lice*. Scabies or lice can be treated with local remedies, or with medicines found in most pharmacies. For more information, see **Where There Is No Doctor**, or another general medical book.

Some itching is caused by soaps or deodorants that have perfume in them. It can also be caused by plants and herbs that are used for douching or washing out the vagina. Wash with plain water to see if the itching goes away.

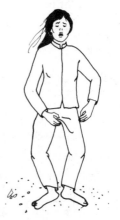

> *Treatment:*
> If you have an abnormal discharge and you **DO NOT** think you have an STD, treat the discharge with these medicines:

Medicines for Discharge <u>if you are **NOT** at risk for an STD</u>
(These medicines will cure yeast, trichomonas and bacterial vaginosis.)

<u>Take 2 medicines:</u> I medicine from Box 1, and also the medicine in Box 2.

Medicine	How much to take	When and how to take
<u>Box 1 (choose 1):</u>		
clotrimazole inserts	500 mg	Put the inserts high into the vagina for 1 night only.
or		
Gentian Violet	1% liquid	Soak clean cotton wool and put high into the vagina each night for 3 nights. Remove the cotton each morning.
<u>Box 2 (also take):</u>		
metronidazole	2 g (2000 mg)	Take all the tablets by mouth at the same time (this will not harm you), unless you are pregnant (see note).

If you are pregnant, do not take all the metronidazole at once. Instead, take 400 mg, 2 times a day for 7 days.

Important: *Do not drink alcohol during the time you are taking metronidazole.*

For other medicines that treat vaginal discharge NOT caused by an STD, see Box 1 on page 277.

> If you have an abnormal discharge and you **DO** think you are at risk for an STD, treat the discharge with these medicines:

Medicines for Discharge <u>if you think you are at risk for an STD</u>
(These medicines will cure gonorrhea, chlamydia and trichomonas.)

<u>Take all these medicines.</u>

Medicine	How much to take	When and how to take
co-trimoxazole	480 mg tablets (80 mg trimethoprim and 400 mg sulfamethoxazole)	10 tablets daily, all at once, by mouth, for 3 days (this will not harm you).
and		
doxycycline	100 mg	By mouth, 2 times a day, for 7 days. Do not take if pregnant or breastfeeding.
and		
metronidazole	2 g (2000 mg)	Take all the tablets by mouth all at the same time (this will not harm you) unless you are pregnant (see above).

Important:
   Co-trimoxazole is cheap and easy to find, but in some countries it no longer works to treat gonorrhea.

For other medicines that treat vaginal discharge caused by an STD, see Boxes 2 and 5 on pages 277 and 278.

Warts are caused by a *virus*. Warts on the genitals look like warts on other parts of the body. It is possible to have genital warts and not know it, especially when they are inside the vagina or inside the tip of the penis. Warts may go away without treatment, but it can take a long time. Usually they continue to get worse and should be treated.

Growths (Warts) on the Genitals

Signs:
- itching
- small, painless, whitish or brownish bumps that have a rough surface.
    - In women, these bumps usually grow on the folds of the *vulva,* inside the vagina, and around the anus.
    - In men, they usually grow on the penis, (or just inside it) and on the *scrotum,* or the anus.

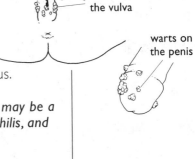

warts on the vulva

warts on the penis

IMPORTANT *Large, flat, wet growths that look like warts may be a sign of syphilis (see the next page). Try to get a test for syphilis, and DO NOT use the following treatment.*

Treatment:
1. Put some petroleum gel or other greasy ointment on the skin around each wart to protect the healthy skin.
2. With a small stick or tooth pick, carefully put on a very small amount of trichloroacetic acid (TCA) until the wart turns white. You can also use bichloracetic acid (BCA).
OR
Apply 20% podophyllin solution in the same way until the wart turns brown. **Podophyllin must be washed off 6 hours later.** Do not use podophyllin while you are pregnant.

➤ *Your partner should use condoms during sex until you both have no more warts.*

If the treatment is working, it will cause a painful sore where the wart used to be. Keep the sores clean and dry. Try not to have sex until they are gone, but if you must have sex, your partner should use a condom. The sores should heal within a week or two. Watch them to make sure they do not get infected.

Several treatments are usually necessary to get rid of all the warts (it does not matter which solution you use). You can repeat the treatment after one week. Try not to get acid on a sore where a wart used to be. If there is too much irritation, wait longer before the next treatment.

➤ *Warts grow faster during pregnancy. If you have a lot of them, this can cause problems with childbirth. Talk with a health worker about this.*

IMPORTANT *Having genital warts can increase your risk of cancer of the opening of the womb (cancer of the cervix). If you have had genital warts, try to have a Pap test done every 1 or 2 years.*

377

cervical cancer Pap test

Sores on the Genitals (Genital Ulcers)

➤ *If you have ever had an open sore on your genitals that was not treated, try to get a blood test for syphilis. Some countries have free testing programs.*

COMMON CAUSES OF SORES ON THE GENITALS

Most sores or *ulcers* on the genitals are sexually transmitted. It can be difficult to know which disease is causing the sores because the ones caused by both syphilis and chancroid often look alike. Sores on the genitals are one of the easiest ways that the AIDS virus passes in to the body.

Syphilis

Syphilis is a serious STD that has effects throughout the body and can last for many years. It is caused by *bacteria* and can be cured with medicine if treated early.

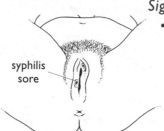

syphilis sore

Signs:

• The first sign is a small, **painless** sore that can look like a *pimple*, blister, a flat, wet wart, or an open sore. The sore lasts for only a few days or weeks and then goes away by itself. But the disease continues to spread throughout the body.

• Weeks or months later, you may have a sore throat, fever, rash (especially on the palms of the hands and soles of the feet), mouth sores, or swollen *joints*. During this time you can infect others.

All of these signs go away by themselves, but the disease continues. Without treatment, syphilis can cause heart disease, *paralysis*, mental illness, and even death.

➤ *If you are pregnant, try to get a blood test for syphilis.*

Pregnancy and syphilis. A pregnant woman can pass syphilis to her unborn baby, which can cause it to be born too early, deformed, or dead. You can prevent this by getting a blood test and treatment during pregnancy. If a pregnant woman and her partner have blood tests that show they have syphilis, they should both be treated with benzathine penicillin, 2.4 million Units, by injection (IM), once a week for 3 weeks.

Chancroid

Chancroid is an STD caused by bacteria. It can be cured with medicine if it is treated early.

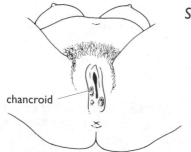

chancroid

Signs:

• one or more soft, **painful** sores on the genitals or anus that bleed easily

• enlarged, painful glands (*lymph nodes*, bubos) may develop in the *groin*

• slight fever

Treatment:

Medicine	How much to take	When and how to take
Medicines for Genital Sores		
(These medicines will cure both syphilis and chancroid.)		

Medicine	How much to take	When and how to take
benzathine penicillin . . . .2.4 million Units		one injection in the muscle (IM)
and		
erythromycin . . . . 500 mg		by mouth, 3 times a day, for 7 days

Important:
- *If you still have a sore after 7 days, continue taking erythromycin for 7 more days.*
- *If you are allergic to penicillin, take only erythromycin, but take 500 mg 3 times a day for 15 days.*

For other medicines that work to treat genital sores, see Box 3 and Box 5 on page 278.

Sores on the genitals should be kept clean. Wash them every day with soap and water, and dry carefully. Do not share the cloth you use to dry yourself with anyone else.

IMPORTANT *The AIDS virus can easily pass through a sore on the genitals during sex. To help prevent the spread of HIV/AIDS, do not have sex when you have a sore, or when your partner has one.*

Genital herpes

Genital herpes is an STD caused by a virus. It can happen on the genitals or on the mouth. It produces sores that come and go for months or years. There is no cure for herpes, but there is treatment to make you feel better.

Not all herpes sores on the mouth are spread by sex. Children and adults often get herpes sores on their mouths when they have a cold or fever.

Signs:

- a tingling, itching, or hurting feeling of the skin in the genital area or thighs
- small blisters that burst and form painful, open sores on the genitals

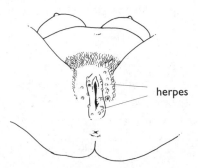

herpes

➤ *A person with AIDS can get herpes infections all over the body that take much longer to go away.*

The first time you get herpes sores, they can last for 3 weeks or more. You can have fever, headache, body ache, chills, and swollen lymph nodes in the groin. The next infection will be milder.

Treatment for genital herpes:

To help you feel better:

• Put ice directly on the sore as soon as you feel it.

• Make a *compress* by soaking some cloth in clean water that has black tea in it and put it on the sore.

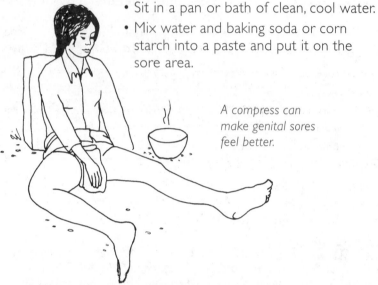

• Sit in a pan or bath of clean, cool water.

• Mix water and baking soda or corn starch into a paste and put it on the sore area.

A compress can make genital sores feel better.

490

acyclovir

• If your signs return again and again, try the medicine acyclovir. Although it cannot cure herpes, it can help the pain and make your signs go away more quickly.

• You can also try the suggestions on page 275.

IMPORTANT

• *Wash your hands with soap and water after touching the sores.*

• **Be careful not to touch your eyes or your children's eyes.** *A herpes infection in the eyes is very serious.*

• *Try not to have sex any time you have herpes sores. You can easily spread herpes to your sex partner.*

Pregnancy and herpes. A pregnant woman who is infected with herpes and has sores at the time of the birth can pass the disease on to her baby. This can cause dangerous problems for the baby. Try to give birth in a hospital. They may be able to do an operation to get the baby out, or give the baby special medicines when it is born.

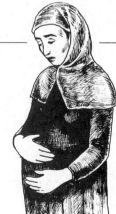

AIDS (Acquired Immune Deficiency Syndrome, HIV, slim disease)

AIDS is a sexually transmitted disease caused by a virus called HIV. It is spread when blood, fluid from the vagina, or semen of someone already infected with the HIV virus gets into the body of another person.

Women can get HIV more easily than men during sex. **You can get HIV from someone who looks completely healthy.**

There is no cure for HIV. If possible, do not have sex with someone who may be at risk for having HIV or AIDS. **To protect yourself, use a *latex* condom every time you have sex.**

Hepatitis B (yellow eyes)

Hepatitis B is a dangerous infection caused by a virus that harms the *liver*. Hepatitis B is spread when the blood, saliva (spit), fluid from the vagina, or semen of someone already infected with the virus gets into the body of another person. It spreads very easily from one person to another, especially during sex.

Signs:

- fever
- no appetite
- tired and weak feeling
- yellow eyes and/or skin
- pain in the belly
- dark urine and whitish stools
- no signs at all

Treatment:

There is no medicine that will help. In fact, taking medicine can hurt your liver even more.

Most people get better from hepatitis B. A small number of people may have liver problems that never go away, including cancer. Rest as much as you can, and eat foods that are easy to digest. **Do not drink any alcohol for at least 6 months.**

Pregnancy and hepatitis. If you have any of these signs when you are pregnant, see a health worker. You may be able to get a vaccination to prevent your baby from getting hepatitis B.

Other STDs

➤ *STDs can make it easier to get AIDS, because HIV, the virus that causes AIDS, can get into your body through open sores or be carried in discharge.*

283

AIDS

➤ *If your partner has had some of these signs, do not have sex until he is completely well. Ask a health worker if you can get vaccinated.*

384

cancer

Complications of STDs

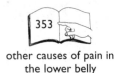

other causes of pain in
the lower belly

PELVIC INFLAMMATORY DISEASE (PID)

Pelvic Inflammatory Disease or PID is the name for an infection of any of the reproductive parts in a woman's lower abdomen. It is often called a 'pelvic infection'.

Pelvic infection can happen if you have had an STD that was not cured, especially gonorrhea or chlamydia. It can also happen if you recently gave birth, or had a *miscarriage* or abortion.

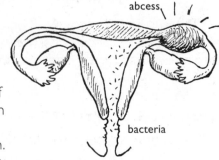

The germs that cause pelvic infection travel up from the vagina through the cervix and then into the womb, tubes, and ovaries. If the infection is not treated in time, it can cause *chronic* pain, serious illness, or death. An infection in the tubes can leave *scars* that make you infertile or at risk for a pregnancy outside the womb (tubal or ectopic pregnancy).

Signs (you may have one or more of these):

- pain in the lower belly
- high fever
- you feel very ill and weak
- green or yellow bad-smelling discharge from the vagina
- pain or bleeding during sex

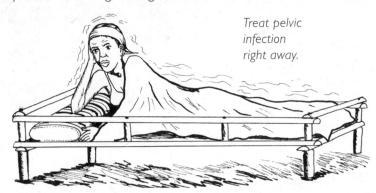

Treat pelvic infection right away.

➤ *To prevent PID, always treat STDs correctly. Be sure to:*

- *take all the medicine.*
- *make sure your partner gets treated.*
- *stop having sex until you and your partner have finished all the medicine and your signs have gone away.*

Treatment:

Start taking the medicines on the next page right away. If you do not feel better after 2 days and 2 nights (48 hours), or if you are very ill with a high fever or vomiting, or if you recently had an abortion or gave birth, **go to a health center or hospital immediately.** You may need strong medicines in the vein (IV).

Medicines for Pelvic Infection (PID)

(This infection is usually caused by a mix of germs, so 3 medicines must be used to cure it.)

Take all these medicines:

Medicine	How much to take	When and how to take
norfloxacin	800 mg	by mouth, once only (do not use if pregnant, breastfeeding, or under age 16).
and		
doxycycline	100 mg	by mouth, 2 times a day, for 10 days (do not use if pregnant or breastfeeding).
and		
metronidazole	500 mg	by mouth, 2 times a day, for 10 days.

For other medicines that work for pelvic infection, see Box 4 on page 278.

My husband taught school in a town far away from our village and returned home to visit me only a few times a year. After one of his visits, I became very ill with fever and a terrible pain in my abdomen. I did not know what was causing my sickness.... I tried remedies from the local healer, but they did not work. I did not want to leave my village to look for help because I did not want to leave my children, and I did not have much money. I got so sick that my neighbors thought I was going to die. So they took me in a truck to the nearest hospital, 90 miles away.

The doctor at the hospital said I had gonorrhea, and that this had caused a bad infection inside my abdomen. He said I would need expensive surgery and many days of medicines to cure me. He also said I would probably not be able to have more children. Now, I only wish I had taken the right medicines when I first became sick.

—*Central African Republic*

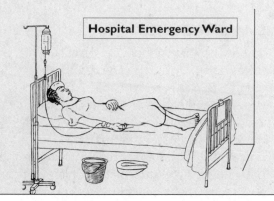

Hospital Emergency Ward

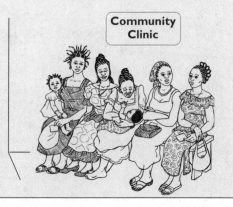

Community Clinic

➤ *Early treatment of STDs can prevent complications.*

In addition to PID, STDs can cause other problems for a woman. A woman with an STD that is not cured is more likely to have problems with infertility (see page 229) and tubal pregnancies (see page 73). STDs can also cause:

SWOLLEN VAGINA (BARTHOLIN GLAND INFECTION)

Just inside the vagina there are 2 small pockets of skin called 'glands'. They make a liquid that helps to keep the vagina wet. Sometimes germs get inside, and one or both glands become infected.

Signs:

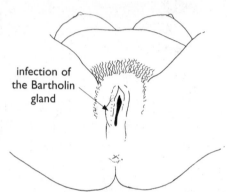

infection of the Bartholin gland

- Swollen, hot, painful vaginal fold that is darker in color. Usually it happens on one side only.
- Sometimes there is swelling with no pain.

Although not always caused by an STD, this infection often happens when a woman has gonorrhea or chlamydia.

Treatment:

1. Soak a cloth in clean, hot water and place it on the swelling. Do not make it so hot that you burn yourself. Do this as often as you can until the swelling opens and *pus* comes out, or until the swelling goes down.

2. Also, you and your partner both need to take medicines for gonorrhea and chlamydia. See the medicine chart on page 266.

3. If the area is painful and stays swollen, see a trained health worker who can cut it open and drain out the pus.

PROBLEMS IN NEWBORN BABIES

83

care of the eyes

Women who have gonorrhea or chlamydia while they are giving birth can pass these diseases to their newborn babies. The babies' eyes become infected with gonorrhea (neonatal conjunctivitis) which can cause blindness. To prevent neonatal conjunctivitis, put antibiotic ointment in the baby's eyes right after birth. Chlamydia can also cause *pneumonia* in newborn babies.

To cure yourself of an STD, you must take the medicine described in this chapter. To get relief from the discomfort of an STD:

How to Feel Better

1. Sit in a pan of clean, warm water for 15 minutes, 2 times a day. Do this until you feel better. If you think you have a yeast infection, you can add lemon juice, vinegar, yogurt or sour milk to the pan of warm water.

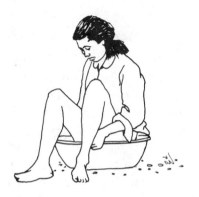

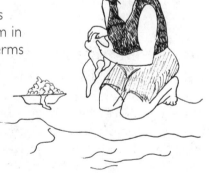

2. Do not have sex again until you feel better.

3. Try to wear underclothes made of cotton. This lets air in around your genitals which will help you heal.

4. Wash your underclothes once a day and dry them in the sun. This kills the germs that cause infection.

5. Take a mild pain medicine.

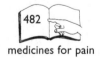

482
medicines for pain

6. If you have genital ulcers and it is painful to pass urine, pour clean water over your genital area while you urinate. Or sit in a pan of cool water while you urinate.

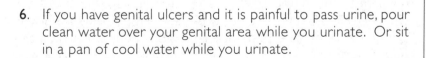

Other Medicines to Treat STDs

On several pages of this chapter (266, 269, and 273) we have recommended medicines to treat STDs and other problems. We selected these medicines because they are:

- effective (they work to cure the problem).
- easy to find.
- not too costly.

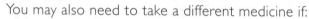

However, different kinds of medicines are sold in different parts of the world, and the prices may vary. So one of these medicines may not be available where you live, or there may be a different medicine that is both effective and less costly.

You may also need to take a different medicine if:

- you are pregnant or breastfeeding and the medicine is not safe to take during those times.
- the STD you are trying to treat has become resistant to the medicine (see below).
- you have an *allergy* to the medicine. Some people are allergic to medicines like penicillin or sulpha antibiotics. See page 480 for how to substitute antibiotics.

In this section we have listed other medicines that will work for each problem. Remember that most people have more than one STD or problem of the genitals at the same time, so it is often necessary to take more than one medicine. Whichever medicines you choose, be sure to take them correctly (see the next page).

➤ Warnings are given in this chapter if pregnant or breastfeeding women should not take a medicine. If a medicine does not have a warning, it is safe to take.

➤ Before you take any medicine, you should read about it in the "Green Pages." There may be more information you should know.

DRUG RESISTANCE AND STD MEDICINES

When using antibiotics for treating STDs and other diseases, it is very important to take all the medicine. If a person does not take enough of the right kind of medicine—or stops taking the medicine before the treatment is finished—the germs causing the infection are not all killed. The strongest germs survive and multiply and create stronger forms of the disease. Then a medicine that once worked against that disease is no longer able to cure it. This is called resistance.

For this reason, in many places gonorrhea has become resistant to the drugs usually used to treat it. Talk with a health worker to find out if there are drug-resistant STDs where you live, and what are the best, locally-available medicines to treat them.

➤ If you are not sure which medicine will work best for a problem, try to check with a health worker or pharmacist who will know which medicines are best where you live.

Box 1 Other Medicines for Vaginal Discharge if you are NOT at risk for an STD

(These medicines are for vaginal infections that are not usually sexually transmitted.)

For yeast infections of the vagina:
- miconazole, 200 mg inserts: put 1 high into the vagina each night for 3 nights.
- nystatin, 100,000 U. inserts: put 1 high into the vagina each night for 7 nights.
- vinegar: mix 3 tablespoons of clear vinegar with 1 liter or quart of boiled, cool water (or 1 tablespoon of vinegar in 1 cup of water). Soak a piece of clean cotton wool in the mixture and put it high into the vagina each night for 3 nights. Remove each morning.

For trichomonas and bacterial vaginosis:
- metronidazole: 2 g (2000 mg) by mouth all at once (this will not harm you). **If you are pregnant**, do not take this medicine all at once. Instead, take 400 mg, 2 times a day for 7 days.
- metronidazole vaginal inserts: put one 500 mg insert high in the vagina, 2 times a day for 10 days.
- tinidazole: use the same dose as for metronidazole (see above).

Box 2 Other Medicines for Vaginal Discharge if you may be at risk for an STD

(This box includes medicines for gonorrhea and chlamydia. Since it is very difficult to tell these infections apart, take medicines for both. These medicines also treat infections in men. Treat for trichomonas by taking metronidazole. See Box 1.)

For gonorrhea:
- norfloxacin: 800 mg by mouth, once only
- ciprofloxacin: 500 mg by mouth, once only

} **(do not use either of these 2 medicines if you are pregnant or breastfeeding or under age 16)**

- ceftriaxone: 250 mg by injection into a muscle (IM), once only
- kanamycin: 2 grams, by injection into a muscle (IM), once only
  (do not use if pregnant or breastfeeding)
- cefixime: 400 mg by mouth, once only

For chlamydia
- tetracycline: 500 mg, by mouth, 4 times a day for 7 days
  (do not use if pregnant or breastfeeding)
- erythromycin: 500 mg, 4 times a day for 7 days
- amoxicillin: 500 mg, 3 times a day for 7 days

Be sure to take medicines correctly

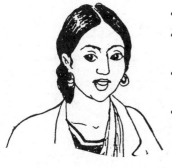

Remember, when treating STDs, always:

- make sure your partner gets treated too.
- take all the medicine.
- stop having sex until your signs have gone away AND you and your partner have finished all the medicine.
- see a health worker if you do not get better by the end of your treatment.
- start practicing safer sex when you do have sex again.

Box 3

Other Medicines for Genital Sores

(These medicines treat early syphilis and chancroid. Since it is very hard to tell the cause of genital sores, treat for both syphilis and chancroid.)

For syphilis:

The best medicine for early syphilis is benzathine penicillin, 2.4 Million Units, by injection into a muscle (IM), once only. If you are allergic to penicillin, you can use instead:

* doxycycline: 100 mg, by mouth, 2 times a day for 15 days
  (do not use if pregnant or breastfeeding)
* tetracycline: 500 mg, by mouth, 4 times a day for 15 days
  (do not use if pregnant or breastfeeding)
* erythromycin: 500 mg, by mouth, 4 times a day for 15 days (erythromycin will also treat chancroid)

For chancroid:

The best medicine for chancroid is erythromycin, 500 mg, by mouth, 3 times a day for 7 days. Other medicines that work for chancroid are:

* ciprofloxacin: 500 mg, by mouth, once only
  (do not use if pregnant or breastfeeding or under age 16)
* ceftriaxone: 250 mg, by injection into a muscle (IM), once only
* co-trimoxazole 480 mg (80 mg trimethoprim and 400 mg sulfamethoxazole) tablets: 2 tablets, by mouth, 2 times a day for 7 days

Box 4

Other Medicines for Pelvic Infection (PID)

(This infection is usually caused by a mix of germs. If possible, 3 medicines should be taken.)

These are the first choice:

* norfloxacin: 800 mg, by mouth, once only **(do not use if pregnant, breastfeeding, or under 16)**
* doxycycline: 100 mg, by mouth, 2 times a day for 10 days **(do not use if pregnant or breastfeeding)**
* metronidazole: 500 mg, by mouth, 3 times a day for 10 days

Instead of *norfloxacin* you can use any of these medicines:

* ceftriaxone: 250 mg, by injection into a muscle (IM), once only
* cefixime: 400 mg, by mouth, once only
* co-trimoxazole 480 mg (80 mg trimethoprim and 400 mg sulfamethoxazole) tablets: 5 tablets, by mouth, 2 times a day for 3 days
* ciprofloxacin: 500 mg, by mouth, once only **(do not use if you are pregnant, breastfeeding, or under age 16)**
* kanamycin: 2 grams, by injection into a muscle (IM), once only **(do not use if pregnant or breastfeeding)**

Instead of *doxycycline* you can use any of these medicines:

* tetracycline: 500 mg, by mouth, 4 times a day for 10 days
  (do not use if pregnant or breastfeeding)
* erythromycin: 500 mg, by mouth, 4 times a day for 7 days
* amoxicillin: 500 mg, by mouth, 3 times a day for 10 days

Box 5

Medicines for Those at Very Great Risk for STDs

(For women who have a very great risk of getting many different STDs—anyone who has unsafe sex with many different partners—this is a medicine that can be useful. It works to treat drug-resistant gonorrhea, as well as chlamydia and genital ulcers. But it is very expensive and can be hard to find.)

* azithromycin: 1 gram, by mouth, once only

For almost all women, 1 gram is enough medicine. In a very few cases, 2 grams may be necessary for effective treatment, but this amount can cause severe nausea and vomiting.

How to prevent STDs

- Practice safer sex (see the chapter on "Sexual Health").

- Use condoms every time you have sex. To learn how to encourage your partner to use condoms, see page 188.

see page 188

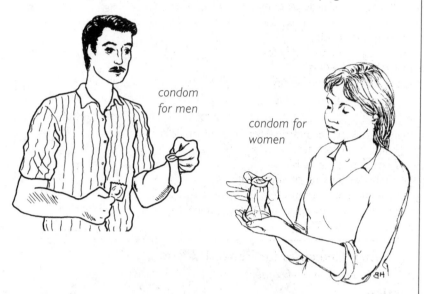

condom for men

condom for women

Working for Change

➤ *Preventing STDs can protect you and your partner from serious illness and infertility.*

- If your partner will not use a condom, use spermicide alone or with a diaphragm. This will give you some protection against gonorrhea and chlamydia.

- Wash the outside of your genitals after sex.

- Pass urine after having sex.

- Do not douche, or use herbs or powders to dry out the vagina. Douching (and washing out the vagina with soap) works against the natural wetness the vagina makes to stay healthy. When the vagina is dry, it can become irritated during sex, making it more likely to be infected with AIDS and other STDs.

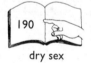

190

dry sex

Use condoms!

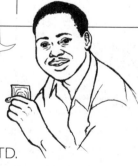

Latex condoms will:

- protect you from STDs including HIV/AIDS.

- protect the health of your partner.

- prevent unwanted pregnancy.

Do not have sex when you or your partner has signs of an STD.

WORKING FOR SAFER SEX IN THE COMMUNITY

Sexually transmitted diseases are a health problem for the whole community. To help prevent STDs in your community you can:

191

bargaining for safer sex

- teach men and women about the risks to their health and the health of their families from STDs. Find opportunities when women are together in groups, such as at the market or waiting at health centers, to explain how STDs are passed, and how to prevent them.

- work with others to find ways to convince men to wear condoms. Practice in the group what to say to your partner to get him to use a condom.

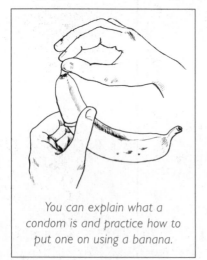

You can explain what a condom is and practice how to put one on using a banana.

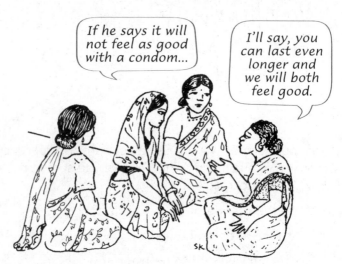

If he says it will not feel as good with a condom...

I'll say, you can last even longer and we will both feel good.

- make latex condoms available in your community. Work to make sure that free or cheap condoms are available at local shops, bars, and cafes as well as from health workers and at health centers.

- train men to teach other men in the community about using condoms.

- organize a community group to talk about health problems and include STDs, HIV, and AIDS. Explain how preventing STDs will also prevent the spread of HIV infection and AIDS.

- support education about sex in your local schools. Help parents understand that teaching children about STDs, including HIV/AIDS, helps the children make safe choices later on when they start having sex.

- encourage teenagers to teach their friends about STDs, including HIV/AIDS.

After a health worker came to speak with a group of women in our community about STDs and AIDs, we began talking about our lives. Some of the women began by saying they did not have anything to worry about. But the more we talked the more we realized that every woman and every man should worry about STDs and AIDS. We thought about how to get men to use condoms and decided that we needed to educate the entire community about the dangers of STDs and AIDS and how to prevent them.

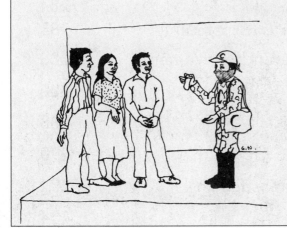

We organized a play and got people from the community to act in it. We created a special character called "Commander Condom" to come to the rescue with condoms. Everyone came to watch the play. People enjoyed it and they also learned. Now the men make jokes about "Commander Condom," but they are also more willing to use them.

— *Oaxaca, Mexico*

To the health worker:

- Find out from your local health center, hospital, or Ministry of Health what medicines work best to treat STDs in your community.

- Try to start a community pharmacy so that it will be easier for people to get medicines, latex condoms, and spermicides.

- Talk to the people you see who have an STD. Give them good information on how to cure their STD, how to keep from infecting others, and how to keep from getting an STD again. Make sure their partners also get treatment.

- Include information about preventing STDs and HIV/AIDS in family planning programs.

- Do not judge or blame those who come to you for help with an STD.

- Respect the privacy of those with STDs or other health problems. Never talk about their problems with others.

See the chapter on "Sexual Health," page 181, for information about:

- sex and *gender roles*
- harmful beliefs about women's sexuality
- how to have safer sex
- feeling pleasure from sex

Chapter 17

In this chapter:

AIDS (<u>A</u>cquired <u>I</u>mmune <u>D</u>eficiency <u>S</u>yndrome)

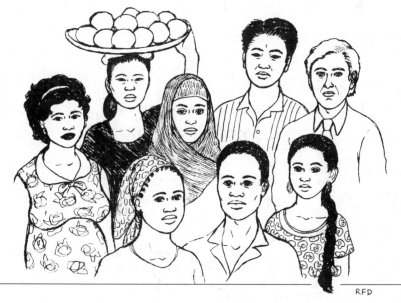

RFD

You must have heard about AIDS by now—on the radio, in the market, from your neighbors, or at the health center. You may think AIDS is not your problem. Yet millions of people are infected with the AIDS *virus*. More and more of them are women.

➤ *AIDS is* **everyone's** *problem.*

We can only protect ourselves from AIDS if we understand what AIDS is, and if we talk about AIDS with our families and friends.

"AIDS is a disease that shines in hush and thrives on secrecy. It was prospering because people were choosing not to talk about it... I wanted to talk about AIDS so that at least my children, and yours, would be spared. They would know and have the information about AIDS before they became sexually active, and be able to talk about it."

—*Noerine Kaleeba, Uganda, whose husband died of AIDS*

WHY SO MANY WOMEN GET **HIV/AIDS**

AIDS is spreading fastest in parts of the world where people are poor and do not have education. If there is famine (not enough food), war, or not enough work, people are often forced to move to cities, away from their families. Traditions often break down and sex with new partners is common.

These conditions are especially hard for women. Poor women have even less power to control their lives. Often laws and tradition keep women from getting an education, skills to support themselves, or information about their bodies.

➤ *Lack of power and information make women more vulnerable to AIDS.*

What Are HIV and AIDS?

HIV (Human Immunodeficiency Virus) is a very small *germ*, called a virus, that you cannot see. AIDS is a disease that develops later, after a person has been infected with HIV, the AIDS virus.

HIV

When a person becomes infected with HIV, the virus attacks the immune system, the part of your body that fights off infection. HIV slowly kills the *cells* of the immune system until the body cannot defend itself against germs anymore. Although a person may feel well for only a short time, many people feel well for 5 to 10 years after getting HIV. But eventually the immune system will no longer have enough cells to fight off germs that normally do not make you sick. Because HIV takes many years to make someone sick, most people with HIV feel healthy and do not know they have it.

➤ *As long as you feel well you have HIV, but you do not yet have AIDS.*

IMPORTANT *You can pass HIV to others as soon as you are infected, even though you look and feel healthy. You cannot tell from looking at a person if he or she has HIV. The only way to know if you are infected is to get the HIV test (see page 288).*

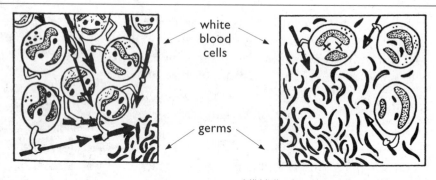

white blood cells

germs

The body has millions of white blood cells that attack germs and fight off infection.

HIV kills the white blood cells until there are not enough cells left to attack the germs. This is when the person has AIDS.

AIDS

A person has AIDS when the immune system gets so weak that it can no longer fight off common infections and illnesses. The signs of AIDS are different in different people, and they can be different for women than for men. Often the signs are lasting infection with other common illnesses (see page 297).

Good *nutrition* and some medicines can help the person's body fight infections caused by AIDS and allow her or him to live longer. But there is no cure for AIDS itself. So after a while, a person infected with HIV will get more and more illnesses until the body is too weak to survive.

How **HIV/AIDS** is spread

HIV lives in body fluids—such as blood, *semen*, and the fluids in the *vagina*—of people infected with HIV. The virus is spread when these fluids get into the body of another person. **This means that HIV/AIDS can be spread by:**

unsafe sex with someone who has the virus.

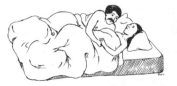

unclean needles or *syringes*, or any tool that pierces or cuts the skin.

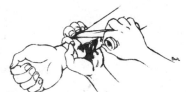

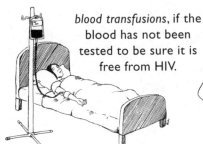

blood transfusions, if the blood has not been tested to be sure it is free from HIV.

an infected mother to her baby through pregnancy, birth or breastfeeding.

infected blood that gets into cuts or an open wound of another person.

How **HIV/AIDS** is **NOT** spread

HIV does not live outside the human body for more than a few minutes. It cannot live on its own in the air or in water. This means **you cannot give or get HIV in these ways:**

by touching, kissing, or hugging.

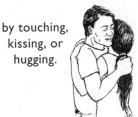

by sharing food.

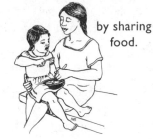

by sharing a bed.

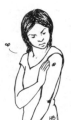

by sharing or washing clothes, towels, bed covers, latrines, or toilets, if you follow the advice on page 295.

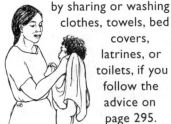

by caring for somone with HIV/AIDS, if you follow the advice on pages 294, 295, and 309.

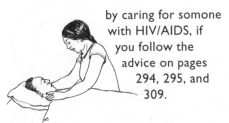

from insect bites.

Why HIV and AIDS Are Different for Women

HIV and AIDS are different for women because:

- women get infected with HIV more easily than men do. A man puts his semen in the woman's vagina, where it stays for a long time. If there is HIV in semen it can pass easily into a woman's body through her vagina or cervix, especially if there are any cuts or sores.

- women are often infected at a younger age than men. This is often because young women and girls are less able to refuse unwanted or unsafe sex.

- women get more blood transfusions than men because of problems during childbirth.

- women become sick with AIDS more quickly after becoming infected with HIV than men do. Poor nutrition and childbearing may make women less able to fight disease.

- women are blamed unfairly for the spread of AIDS. But men are just as responsible as women (if not more). For example, they are the ones who buy sex, which is a common way that AIDS spreads.

- a pregnant woman infected with HIV can pass it to her baby.

- women are usually the caretakers for family members who are sick with AIDS, even if they are sick themselves.

Preventing HIV/AIDS

safer sex

You can prevent AIDS in these ways:

- If possible, have sex with only one partner who has sex only with you.

- Practice safer sex—sex that prevents the germs in a man's semen from getting into your vagina, anus, or mouth.

- Avoid piercing or cutting the skin with needles or other tools that have not been disinfected between uses (see page 521).

- Avoid blood transfusions except in emergencies.

- Do not share razors or toothbrushes.

- Do not touch someone else's blood or wound without protection (see page 295).

Women and girls should have a right to protect their lives against AIDS. To do this we need:

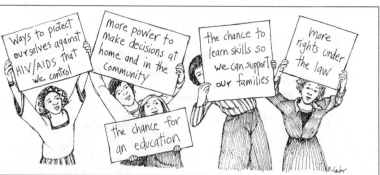

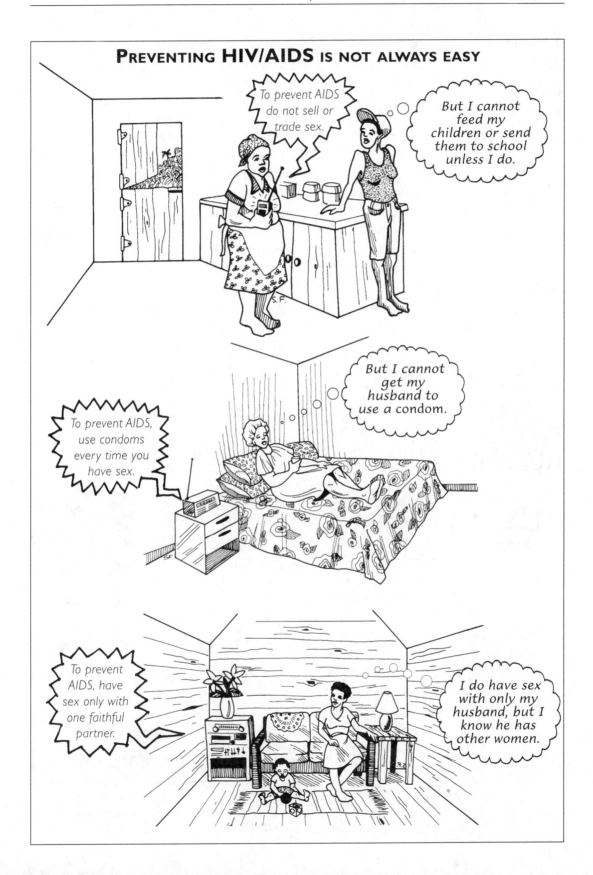

The HIV Test

➤ *Your local Red Cross or Red Crescent may offer testing and counseling at a low cost. Check with your national AIDS control program to find out where you can be tested in your country. It can take about 2 weeks to get the test results.*

➤ *If possible, have someone you trust go with you to get your HIV test results.*

When HIV enters the body, the body starts to make antibodies right away to fight the virus. These antibodies usually show in the blood 4 to 8 weeks later, but it can take as long as 6 months for the body to make enough of them to show up in a test. This time between infection and when the antibodies appear in the blood is called the 'window period'.

The HIV test looks for these antibodies in the blood. It is the only way to know if a person has been infected with HIV. **It is not a test for AIDS.**

A positive HIV test means that you are infected with the virus and your body has made antibodies to HIV. Even if you feel completely well, you can spread the virus to others.

A negative HIV test means 1 of 2 things:
  • you are not infected with HIV, or
  • you are infected but have not yet made enough antibodies to HIV to test positive (the window period).

If you have tested negative for HIV but think you might be infected, you should take the test again in a few months. Sometimes a positive test also needs to be repeated. A health worker can help you decide.

THE WINDOW PERIOD

This is different for different people. Here is an example of how long the window period was for one woman:

1. *He was HIV-infected.*

They had unprotected sex.

She became infected too.

2. *Three weeks later, she tested negative for HIV. But she was still infected and could give the virus to others. She was in the 'window period'.*

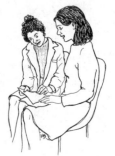

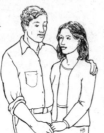

3. *Nine weeks later she tested positive for HIV.*

4.

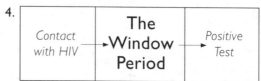

| Contact with HIV | The Window Period | Positive Test |

*The time between her first contact with HIV, and when **antibodies** appear in her blood is the **window period**.*

Since the window period can be as long as 6 months, it is best to wait that long after being exposed before getting the HIV test. If you think you may have come into contact with HIV again during that 6-month window period, you will need to get another test in 6 months from the date of the new contact.

WHEN SHOULD YOU HAVE THE HIV TEST?

It is usually more important to change unsafe behavior than to have an HIV test. But you and your partner may want to be tested if:

- you want to get married (or start a faithful sexual relationship with one person) or have children.
- you, your partner, or your baby have signs of AIDS.
- you or your partner have had unsafe sex.

The advantages of knowing the test results

If your test is negative, you can learn how to protect yourself so that you stay negative and never get HIV/AIDS.

If your test is positive, you can:

- prevent the spread of HIV to your partner.
- get treatment early for health problems.
- make changes in how you live so you can stay healthy longer.
- get support from other HIV-infected people in your community.
- plan for yourself and your family's future.

The disadvantages of knowing the test results

You may have many different feelings if you find out you are infected. It is normal at first to be shocked and deny that your test results are positive. You may also feel anger and despair, and blame yourself or others.

It often helps to talk with someone, such as the health worker who gave you the test results or someone close to you. But be careful who you tell. Your husband or partner may blame you, even if he is also infected with HIV. Other people may act afraid and shun you, because they do not understand HIV/AIDS or how it is spread. If possible, see a trained HIV/AIDS counselor, who can help you decide who to tell and how to face this change in your life.

> *The HIV test should always be done:*
> - *with your permission.*
> - *with counseling before and after the test.*
> - *with privacy. No one should know the results except you and those you want to know.*

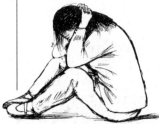

AIDS is not a curse or a punishment.

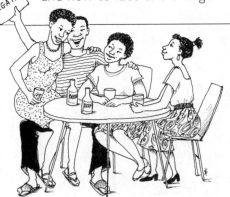

IMPORTANT *A negative test does not mean that you will never become infected with HIV. If you practice unsafe sex, you can still get infected.*

Practice safer sex.

➤ *Counseling for HIV-positive people and their families can mean the difference between hope and despair. As an HIV-positive woman from Kenya says, "When you meet a good counselor, you feel as if you have healed."*

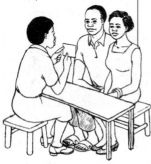

Counseling

A counselor is someone who listens and talks with a person and his or her family to help them to cope with their worries, concerns, and fears, and to make their own decisions.

Counseling is important throughout the life of a person with HIV, not only when they first discover they are infected. If you are infected, a skilled counselor may be able to help you:

- decide who to tell about being HIV-infected.
- find the support of others who are also HIV-infected.
- get the care you need from health centers.
- explain to your family what it means to be HIV-infected, and how HIV is spread. This will help them to accept and care for you without being afraid.
- understand how to stay healthy for as long as possible.
- plan for your future.
- learn how to be sexual in a safe way.

If you are a health worker or a leader of a religious group, you are in an ideal position to get training to help those suffering with the problems of HIV. Some people who have lost family members to AIDS have learned to counsel others about living with HIV.

Living Positively with HIV and AIDS

➤ *Most people with HIV can be healthy for many years.*

Modern medicine and traditional healers still do not have a cure for AIDS. But most people with HIV can be healthy for many years. During this time it can help to:

- **make the best of every moment of your life.**
- **spend time with friends and family.**
- **try to keep active by doing your daily work.**
- **be sexual if you want to.** Enjoying sexual touch can help you stay healthier longer.

If your partner is HIV infected

Although it is risky, if you practice safer sex carefully, you can continue to have sex with an HIV infected partner without becoming infected yourself. Besides using safer sex methods (see page 188), watch your own health carefully. Watch for breaks in the skin or other places where infection could occur. And remember, there are other ways to be sexual besides having sex. It is safe to hug, to hold someone in your arms, and to kiss them.

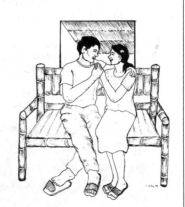

- **Try joining or starting a group of people with HIV and AIDS.** Some people with HIV and AIDS work together to educate the community, to provide home care to those who are sick with AIDS, and to support the rights of people with HIV and AIDS.

support groups

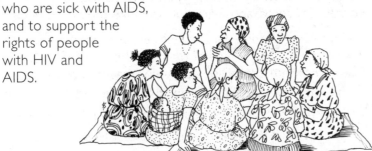

- **Look after your spiritual and mental health.** Your faith and traditions can bring you hope and strength.
- **Think about the future.** If you have children:
  - spend time with them now, and give them care and guidance.
  - make arrangements for family members to look after them when you are no longer able to do so.
  - make a *will*. If you have some money, a house, or property, try to make sure that they will go to those whom you want to have them. Sometimes women who are not legally married cannot leave their possessions to their children and other family members. So it may be helpful to get legally married in order to leave your possessions to those you want to have them.

mental health

➤ *If you have children, make staying healthy for them a goal.*

Take care of your health

- **Take care of medical problems early.** Each infection can weaken your immune system more.
- **Eat nutritious food to keep your body strong.** The same foods that are good to eat when you are healthy are good for you when you are sick. Buy nutritious food instead of spending money on *vitamin* tablets or *injections* (see page 165).
- **Avoid tobacco, alcohol, and other drugs** (see page 435).
- **Practice safer sex** for your own health as well as your partner's. Safer sex can prevent new infections and unplanned pregnancies that could weaken the immune system even more.
- **Try to get enough rest and exercise.** This will help your body stay strong to fight infection.
- **Prevent infection by washing often.**

Pregnancy, Childbirth, and Breast-feeding

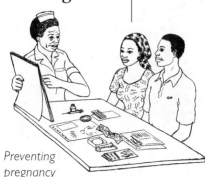

Preventing pregnancy may keep you healthier and help you live longer. If you are HIV infected and already pregnant, it is especially important to take good care of yourself.

your fertile time, 220 and 233

PREGNANCY

Pregnancy can be dangerous for a woman with HIV or AIDS. During pregnancy and childbirth she is more likely to have some of the following problems than a woman who does not have HIV or AIDS:

- lose the baby during pregnancy (miscarriage)
- fevers, infections, and poor health
- serious infections after giving birth, which are hard to treat and may threaten her life

In addition, her baby may:

- be infected with HIV.
- be born too soon, or be sickly and die.

Some women who become infected with HIV may still want to get pregnant. Or they may have no way to prevent pregnancy.

If you want to get pregnant

If you are not sure whether you or your partner are infected with HIV and you can get a test for HIV, both of you should wait 6 months before having the test. While you wait, use condoms every time you have sex, and have sex with only each other.

If you cannot get an HIV test, you can reduce your risk by following this advice:

- Have sex with a condom, except during your *fertile time*.
- When you are not fertile, practice safer sex.
- Never have sex when there are signs of an STD.

About 1 out of 3 babies born to HIV-infected mothers becomes infected.

This baby is HIV positive.

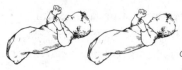

These 2 babies are HIV negative.

A baby can become infected while it is in your *womb*, or during birth, or while breastfeeding. Some anti-viral drugs (like AZT) are being tested that may reduce the risk of passing HIV to your baby. Check with a health worker who has been trained to treat HIV/AIDS during pregnancy.

An HIV-positive mother always passes antibodies (but not always HIV itself) to her unborn baby. This means that a new baby will always test positive for HIV because the mother's antibodies show up in the baby's blood. But many babies later have a negative test. This means they were not actually infected with HIV itself. It is impossible to tell from the usual HIV test if the baby has the virus or just the antibodies until the baby is 18 months old. At that time, the mother's antibodies will disappear from its blood.

CHILDBIRTH

If you think your midwife or birth attendant would be understanding, tell her that you are HIV infected so she can protect both of you from infection.

After the birth, wash your genitals 2 times a day with mild soap and clean water. Learn the signs of infection after birth and get treated immediately if necessary.

infection after
childbirth

BREASTFEEDING

HIV infection is sometimes passed to the baby in breast milk. No one knows yet how often this happens or why it happens to some babies and not others. There is more HIV in the breast milk of mothers who have become infected recently, and in those who are very sick with AIDS.

when the mother
is sick

Some mothers find a friend or relative who is not HIV infected who can breastfeed their baby for them. This can be the safest choice for your baby. But even if you are HIV infected, it is usually better to breastfeed than to use other milks or *formula*. In many communities the *risk* of *diarrhea* and *malnutrition* from other milks is greater than the risk of HIV, especially in the baby's first 6 months of life.

After 6 months, when your baby is bigger and stronger, there is less danger of diarrhea and infection. You can then switch to other milks and feed your baby other foods. This way your baby has many of the *benefits* of breastfeeding with less risk of getting HIV.

other foods

Talking with a trained health worker about breastfeeding and HIV can help you answer some of the following difficult questions and make a decision about whether to breastfeed your baby:

* Are you certain you have HIV or AIDS? Perhaps you should be tested.
* Do children in your area often get sick or die from infections, diarrhea, or poor nutrition? If the answer is yes, then breastfeeding may be best.
* Are other clean, nutritious milks or formula available? You will need to buy them for at least 6 months, which is very costly. You will also need enough clean, boiled water and some training in how to feed other milks or formula with a cup or spoon.
* Is there another woman who can breastfeed your baby? Are you certain she is not infected with HIV?

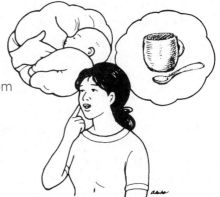

Whatever you choose to do, do not blame yourself if your baby becomes infected with HIV. There is no way to know for sure how to protect your baby.

Care for Persons with AIDS

The health and medical problems of AIDS may last a long time. These problems can take a lot of the energy and resources of the sick person and her or his family.

If you have AIDS, you will probably need to see a health worker or go to a clinic from time to time to have an infection treated. But you may never need to stay in the hospital. You may be more comfortable at home, cared for by family members in familiar surroundings.

If you have a problem that does not get better with home treatment, try to find a health worker, clinic, or doctor you trust who is experienced with AIDS. Then go to the same person whenever you have a problem. Going from clinic to clinic wastes time, energy, and money.

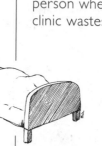

➤ *A good counselor is key to helping you care for someone with AIDS at home.*

A stay in the hospital usually costs more than the food and medicine needed for good care at home.

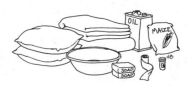

Much of the work in caring for sick people at home is done by women, who are usually the family's caregivers. **If you are caring for someone with AIDS,** be sure to take care of your own needs, too. Try to get help from other family members, friends and people in the community. Community clubs, religious groups, youth clubs, and AIDS self-help groups may assist you.

When Rosa was in bed because of AIDS *complications*, her mother kept a cheerful attitude. Every day she bathed her daughter, dressed her with nice clothes, and put a little flower next to her bed. Rosa was not hungry but her mother arranged the food in a way that could make her want to eat. The family would talk to Rosa about daily life, and their work and community. With their good humor and positive comments, Rosa felt that she was not cast aside. Even though Rosa was often tired or didn't feel well, the family arranged for her friends to visit her in the moments she felt better. Music, conversation, and good spirit made the house full of life. Rosa felt that she was loved and needed, and that AIDS could not ruin her closeness and her time with her family.

PREVENTING HIV INFECTION AT HOME

If you follow these rules, there is no risk of spreading HIV from an infected person to others around her, or of getting HIV yourself:

- Avoid touching body fluids, like blood, *vomit*, *stool*, and *urine*.

- Do not share anything that touches blood. This includes razors, needles, any sharp instruments that cut the skin, and toothbrushes. If you must share such things, *disinfect* them before another person uses them. If you are unable to disinfect them, boil them in water for 20 minutes.

disinfecting

- Keep wounds covered. Both caregivers and persons with HIV or AIDS should cover all open wounds with a clean bandage or cloth.

- Use a piece of plastic or paper, gloves, or a big leaf to handle dirty bandages, cloths, blood, vomit, or stool.

- Wash your hands with soap and water after changing dirty bedding and clothes.

➤ *Burn or bury soiled bandages that cannot be rewashed.*

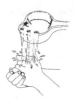

- Keep bedding and clothing clean. This helps keep sick people comfortable and helps prevent skin problems. To clean clothing or sheets stained with blood, *diarrhea*, or other body fluids:

  - keep them separate from other household laundry.

  - hold an unstained part and rinse off any body fluids with water. Be especially careful if there are large amounts of blood, such as after childbirth.

  - wash the bedding and clothing in soapy water, hang to dry—if possible in the sun—and fold or iron as usual.

➤ *The following things are helpful but not necessary:*

- *Add bleach to the soapy water and soak 10 minutes before washing.*

- *Wear gloves or plastic bags on your hands.*

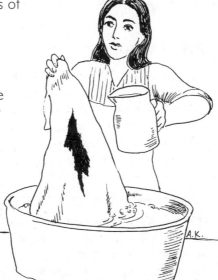

You will not get HIV from washing the clothes of an infected person if you follow the advice above.

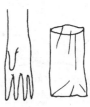

Staying Healthy for as Long as Possible

When a person has AIDS, the body's immune system is no longer able to fight off common infections and illnesses. The immune system gets weaker with each illness, making it even less able to fight infection the next time. This continues until the person's body is too weak to survive.

Preventing infections and illness is the best way to slow down the weakening of the immune system. It is also important to treat any infections to keep them from spreading or getting worse. This way a person with AIDS can stay healthy for as long as possible.

Preventing some infections with medicines

For persons with AIDS, regular use of the *antibiotic* co-trimoxazole may help prevent some kinds of *pneumonia* and diarrhea. You can start taking it as soon as you begin to fall ill from serious *lung* infections, diarrhea, and skin infections.

Take: co-trimoxazole 480 mg (80 mg trimethoprim and 400 mg sulfamethoxazole), 1 tablet by mouth daily, **or** 2 tablets by mouth 2 times a week. Drink a lot of water every day if you take co-trimoxazole.

IMPORTANT *Allergic reactions to co-trimoxazole are more common in persons with AIDS. Stop taking it if you get a new skin rash or any other sign of drug allergy. Taking antibiotics regularly usually causes problems with fungal infections of all kinds: in the mouth, on the skin, in the vagina. You may be able to prevent some of these infections by eating yogurt or sour milk products every day.*

Women will usually have more problems with *yeast infections* of the vagina when they take antibiotics. Eating yogurt or sour milk, or sitting in a bowl of water with yogurt or vinegar in it can help.

For more information on yeast infections of the vagina, see page 264; for yeast of the skin, see page 300; and for yeast of the mouth, see page 305.

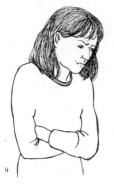

signs of anxiety and depression

MENTAL HEALTH

Good mental health is very important for staying healthy and avoiding illness. AIDS places a heavy stress on the mind and the emotions. Often people feel very afraid and tense (anxiety), or feel sadness or have no feelings at all (depression). Sometimes these feelings are so strong they cause physical signs. Anxiety and depression can also weaken the body and make a person more likely to get sick.

It is important to try to tell the difference between signs of illness that are caused by physical problems, and signs that are caused by anxiety or depression. Knowing the cause of a problem may make it easier to treat. It is also important to try and overcome these feelings so that they do not contribute to making a person with AIDS become sicker.

A person with AIDS can get sick very easily from many different common medical problems. The rest of this chapter has information about the most common of these problems and how an individual or family may care for them.

Just because someone has one of these problems does not mean she has AIDS. This information will be helpful to anyone suffering from one of these illnesses.

FEVER

Fevers often come and go. It is hard to know if the fever is from an infection that can be treated, like *tuberculosis*, *pelvic inflammatory disease (PID)*, or *malaria*, or if it is from HIV itself. If the fever is caused by an infection, then make sure the infection itself is also treated.

To check for fever, use a *thermometer*, or put the back of one hand on the sick person's forehead and the other on your own. If the sick person feels warmer, she probably has a fever.

Treatment:

- Remove extra clothing and let fresh air into the room.
- Cool the skin by pouring water over it, wiping the skin with wet cloths, or putting wet cloths on the chest and forehead and fanning them.
- Give plenty of liquids even if the person is not thirsty. With fever it is easy to become dehydrated (lose too much water).
- Take a medicine like paracetamol, aspirin, or ibuprofen to help reduce fever.
- Keep the skin clean and dry. Use lotion or corn starch to help prevent sores and rashes.

Get help when:

- the temperature is very high.
- the fever goes on for many days.
- there is coughing, difficulty breathing, and loss of weight.
- there is a stiff neck, severe pain, or sudden, severe diarrhea with the fever.
- the person with the fever is pregnant or recently had a baby, miscarriage, or *abortion*.
- the person is being treated for malaria, and the fever has not gone away after the first treatment.
- there is discharge from the vagina and pain in the belly with the fever.

Common Medical Problems

➤ *For the medical problems mentioned in this chapter, also see* **Where There Is No Doctor** *or another general medical book.*

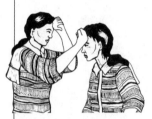

taking the temperature

pneumonia, 304
tuberculosis, 303 and 387
infection after abortion, 255
pelvic infection, 272

DIARRHEA

Diarrhea is passing 3 or more loose or watery stools in a day. Passing many normal stools is not the same as having diarrhea. Diarrhea may come and go and can be hard to cure. The most common causes of diarrhea in persons with AIDS are infections in the *intestines* from unclean food or water, infection because of HIV, or the *side effects* of some medicines.

Diarrhea can cause:

- *malnutrition*, if the food passes through the body so quickly that the body cannot use it. Also, people with diarrhea often do not eat because they are not hungry.

- **dehydration**, if the body loses more liquid in the stools than you take in. Dehydration happens faster in hot climates and in people who have fever.

Signs of dehydration:

- thirst
- little or no urine
- dry mouth
- loss of stretchiness of the skin
- feeling *dizzy* when standing up

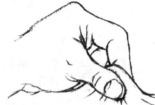

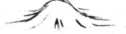

Lift the skin between two fingers...

...if the skin fold does not fall right back to normal, the person is dehydrated.

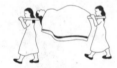

TRANSPORT!

IMPORTANT *If someone has these signs and is also vomiting, she needs liquids in the vein (IV) or in the rectum (see page 537). Get medical help fast. Severe dehydration is an emergency.*

Treatment:

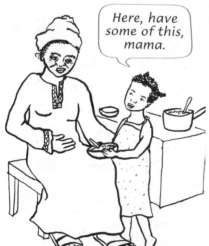

Here, have some of this, mama.

- **Prevent dehydration by drinking more liquids than usual.** Fruit juices, coconut milk, sweetened weak tea, gruel, soup, rice water, and rehydration drink (see page 536) are good for fighting dehydration. Even if the person does not feel thirsty, she should still sip something every 5 to 10 minutes.

- **Keep eating.** Try to eat small amounts of foods that are easy for the body to digest. Cook food well, and then mash and grind it. Some good foods are cereals mixed with beans, meat, or fish; dairy products, such as milk, cheese and yogurt; and bananas. Do not eat uncooked vegetables, whole grains, fruit peels, hot peppers, or food or drink with a lot of sugar. These make diarrhea worse.

Take medicine only for these kinds of diarrhea:

- Sudden, severe diarrhea with fever (with or without blood in the stool). Take co-trimoxazole 480 mg (80 mg trimethoprim and 400 mg sulfamethoxazole), 2 tablets twice a day for 10 days. If you are allergic to sulfa drugs, take norfloxacin instead, 400 mg, one time only. If you are no better after 2 days, see a health worker.
- Bloody diarrhea without fever, which can be caused by amoebas (tiny animals that live in water or in the intestines). Take metronidazole 500 mg, 3 times a day for 7 days. If you are not better after 2 days, see a health worker.
- **When someone has diarrhea for a long time,** she may get a red, sore area around the *anus*. It may help to apply petroleum gel or zinc oxide cream each time after passing stool. The person may also get piles *(hemorrhoids).*

➤ *If you are pregnant or breastfeeding, do not take norfloxacin. For more information about these medicines, see the "Green Pages."*

70

piles

Get help if the person:

- has the signs of dehydration (see page 298).
- cannot eat or drink as usual.
- does not seem to be getting better no matter what she does.
- has a high fever.
- passes many watery stools in a day.
- passes bloody stools that do not go away with medicine.
- is also vomiting.

Prevention:

- **Drink clean water.** Purify your water before using it in food or drink.
- **Eat clean, safe food.** Make sure raw foods are washed or peeled, and that meat is well cooked. Protect food from dirt, flies, crawling insects and animals, which can give you germs.
- **Always wash your hands:**
  - after using or helping someone use the *latrine* or toilet.
  - after cleaning soiled children or sick people.
  - before making food or drink.
- **Protect your community's water source.**

clean water, 155

safe food, 156

washing your hands, 522

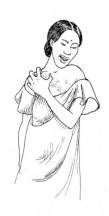

SKIN RASHES AND ITCHING

It is often difficult to know what causes skin rashes and itching. Many skin problems can be helped by keeping the body clean. Try to wash once a day with mild soap and clean water.

If the skin becomes too dry, wash less often and do not use soap. Try rubbing petroleum gel, glycerin, or vegetable oils into the skin after bathing. Wear loose cotton clothing.

Allergic reactions

Allergic reactions, which often cause an itchy rash, are more common in people with AIDS. Medicines that contain sulfa (like co-trimoxazole) may cause especially bad reactions. If you are using these medicines and you get an itchy rash, itchy eyes, vomiting or dizziness, **stop taking them immediately** and see a health worker. She may be able to give you a non-sulfa medicine that will work.

Fungal infections (yeast, candida)

Fungal infections are difficult to describe because they can look like many different things. Some fungal infections look like round, red, or scaly patches that itch. Women with AIDS can also get frequent yeast infections in the vagina.

You may have a fungal infection if you have a skin problem in one of these areas:

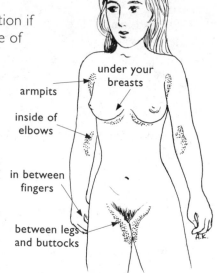

under your breasts

armpits

inside of elbows

in between fingers

between legs and buttocks

Treatment:

- If you have red, itchy patches, keep the area clean and dry. If possible, keep the area uncovered and open to the air and sunlight.

- Apply nystatin cream 3 times a day or Gentian Violet 2 times a day until the rash is completely gone.

- If you have a very bad fungal infection, taking ketoconazole by mouth may help. Take one 200 mg tablet each day for 10 days (but do not take this medicine if you are pregnant).

Brown or purple patches on the mouth or skin

These patches are caused by a cancer of the blood vessels or *lymph nodes* called Kaposi's sarcoma. Medicines are not helpful. If you are having problems, like difficulty eating because of patches in your mouth, see a health worker.

Itching

Treatment without medicines:

- Cool the skin or fan it.
- Avoid heat and hot water on the skin.
- Avoid scratching, which causes more itching and sometimes infection. Cut the fingernails short and keep them clean to avoid infection.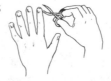
- Use cool cloths soaked in water from boiled and strained oatmeal, or plant medicines from local healers.

These can also help itching:

- tincture of tea tree from Australia
- juice from aloe vera plants

Treatment with medicines (use any one of these):

- Apply calamine lotion with a clean cloth as needed.
- Apply small amounts of 1% hydrocortisone cream or ointment 3 times a day.
- Take an antihistamine, such as diphenhydramine or hydroxyzine, by mouth. Take 25 mg 4 times a day. Antihistamines may make you sleepy.

➤ *Antihistamines should be used with caution by women who are pregnant or breastfeeding (see the "Green Pages").*

Herpes zoster (shingles)

Shingles is an infection caused by a herpes virus. It usually begins as a painful rash with blisters, which may then break open. It is most common on the face, back, and chest. The area may burn and be very painful. The rash may start to heal in a few weeks, but the pain may last longer.

Treatment:

- Apply calamine lotion 2 times a day to help with pain and itching.
- Keep sores dry. Cover with a loose bandage if clothing rubs the sores.
- To prevent infection, apply Gentian Violet liquid. If the sores do become infected, see page 307.
- Pain medicine is often needed (see page 482).
- The medicine acyclovir may help.

Do not touch your eyes because shingles can damage your eyesight and can cause blindness.

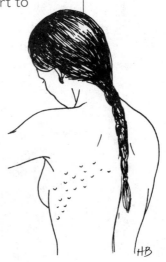

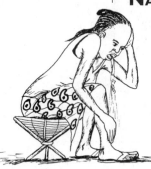

NAUSEA AND VOMITING

If nausea and vomiting prevent a person from eating or drinking, she can become weak, malnourished, and dehydrated. For some people nausea or vomiting may go on day after day. Nausea and vomiting may be caused by:

- infections.
- some medicines.
- problems with the *stomach* and intestines.
- HIV infection itself.

Treatment:

- Take small bites of dry food (bread, crackers, chapati, tortilla) when you wake up in the morning.
- Try to avoid the smell of food as it cooks. If a food or smell seems to cause nausea, avoid that food.
- Drink small amounts of mint, ginger, or cinnamon tea.
- Lick a lemon.
- Clean the teeth and rinse the mouth often to get rid of the bad taste after *vomiting*.
- Let fresh air into the house or room often.
- Soak a cloth in cool water and put it on the forehead.
- If the problem is caused by a medicine, see if another medicine can be used instead.

other medicines

If vomiting is severe:

1. Do not drink or eat for 2 hours.
2. Then, for the next 2 hours, sip 3 tablespoons of water, rehydration drink, or other clear liquid every hour. Slowly increase the amount of liquid to 4 to 6 tablespoonfuls every hour. If the person does not vomit, keep increasing the amount of liquid.

rehydration drink

4. If the person cannot stop vomiting, use promethazine 25 mg to 50 mg every 6 hours as needed.
5. As nausea gets better, start to eat small amounts of food again. Start with plain foods such as bread, rice, *cassava*, or porridge.

When to get help:

- The person cannot keep any food or drink in her body for 24 hours.
- The person vomiting has pain in the belly or a high fever.
- The vomiting is very strong, it is dark green or dark brown, it smells like stool, or has blood in it.
- The person has signs of dehydration.

COUGH

Coughing is the body's way of cleaning the breathing system and getting rid of *mucus*. Coughing is also a common sign of lung problems, such as pneumonia or tuberculosis. The lungs make more mucus when they are irritated or infected.

When a cough produces mucus, do not take medicine to stop the cough. Instead, do something to help loosen and bring up the mucus. This will make the cough heal faster.

Treatment:

- Drink lots of water. Water is better than any medicine. It loosens the mucus so you can cough it up more easily.

- Cough several times during the day to clear the lungs. Be sure to cover your mouth.

- Keep active by walking, or by turning in bed and sitting up. This helps the mucus come out of the lungs.

- Soothe the throat by drinking tea with lemon and honey, or your own herbal remedy. Cough syrups that you buy are more expensive and no more helpful.

- If the cough is very bad and keeps you awake at night, take codeine, 30 mg, or codeine cough syrup (see page 497).

IMPORTANT *If you cough up yellow, green, or bloody mucus, the cough could be caused by pneumonia or TB, and you will need special medicines (see the next page).*

➤ *DO NOT smoke if you have a cough.*

➤ *Persons with AIDS often get pneumonia or TB. For more information, see below and the next page.*

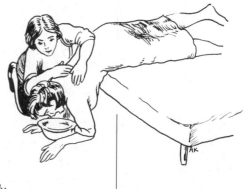

Have someone hit you on the back of the chest (postural drainage). This can make it easier to cough up the mucus.

Tuberculosis (TB)

Tuberculosis (TB) is a serious infection caused by a germ that usually affects the lungs. The signs of AIDS and TB are similar, but they are different diseases. **Most men, women, and children with TB do not have AIDS.**

But someone with AIDS can get TB very easily because the person's body is too weak to fight it. In 1 out of every 3 people who die from AIDS, it is TB that actually kills them.

A woman infected with HIV/AIDS is even more likely to get TB if her body is also weak from many pregnancies, poor nutrition and weak blood *(anemia)*.

TB can be cured, even in persons with AIDS, so it is important to get treatment early. **But people with AIDS should never take thiacetazone for TB.** For complete information, see the chapter on "Tuberculosis," page 387.

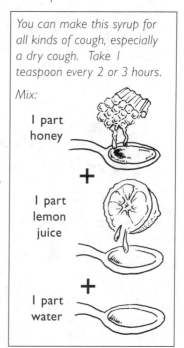

You can make this syrup for all kinds of cough, especially a dry cough. Take 1 teaspoon every 2 or 3 hours.

Mix:

1 part honey

+

1 part lemon juice

+

1 part water

Pneumonia

Pneumonia is caused by germs that infect the small breathing tubes deep in the lungs. Old people and very sick or weak people often get pneumonia.

Pneumonia can be very serious for people with AIDS. It should be treated with antibiotics right away. Sometimes pneumonia must be treated in the hospital with medicines in the vein (IV).

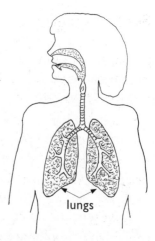

lungs

Signs:

- Breaths are small and fast (more than 30 breaths a minute in an adult). Sometimes the nostrils open wide with each breath.
- You feel as if you cannot get enough air.
- You have a sudden, often high, fever.
- You cough up mucus that is green, rust-colored, or bloody.
- You feel very ill.

Treatment:

- Take co-trimoxazole for 10 days or more (see the "Green Pages").
- Drink plenty of liquids.
- Try to bring the fever down.
- If you are no better in 24 hours or if you are getting worse, get medical help right away.

PROBLEMS WITH THE MOUTH AND THROAT

Problems with the mouth, or with other parts of the body that food passes through, can keep a person from eating normally. She may then become weak, malnourished, and have a harder time fighting infections. She should try to:

- eat small amounts of food often.
- add vegetable oil or groundnut paste (peanut butter) to foods to give more energy.
- avoid uncooked vegetables. They are hard for the body to digest and may have germs.
- drink a lot of liquids and watch for dehydration.

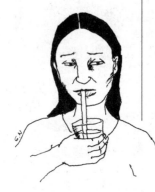

Using a straw to drink can help with painful mouth problems.

Soreness in the mouth and throat

Many people with AIDS have soreness in the mouth, and problems with their teeth and gums. Try to:
- eat soft foods—not hard or crunchy foods.
- eat plain foods—not spicy foods.
- use a straw to drink liquids and soups.
- try cold foods, drinks, or ice to help ease pain.

Sores, cracks, and blisters around the mouth

Painful blisters and sores (also called *cold sores* or fever blisters) on the lips can be caused by the *herpes* virus. A healthy person can get these sores after a cold or fever. Someone with AIDS can get these sores at any time. The sores may last a long time, but they usually go away on their own. To help prevent infection, apply Gentian Violet to the sores. A medicine called acyclovir may also help (see the "Green Pages"). Wash your hands after touching the sores.

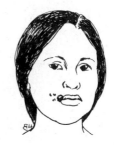

➤ *Cracks and sores in the corner of the mouth can also be caused by malnutrition.*

White patches in the mouth (thrush)

Thrush is a fungal infection that causes white patches and soreness on the skin inside the mouth, on the tongue, and sometimes down the tube that connects the mouth and stomach (esophagus). This can cause pain in the chest.

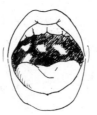

The patches look like milk curds stuck to the cheek or tongue. If the patches can be scraped off, it is probably thrush. Thrush happens more often when someone is taking antibiotics.

Treatment:

Gently scrub the tongue and gums with a soft toothbrush or clean cloth 3 or 4 times a day. Then rinse the mouth with salt water or lemon water and spit it out (do not swallow). In addition, use any ONE of these remedies:

1. Suck a lemon if it is not too painful. The acid slows the growth of the fungus. **Or,**

2. Rinse the mouth with 1% Gentian Violet liquid 2 times a day. Do not swallow. **Or,**

3. Put 1 ml of nystatin solution in the mouth and hold it there 1 minute and then swallow it. Do this 3 or 4 times a day for 5 days. **Or,**

4. If thrush is very bad, ketoconazole may help. Take one 200 mg tablet, 2 times a day for 14 days (but do not take this medicine if you are pregnant).

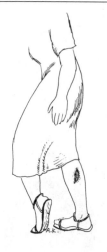

WOUNDS AND SORES

Wounds are caused by an injury that breaks the skin. Sores are often caused by *bacteria* or pressure on the skin *(pressure sores)*. They can happen very easily to people who stay in bed a long time. Take special care of any cut, wound, or open sore so that it does not become infected.

General care of open wounds and sores:

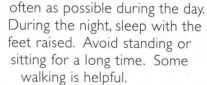

1. Wash the wound or sore with clean water and mild soap at least once a day. Wash around the edge of the wound first, then wash from the center out to the edges. If possible, use separate pieces of cloth for each wipe.

2. If the wound has pus or blood in it, cover the area with a clean piece of cloth or bandage. Leave the bandage loose, and change it every day. If the wound is dry, it can be left open to the air. It will heal more quickly that way.

3. If the wound is on the legs or feet, raise the leg above the level of the heart. Do this as often as possible during the day. During the night, sleep with the feet raised. Avoid standing or sitting for a long time. Some walking is helpful.

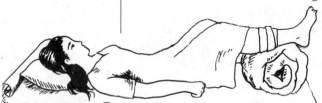

4. Wash soiled cloth and bandages in soap and water, then put them in the sun to dry. Or boil them for a short time and hang them to dry. If the cloths and bandages will not be used again, burn them or throw them in a pit latrine.

Home treatments for pressure sores

Papaya (paw paw): This fruit contains *chemicals* that help make the old flesh in a pressure sore soft and easy to remove.

Soak a sterile cloth or piece of gauze in the 'milk' that comes from the trunk or green fruit of a papaya plant. Pack this into the sore. Repeat this 3 times a day.

Honey and sugar: These will kill germs, help prevent infection, and speed healing. Mix honey and sugar together into a thick paste. Press this deep into the sore, and cover with a thick, clean cloth or *gauze* bandage. (Molasses or thin pieces of raw sugar can also be used.)

IMPORTANT *Clean out and refill the sore at least 2 times a day. If the honey or sugar becomes too filled with liquid from the sore, it will feed germs rather than kill them. For more information on pressure sores see page 142.*

Treatment of open wounds and sores that are infected:

Wounds and sores are infected if they:
- become red, swollen, hot, and painful.
- have pus in them.
- begin to smell bad.

Treat the infected area as in steps 1 through 4 on the previous page, **and** also do the following:

1. Put a hot *compress* over the wound 4 times a day for 20 minutes each time. Or try to soak the wound in a bucket of hot water with soap or potassium permanganate in the water. Use one teaspoon of potassium permanganate to 4 or 5 liters (or quarts) of water. When you are not soaking the infected part, keep it raised up above the level of the heart.

2. If part of the wound looks gray or rotten, rinse it with hydrogen peroxide after soaking it. Try to pick off the gray parts with a clean piece of gauze or tweezers that have been properly cleaned.

3. If you can, put Gentian Violet on the wound before putting on the dressing.

4. If there are many infected sores at the same time, especially with a fever, treat with antibiotics. Use erythromycin, dicloxacillin or penicillin for 10 days (see the "Green Pages").

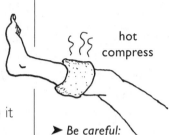

hot compress

➤ *Be careful:*
If you use too much potassium permanganate or very hot water, you will burn the skin.

Treatment of closed wounds that are infected (abscesses and boils):

Abscesses and boils are raised, red, painful lumps on the skin. They are most common in the *groin* and armpits, and on the *buttocks*, back, and upper legs.

If you notice a lump, start using warm compresses right away for 20 minutes, 4 times a day. Often this will make the lump open and the pus inside will come out. Keep applying clean, warm cloths until the pus stops coming out and the area begins to heal. Cover the lump with a loose, clean bandage. If it becomes too large and painful, see a health worker who has been trained to drain abcesses using sterile equipment.

When to get help:

See a health worker trained to treat the signs of AIDS if you have a wound and:
- a fever.
- a red area around the wound is getting bigger.

Get medical help if you have a wound and:
- you can feel swollen *glands* in your neck, groin, or armpits.
- the wound has a bad smell, or brown or gray liquid comes out, or it turns black and bubbles, or blisters form. This could be gangrene.
- you are taking antibiotics and not getting better.

MENTAL CONFUSION (DEMENTIA)

Some mental confusion or mental change is common among people with AIDS, especially if a person has been sick for a long time. These changes may be caused by HIV infection in the brain, by other infections, by depression, or by the side effects of a medicine (see page 478).

PAIN

In the later stages of AIDS (and other serious illnesses like cancer), pain may become a part of daily life. Pain can be caused by many things, such as:

- not being able to move.
- pressure sores (see page 142).
- swelling of the legs and feet.
- infections, like herpes.
- headache.
- nerve pains.

Treatment for pain, without medicines:

- Try relaxation exercises, meditation, or prayer (see page 423).
- Try to think about other things.
- Play music, or have someone read aloud or tell stories.
- For pain from swelling in the hands and feet, try raising the swollen part.
- For a burning feeling in the hands and feet caused by nerve pain, put the body part in water.
- For skin that hurts to touch, line the bed with soft covers and pillows or animal skins. Be gentle when touching the person.

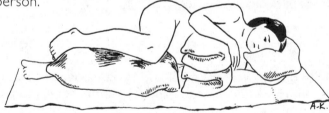

- For headache, keep the room dark and quiet.
- Acupressure may help some kinds of pain (see page 542).

Treatment for pain, with medicines:

The following medicines may be used to control pain that comes day after day (chronic pain). Take the medicines regularly, according to instructions. If you wait until the pain has become very bad, the medicines will not work as well.

- mild pain medicine, like paracetamol
- ibuprofen—if you need something stronger
- codeine—if the pain is very bad

➤ *Pain medicines work best if you take them before the pain gets very bad.*

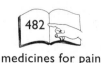

482

medicines for pain

At some point there is nothing more that can be done for a person with AIDS. You may know this time has come when:

- the body starts to fail.
- medical treatment is no longer effective or is not available.
- the person says she is ready to die.

If the sick person wants to remain at home, you can help her die with dignity by:

- giving comfort.
- having family and friends stay with her.
- allowing her to make decisions.
- helping her prepare for death. It may help her to talk about death, about fears of dying, and about worries for the family's future. It does not help to act as if she is not dying. Assure her that you will do what you can to prevent pain and discomfort. Talk about funeral arrangements if she wishes.

Caring for Someone Who Is Near Death

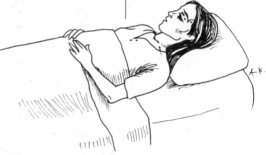

As she nears death, she may be unconscious, stop eating, breathe very slowly or very fast and unevenly, stop passing urine, or lose control of passing urine or stool.

Care of the body of someone who has died of AIDS

The AIDS virus can live up to 24 hours in a person's body after death. During that time, take the same precautions with the body as you did when the person was alive (see page 295).

AIDS IS EVERYONE'S PROBLEM

It is important that everyone in the community know how AIDS is spread and how to prevent it. But this information will not help them unless they also realize that AIDS can happen to anyone—even them. If people think that AIDS can not touch them, they will not act to prevent infection.

Placing the blame on any group of people (such as sex workers, homosexuals, or drug users) makes others think that only that group is at risk. It is true that some people, like sex workers, may be more likely to get AIDS (because their work requires that they have sex with many men). But everyone— especially young women—is at risk for AIDS. And every person in the community needs to take responsibility for fighting it.

It is also important to remember to fight against the conditions that lead to the spread of AIDS, and not against the people who have AIDS.

Working for Change

➤ *Fight AIDS, not the people who have it.*

How you can help prevent AIDS

In the community

Education is one of the main ways a community can work to keep AIDS from spreading. Here are some ideas:

- Train girls and women to work as peer educators. They can talk with others alone or in groups to help girls and women understand their bodies and sexuality, and gain the self-confidence and skills to demand safer sex.
- Tell the truth about women's risk of AIDS. Help people see that AIDS has roots in poverty and in women's lack of control over their sexual relations.
- Use theater and media to help women feel it is OK to know about and to prevent AIDS. For example, use a play or comic book to show that 'good' girls or women can discuss AIDS with their partners, or can buy condoms and ask their husbands or boyfriends to use them.

sexual health

Train men as outreach workers. They can go to the places where men gather and talk to them about AIDS.

At the same time, you can show different ideas about what it means to be a man or a woman. Help people question the idea that men should have many sex partners and that women should be passive about sex. Show how these ideas are dangerous to both men's and women's health.

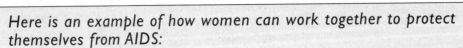

- Help parents, teachers, and other adult role models become more comfortable talking about sex and AIDS with young people.
- Make sure that all people have access to information and sexual health services, including condoms, to keep AIDS from spreading in the community.
- Bring education about AIDS to community meeting places—like bars, schools, religious meetings, and military bases.

Here is an example of how women can work together to protect themselves from AIDS:

To help fight the spread of AIDS, the women of Palestina, a small town in northeastern Brazil, began a 'sex strike'. After women in the community learned that a man infected with HIV had unsafe sex with at least two women in the town, they decided to stop having sex with their husbands and boyfriends. They demanded that their partners take the test for HIV before they would begin to have sex again and then insisted upon safer sex practices.

The women will now demand safer sex and proof of an HIV test before they have sexual relations with a partner. One woman said, "If he won't practice safer sex, we won't go together anymore."

If you are a health worker

Health workers can play a very important role in helping to stop the spread of AIDS. You can do this if you:

- give information about how AIDS is spread and how it is not spread to **every** person you see—especially if they already have other STDs.

- encourage both men and women to use condoms, even if they are already using another form of family planning.

- use precautions against HIV infection with every person you see. Since most people with HIV appear healthy, it is best to act as if everyone you care for is HIV-infected. Any time you have to cut the skin or touch body fluids, follow the advice on page 295. This includes any time you must give an injection, stitch skin or tissue, help with childbirth, or examine a woman's vagina.

- make health services private, confidential, and accessible to all members of the community, including young people.

- invite someone from a regional AIDS organization to meet with health workers in your area. He or she can help you learn about the best ways to treat the infections that people with AIDS often get. Discuss the other problems that people with AIDS face. Try to decide how you can help people using the resources you have, and think about where you might find more resources to help meet people's needs. If health workers can work together and share resources, they will not have to confront this huge problem alone.

➤ *If every health worker can offer the same information and services, it will save people time, money, and energy because they will not have to search for the best treatment.*

Fight the fear and negative attitudes that many people have about AIDS

A good way to begin is to plan a meeting with other health workers in your area to discuss AIDS. Help all the health workers learn about AIDS so they will be able to provide accurate, consistent information to the people in their communities. If all health workers can give the same information, it will help prevent the fear caused by wrong ideas about AIDS. With less fear from their neighbors, people with AIDS—as well as those who care for them—can become more accepted in the community. Then they can help others understand every person's real risk of getting AIDS.

A health worker's sympathy and compassion can also help others change their attitudes toward people with AIDS. Then she can fight HIV/AIDS together with the community.

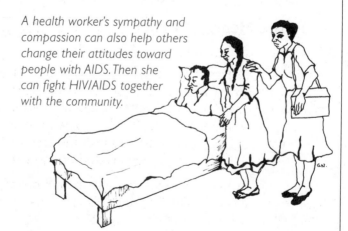

Chapter 18

In this chapter:

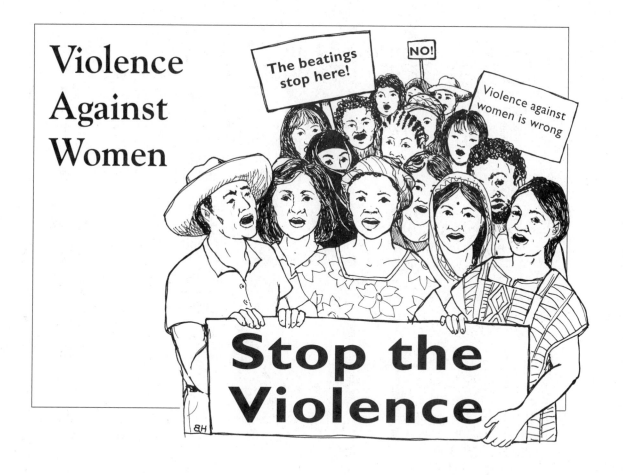

Violence Against Women

The beatings stop here!

NO!

Violence against women is wrong

Stop the Violence

Every day, women are slapped, kicked, beaten, humiliated, threatened, sexually *abused*, and even murdered by their partners. But often we do not hear about this violence, because the women who are abused may feel ashamed, alone, and afraid to speak out. Many doctors, nurses, and health workers do not recognize violence as the serious health problem it is.

This chapter is about the violence that occurs between a woman and her male partner. It can help you understand why violence happens, what you can do about it, and how you can work for change in your community.

➤ *There is no reason why a person should be beaten or abused in any way.*

rape by someone the woman knows

Although this chapter talks about violence between a woman and a man, violence can happen in any close relationship: for example, between a mother-in-law and her son's new wife, between parents and their children, between an older and younger child, between family members and an older person living in the home, and between partners of the same sex.

The Story of Laura and Luís

Luís was 12 years older than Laura and was already a successful merchant when they met. He sold his goods to the store where Laura worked as a clerk to help her family pay the rent. Luís was charming and would talk about the kind of life they could have together. He told Laura he would buy her anything she wanted and she would be his "best woman." He often bought her new clothes that he liked to admire her in, telling her how pretty she would be if she stopped dressing the way she did. He eventually began to see her every day, and soon asked her to quit her job and marry him.

After they married, Laura expected Luís to keep his promises. Instead, things began to change. He would not allow her to go out, because she "looked so ugly." In fact, he took all the beautiful clothes he had bought her and burned them, saying, "That stupid, ugly woman didn't deserve such clothes."

One day Luís came home in the middle of the day and tore all the clean wash down from the line, accusing Laura of sleeping with his friend. When she said that she had just gone to visit her mother, Luís called her a lying whore and hit her. He said she would not go to visit her family—they did not want her either. He never said anything more about it, but when he came home later that night, he brought her a present and told her how much he loved her and wanted to take care of her.

When Laura got pregnant, she thought Luís would start treating her better. But it seemed to give him more excuses to hurt her. When he got angry, he started hitting and kicking her in the stomach. She was terrified she would lose the baby, but she had no place to go. She believed Luís when he said her family did not want her, and besides, she had no money of her own. There were times when Luís would go several weeks without losing control, and Laura would convince herself that everything was OK. He really did love her, after all. If only she could learn how to avoid setting him off. She would try even harder than before, but nothing helped.

Through the years, Luís drank too much, threw her against walls, and would force her to have sex even when her body ached from his beatings. Laura awoke one night to find him holding a knife to her throat. The next day, he told her she was imagining things, that she was crazy. He always said that if she told anyone "lies" about him he would kill her. She didn't tell anyone and she went out as little as possible. She hated the thought of anyone seeing her bruises and knowing what he did to her. Laura often thought about leaving, but she did not know where to go.

After 12 years of being his wife, not only was Laura afraid of what he would do to her, but without him she would have no home, no money, no father for her children. Luís had said bad things about her to the people at the store where she used to work, and she knew that, because of her children, no one would take her in as a domestic servant. Laura felt so alone.

Laura's father was dead now and her mother lived with her brother's family. They did not have room for her and her children. Her sister was deeply religious and told Laura it was her duty to stay with her husband, even if she were killed. "That is the way it is meant to be." She had so much work to do at home she was always busy. And since Luís got mad when she went out or when someone came to visit, Laura stopped seeing her friends. She was sure they had long since given up on her. Besides, most people thought that it was okay for men to 'punish' their wives.

Then came the night when Laura's oldest daughter was 11. She came to Laura crying, saying Luís had hurt her "down there." Laura was shocked. She had thought the children would not be affected by Luís' behavior. She knew it would do no good to confront him, but she would NOT let it happen again.

When Laura lost her last pregnancy, the health worker who examined her asked about her injuries. Laura had made some excuse. The health worker nodded her head and gave Laura a card with an address in the next town. She told her if Laura ever needed to leave, she and her children could go there, but to make sure that she was ready to leave when she did. Laura was ready now.

Why did Luís hit Laura? These are some of the wrong ideas that people have:

A man can do whatever he wants to his wife.

The truth: No man has the right to beat his wife. Nothing a woman does gives a man the right to hurt her, even if he thinks she deserves it—even if she herself thinks she deserves it.

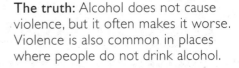
It's just because he drinks...

The truth: Alcohol does not cause violence, but it often makes it worse. Violence is also common in places where people do not drink alcohol.

He wouldn't beat her if he didn't love her so much.

The truth: Beating is not a sign of love. Love means showing respect and kindness.

It's their business. It's not right to interfere with the private affairs of a couple.

The truth: Violence is not just a family matter. Many women are hurt or killed. Violence is a social and community health problem.

Only poor, ignorant men beat their wives.

The truth: Violence is not just a problem of poverty or ignorance. Violence can happen in any home: rich or poor, educated or less educated, in the city or in rural areas.

It is best for the children if she stays with him. He can still be a good father to them.

The truth: It is not always better for the family when a woman stays with a violent man. He is teaching the children terrible, wrong ways to deal with their feelings, and about how women should be treated. He is not being good to his children if he is beating their mother—or them.

Why Does a Man Hurt a Woman?

➤ *These reasons may explain why a man abuses his wife, but they do not give him permission to do so.*

➤ *Violent or abusive relationships often happen when one person has more power over the other.*

sex and gender roles

A man may offer many excuses for hurting a woman—that he was drunk, that he lost control, or that she 'deserved it'. But a man **chooses** to use violence because it is a way he can get what he needs or what he feels is rightfully his as a man.

When a man does not feel that he has power over his own life, he may use violence to try and control another person's life. It is natural for someone to want to control his or her own life in normal ways, but it is wrong to try and control someone else's life, especially with violence. Here are some of the reasons why some men hurt women:

1. **Violence works.**
   - It offers the man a quick end to a disagreement without having to talk about the real problem or find a real solution.
   - A man may find the fight exciting, and have lots of energy afterward. He may want to have these feelings again.
   - If a man uses violence, he 'wins' and gets his way. The victim is likely to give him his way again the next time to avoid being hurt. This gives the man even more power.

2. **The man has a wrong idea about what it means to be a man.**
   - If a man believes that to be a man, he must control what a woman does, he may feel it is OK to hurt her.
   - Some men think that they have a 'right' to certain things— to a 'good' wife, to sons, to making all the decisions in the family—just because they are men.

3. **The man feels that the woman belongs to him, or that he needs her.**
   - If the woman is 'strong', the man may feel afraid that he will lose her, or that she does not need him. He will take steps to make her more dependent on him.

4. **He does not know any other way to be.**
   - If a man has seen his father or other people in his life react with violence when life is difficult and stressful, then he may have never learned any other way to behave.

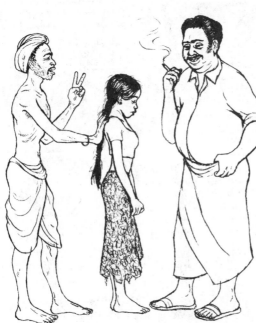

If men think of women and girls as their property—something they own—they are more likely to feel as though it is their right to treat them however they want.

There are many different ways that a man tries to gain power over a woman. Beating is only one of them. But all of them can hurt a woman.

Imagine that the circle below is a wheel. Power and control are at the center of the wheel because they are the reasons behind all of the actions. Each section of the wheel is a behavior that a violent man may use to control a woman. Violence is the rim of the wheel—what holds it together and gives it strength.

Kinds of Violence

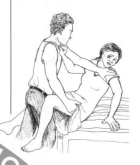

VIOLENCE

Emotional Abuse
The man insults the woman, puts her down, or makes her think she is going crazy.

Sexual Abuse
The man makes the woman do sexual things against her will, or physically attacks the sexual parts of her body. He treats her like an object.

VIOLENCE

Isolation
The man controls everything the woman does—who she sees and talks to, and where she goes.

Controlling Money
The man tries to keep the woman from getting a job or making her own money. He makes her ask him for any money she needs. Or he may force her to work and then take the money she earns.

Power and Control

Making Threats
The man uses a look, action, tone of voice, or makes threats, that make the woman feel afraid that he will hurt her.

Because he is a 'Man'
The man uses the fact that he is a man as an excuse to treat the woman like a servant. He makes all the decisions and tells her that, as a woman, she has no right to object.

Using Children
The man uses the children to make the woman feel guilty, or to hurt her.

Blaming Her
The man says that the abuse did not really happen, that it was not serious, or that it was the woman's fault.

VIOLENCE

VIOLENCE

One form of abuse often turns into another

In many cases, verbal abuse becomes physical abuse after a while. It may not seem like it at first, but the man may slowly begin to 'accidentally' push or bump the woman, or begin to sit down in the place the woman usually sits, so that she has to move. If this behavior works for him, it may get worse until he becomes violent. Not all women who suffer other forms of abuse are beaten, but all women who have been beaten have suffered from other forms of abuse.

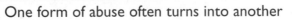

Warning Signs

➤ *It does not matter how much you love a person. Love cannot change someone. Only that person can choose to change himself.*

When an abusive relationship becomes violent, it is much harder to leave. The longer a woman stays, the more control the man has over her, and the less faith she may have in herself. Some men are more likely to become violent than others. There are certain signs that may mean a man will become violent. If you see these signs, and have a way to get out of the relationship, think carefully.

Ask yourself these questions:

• Does he act jealous when you see other people, or accuse you of lying to him? If you find you change your behavior to keep him from acting jealous, then he is controlling you.

• Does he try to keep you from seeing your friends and family, or from doing things on your own? It does not matter what reason he uses. He is trying to keep you from having their support. It will be easier for him to abuse you if you have nowhere else to go.

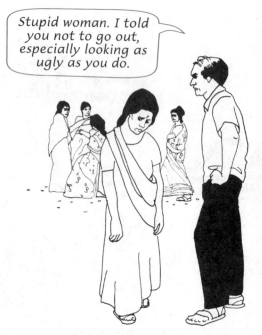

Stupid woman. I told you not to go out, especially looking as ugly as you do.

• Does he insult you or make fun of you in front of other people? You may start to believe what he says. This can make you feel as though you deserve to be treated badly.

• What does he do when he gets angry? Does he break or throw things? Has he ever physically hurt you or threatened to hurt you? Has he ever hit another woman? All of these things show that he has trouble controlling the way he acts.

• Does he feel insulted by people with authority, such as his teachers, bosses, or his father? He may feel he has no power. This can make him try to gain power over other people in other areas of his life by using violence.

• Does he claim that alcohol, drugs, or *stress* are the reasons he acts the way he does? If he puts the blame on something else, he may say things will get better if he gets a new job, moves to a new town, or stops using drugs or alcohol.

• Does he blame you or someone else for the way he acts, or deny that he is doing anything wrong? He is less likely to want to change himself if he thinks that the way he acts is your fault.

Some women are more likely to be abused

In many couples, the man becomes violent for the first time when the woman is pregnant. He may feel as though he is losing control because he cannot control the changes in her body. He may feel angry because she is paying more attention to the baby and less to him, or because she may not want to have sex with him. Also, many couples feel extra worried about money when they are expecting a new baby.

Women with disabilities are also more likely to be abused:

- Some men may feel angry that they did not get a 'perfect' woman.
- Men may think a woman with a disability is easier to control because she may be less able to defend herself.

The Cycle of Violence

The first violent attack often seems like an isolated event. But in many cases, after the violence first happens the following pattern, or cycle, develops:

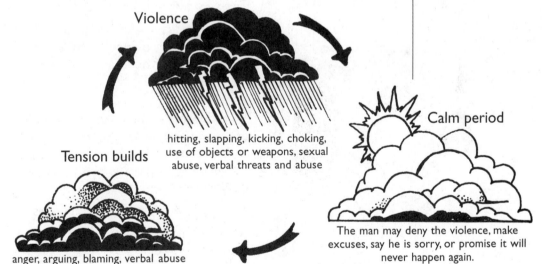

Violence

hitting, slapping, kicking, choking, use of objects or weapons, sexual abuse, verbal threats and abuse

Tension builds

anger, arguing, blaming, verbal abuse

Calm period

The man may deny the violence, make excuses, say he is sorry, or promise it will never happen again.

➤ *Some women try to make the violence happen so that it will be over with more quickly, and to get to the calm period sooner.*

As the violence goes on, the calm period gets shorter and shorter for many couples. As the woman's will is broken, the man's control over her becomes so complete that it is no longer necessary for him to make promises that things will get better.

Harmful Effects of Violence

413
mental health

STDs, 261
AIDS, 283
lack of desire, 193

When a woman is abused at home, her children believe that this is how girls and women should be treated.

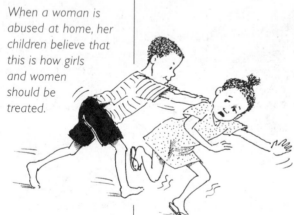

Violence not only hurts women. It also affects their children, and the whole community.

Women

In women, men's violence can cause:

- lack of motivation or lack of a sense of self-worth.
- mental health problems, like *anxiety* and problems eating and sleeping. As a way to cope with the violence, women may begin harmful or reckless behavior—such as using drugs or alcohol, or having many sex partners.
- serious pain and injuries: broken bones, burns, black eyes, cuts, bruises, as well as headaches, belly pain, and muscle pains that may continue for many years after the abuse happens.
- sexual health problems. Many women suffer *miscarriages* from being beaten during pregnancy. They may also suffer from unwanted pregnancies, *sexually transmitted diseases (STDs)* or *HIV/AIDS* as a result of sexual abuse. Sexual abuse often also leads to a fear of having sex, pain during sex, and lack of desire.
- death.

Children

In children, seeing their mothers abused can often cause:

- angry or aggressive behavior—copying the violence. Or they may become very quiet and withdraw to escape notice.
- nightmares and other fears. Children in abusive families often do not eat well, grow and learn more slowly than other children, and have many illnesses, like stomach aches, headaches, and *asthma*.
- injury and death if the violence is turned on them.

Community

In a community, violence can cause:

- the cycle of violence to continue into new generations.
- the continued false belief that men are better than women.
- everyone's quality of life to suffer because women take part less in their communities when they are silenced or killed by the violence.

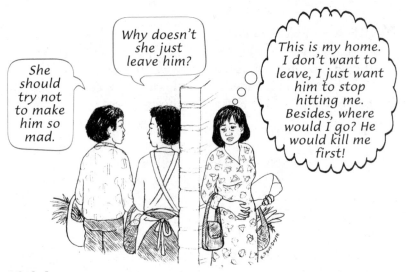

➤ If we ask why she does not leave, it says that we think the violence is her personal problem to solve. The whole community needs to be responsible for the health and well-being of every person in that community.

"**W**hy does she stay?" is the first question most people ask when they hear about a woman who is being abused. There are many reasons why a woman might choose to stay in an abusive relationship. They include:

- **fear and threats.** The man may have told her, "I will kill you, kill the children, kill your mother... if you try to leave." She may feel she is doing everything she can to protect herself and others by staying.

- **no money, and no place to go.** This is especially true if he has controlled all the money and not allowed her to see her family and friends.

- **no protection.** There may be nothing to stop him from coming after her and killing her.

- **shame.** She may feel the violence is somehow her fault, or that she deserves it.

- **religious or cultural beliefs.** She may feel it is her duty to keep the marriage together, no matter what it costs her.

- **hope for change.** She may feel she loves the man and wants the relationship to continue. She may think there is some way to make the violence stop.

- **guilt about leaving the children with no father.**

But perhaps a better question to ask is, "Why doesn't **he** go?" If we ask why **she** does not leave, it says that we think it is **her** personal problem to solve. It is wrong to think of the violence as only her problem.

- The whole community needs to be responsible for the health and well-being of every person in that community.

- It is the **man** who is committing a crime by violating the woman's right to live free from physical harm, or by killing her. His actions should be challenged and stopped.

What to Do

➤ *Think about these things even if you do not think the violence will ever happen again.*

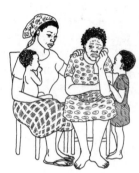

Find someone you trust who can help you sort out your feelings and think about your choices.

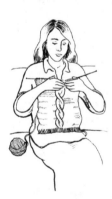

Do you have skills that you can use to earn extra money?

MAKE A SAFETY PLAN

A woman does not have control over her partner's violence, but she does have choices about the way she responds to him. She can also try to plan ahead how she can get herself and her children to safety until the man stops being violent.

Safety before the violence happens again

- Tell someone nearby about the violence. Ask that person to come or to get help if the person hears that you are in trouble. Perhaps a neighbor, male relative, or a group of women or men can come before you are seriously hurt.
- Think of a special word or signal that will tell your children or someone else in your family to get help.
- Teach your children how to get to a safe place.

Safety during the violence

- If you can tell that he is going to become violent, try to have it happen where there are no weapons or objects that he can use to harm you, and where you can get away.
- Use your best judgement. Do whatever you need to do to calm him down so that you and your children are safe.
- If you need to get away from him, think about how you can escape. Where is the safest place to go?

Safety when a woman gets ready to leave

- Save money any way that you can. Put money in a safe place (away from the house) or open a bank account in your own name so you can become more independent.
- If you can do so safely, think of other things you can do to become less dependent on him, such as making friends, joining a group, or spending more time with your family.
- See if there are 'safe houses' or other services for women who have been abused. These are special places in some towns and cities where abused women and their children can stay for a while. Try to find out before you leave if there is one that you can get to.
- Ask friends or relatives you trust if they would let you stay with them or lend you money. Be sure they will not tell your partner that you asked.
- Get copies of important documents, such as your identification or your children's *vaccination* records. Keep a copy at home and give a copy to someone you trust.
- Leave money, copies of your documents, and extra clothes with someone you trust so that you can leave quickly.
- If you can do it safely, practice your escape plan with your children to see if it would work. Make sure the children will not tell anyone.

IF YOU LEAVE

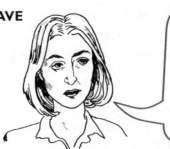

I wanted to leave my husband, but I did not have any money of my own. So my aunt let me help her sell things in the market. I also made some money by taking care of other people's children. After 2 years I had some money saved. So one day I took the children and left. Sometimes it is hard to live on the money I make, but not as hard as living with all the beatings.

If you decide to leave, you will need to be prepared for some of the new difficulties you will face:

Safety. The most dangerous time for a woman is after she leaves. The man has lost control over her and will usually do anything to get it back. He may even try to follow through on his threat to kill her. She must make sure she is staying in a safe place that he does not know about or where she is protected. She should not tell anyone where she is staying. He may be able to force them to tell him where she is.

Surviving on your own. You need to find a way to support yourself and your children. If you can stay with friends or family, use that time to get more education or learn job skills. To save money, maybe you can share a place to live with another woman who also was abused.

Feelings. All the things you need to do to set up a new life may feel like too much to face. You may feel scared and lonely because you are not used to being alone in a strange place. You may miss your partner—no matter what he did to you. When things seem very difficult, you may not remember how bad it really was before you left. Give yourself time to feel sad about the loss of your partner and your former life. Try to stay strong. See if you can find other women in the same situation as you. Together you can support each other.

424

starting a support group

Ｆor change to happen, people must stop thinking of violence against women as something that 'is just the way things are' or that is the woman's fault. Here are some ideas for helping stop violence in your community.

TALK ABOUT IT

Talking about the abuse is the first step to changing it. Try to find other women who have the same problems with violent and abusive men and share ideas with each other. Find men who believe that violence is wrong. Make violence something people talk about. Make it into something that people think is wrong.

Working for Change

➤ *Be careful! In some communities, working against violence can be dangerous.*

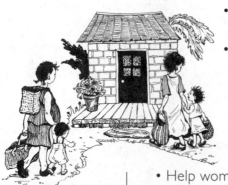

SET UP SERVICES TO HELP WOMEN WHO LEAVE

- Set up a 'safe house' or shelter as soon as possible. Keep the place hidden and secret.

- Get support from others—especially larger, more powerful organizations. For example, see if there is a network of health organizations in your country that can help. You can also talk with respected community members whom you trust. Get as many men as possible to work with you.

- Help women learn about their rights under the law. There may be special laws about families and violence that women can use.

- Find ways to train women in new skills, so that abused women have a way to support themselves.

USE SOCIAL PRESSURE

What are the pressures that prevent people where you live from doing things that most people believe are wrong? In some places, it is the police. In others it may be the military, the family, or religion. In most places, it is a combination of these things.

In some communities in Central America, men volunteer to patrol their communities to warn the people of attacks, and to keep them safe from crime.

In these communities, violence against women is not tolerated. If a man is caught beating his wife, he knows the other men in the town will punish him.

Encourage community leaders and other men to speak out against violence against women and to show their disapproval of men who beat women. Try and use all of the pressures that work where you live to keep men from abusing women.

In some countries, women have organized to get laws passed that punish men who abuse their wives. But laws do not always work well for abused women. In some places, the people who are supposed to enforce the laws—especially the police, the lawyers, and the judges—cannot be trusted to help. But if the legal system and the police both work to protect women where you live, try to learn as much as you can about the laws and about women's rights.

Raise your children to lead non-violent lives. You can work for change at home by helping your children find peaceful ways to solve problems. Teach boys to respect themselves and to respect girls and women.

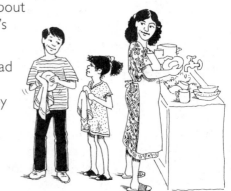

Health workers can take a more active role in stopping violence against women. It is not enough just to take care of a woman's wounds.

When you examine a woman, look for signs of abuse. Men often beat their wives where the marks will not show. Women who have been beaten may wear clothing to hide it. As a health worker, you are one of the few people who sees the private parts of her body.

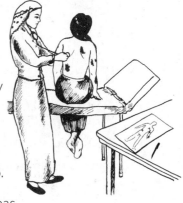

If you see an unusual mark, bruise, or scar, ask her how it happened. Or if a woman comes to you in pain, bleeding, or with broken bones or other injuries, ask her if she has been beaten. Remember that many beaten women will say they got injured by accident. Assure her that you will not do anything she does not want you to do.

Write everything down. When you see a woman who has been abused, draw a picture of the front and back of her body and mark the places where she has been injured. Write down the name of the person who abused her. Try to find out how many times this has happened before. Ask if other family members, such as her sisters or her children, have also been abused. If she is in danger, help her decide what she wants to do. Whether or not she wants to leave, you can help her make a safety plan. If she wants to go to the police, go with her. You can help make sure they take her claim seriously. Also, you can put her in contact with other women who have been abused. Together they may be able to find solutions.

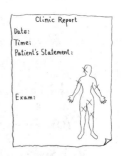

> For information about how to treat a woman's injuries, see **Where There Is No Doctor** or another general medical book.

What resources are available in your community or nearby for abused women? Look for:

- legal help.
- safe houses.

- money-earning projects for women.
- mental health services.

- programs that teach adults to read and write, or other education services.

Help the man. Men who are violent need help themselves. Talk to community or religious leaders to see if they can help find a way for men in your community to take responsibility to stop violence against women.

> Help your community to see the harmful effects of violence.

Chapter 19

In this chapter:

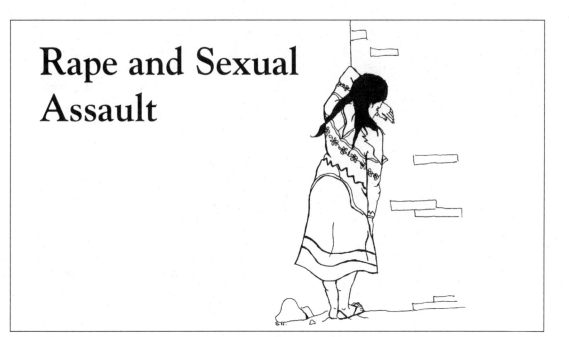

Rape and Sexual Assault

Rape and sexual assault both mean sexual contact that a woman does not want. Rape is any time a man puts his *penis*, finger, or any object into a woman's *vagina*, *anus*, or mouth without her consent.

Rape is sometimes called sexual 'assault' because it is an act of violence, using sex as a weapon. Sexual assault can include rape as well as other kinds of unwanted sexual attention.

Some people think that forced sex is rape only if the man beats up a woman or leaves her *unconscious*. They think she must try hard to get away and risk being killed rather than be raped. But even if a woman does not fight back, it is still rape. No matter what she decides to do, if it was not her choice, it was rape, and it is **never** her fault.

➤ *Rape is sexual violence. Women are not to blame for it.*

➤ *As with other kinds of violence, the goal of the rapist is to gain power over and control his vicitim. For more information, see page 316.*

Any woman can be raped, but there is an even greater risk if she:
- has a *disability*—if she is in a wheelchair, deaf, blind, or mentally slow.
- is a refugee, migrant, or displaced person, or has lived in war situations.
- lives on the streets or is homeless.
- is a *sex worker* (prostitute).
- has been arrested or in prison.
- is being *abused* by her husband or boyfriend.

A rapist may see these women as easy victims—because of their disabilities, or because they have lost the protection of a community.

Kinds of Rape and Sexual Assault

➤ *A woman often finds it harder to ask for help if the man is someone she knows. It is also harder to feel safe if she must see him again.*

sexual abuse

317

62

date rape

There are many different kinds of sexual assault. But only a few of them are seen by most people as rape. For example, sometimes life events can push a woman into having sex when she does not really want to. This can happen in a marriage. Some married women are made to feel that having sex is their duty, whether they want to or not. Although society does not punish this type of forced sex, it is still wrong.

For other women, having sex is a way to survive—to get support for their children, to have a place to live or some money, or to keep a job. No matter what the reason is, a woman should not be forced to have sex if she does not want to.

In any relationship, a woman can choose to accept or refuse a sexual approach. If she refuses, the man then has a choice to either respect her and accept her decision, to try and change her mind, or to force her. Even if the woman knows the man and says "yes," if saying "no" was not really an option, then it is rape.

Any time a woman is forced to have sex, whether or not there is other violence too, it can cause many problems with her health and emotions.

RAPE BY SOMEONE THE WOMAN KNOWS

Most women who are raped know the man who rapes them. If the woman must continue to have contact with him, it can make it very hard for her to recover from the rape and to tell others about it.

Rape by a husband or ex-husband. If the law or traditional custom treats a woman as the property of her husband, he may think he has the right to have sex whenever he wants, even if the woman does not want it.

A woman can be raped by her boyfriend. Her boyfriend may say he has the right to have sex because he has spent money on her, because they have had sex before, because she has teased him sexually, or because he has offered to marry her. **But if he forces her, it is still rape.** A woman may find it hard to talk about this kind of rape, because she fears others will blame her.

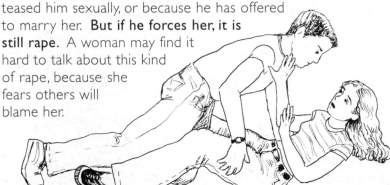

Sexual harassment. A woman may be forced to have sex by a co-worker or by her supervisor or boss so that she can keep her job. She may be threatened with losing her job or other punishment if she tells anyone.

407

sexual harassment

Sexual abuse of children. A girl or boy can be raped by a man in the family or any adult. If a father, stepfather, uncle, brother, cousin, or any other family member makes a child have sex, or touches her or him in a sexual way, this is rape. It is important to realize that children may be confused and may not understand what is happening to them, especially if they trust the person who is abusing them. Other members of the family may not know of the abuse, they may deny that it happens, or they may say it is the child's fault. It is never right to blame the person who has been raped, but especially not a child.

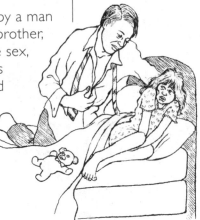

Touching a child sexually is rape.

RAPE BY A STRANGER

This is the kind of sexual assault that most people think of when they hear the word 'rape.' A woman may be grabbed on the street, or attacked in her home. This kind of rape is very frightening, but it is much less common than rape by someone the woman knows.

Gang rape. A woman can be raped by more than one man. Sometimes a man starts raping a woman and other men see it and join in. Or sometimes young men and boys get together and rape a woman to prove their 'manhood' to one another.

Prison rape. Many women are raped by police or prison guards after they have been arrested. Also, rape is common between male prisoners as a way to establish who has more power.

War. Soldiers or fighters often use rape to terrorize women and their community, and to make people feel ashamed. Soldiers may gang rape women and girls in front of their families to show the enemy's power. Women may be held in camps, and forced into prostitution or sexual slavery in order to stay alive, to keep their children safe, or to get food.

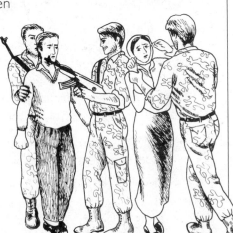

➤ *Those who survive war rape need special care. If a woman gets pregnant, she and her child may suffer from the reminder that she was raped by an enemy.*

Rape is a form of torture when it is used in war.

How to Avoid Rape

There is no one right or wrong way to behave to avoid rape. But there are some things a woman can do that may make her less likely to suffer some kinds of rape. What a woman does depends on how well she knows the man, how afraid she is, and how much danger she thinks she is in. Remember, if a woman is raped, it is not because she failed to avoid the rape, but because **someone stronger forced himself on her.**

THESE IDEAS MAY HELP ANY WOMAN AVOID RAPE

- Do your work with other women. You will be safer and stronger if you work together in groups.

- Do not let anyone who makes you feel nervous into your home. Do not let him know if you are there alone.

- Try not to walk alone, especially at night. If you must go alone, hold your head up and act as though you feel confident. Most rapists will look for a woman who looks easy to attack.

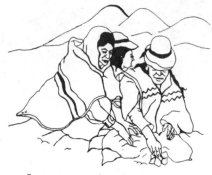

Protect yourselves. Work with others.

332

self defense

- If you think you are being followed, try walking in another direction, or go up to another person, a house, or a store. Or, turn around and ask him very loudly what he wants.

- Carry something with you that will make a loud noise, like a whistle. Also, carry something that you can use to defend yourself. This could be a stick, something you can spray in his eyes, or even some hot spicy powder—like hot pepper or chili powder—to blow in his eyes.

- If you are attacked, scream as loudly as you can or use your whistle. If this does not work, hit back quickly to hurt him, so that you may be able to get away.

AVOIDING RAPE BY SOMEONE YOU KNOW

Learn to trust your feelings. A woman can learn to recognize when she feels good about a person or a situation, and when she does not. When a woman feels good about someone, she may feel warmth, caring, or attraction toward him. If she can learn to act on these good feelings, it can make her more confident that she will know when she does **not** like someone.

Be aware if you:
- have a lasting feeling that something is not right.
- feel afraid, or like you want to leave.
- feel uncomfortable with comments or suggestions the person is making.
- dislike the physical contact he makes.

It can be hard to act on these feelings because you may be afraid of what other people will think. In addition, if the person is someone you know or care about, you may not want to admit that he would do you harm. But it is always best to trust your feelings and get out of a situation that feels uncomfortable **before** anything bad happens.

I don't want to look stupid by running away from him... It's probably nothing anyway.

Trust your feelings. It is better to offend someone if you are wrong than to be raped.

Be prepared to get away:

- Avoid going somewhere alone with a person who makes you feel uncomfortable or who you do not know well.
- Always have a way to get home if you decide you need to leave. It is better not to go somewhere if you will not be able to get back without the person's help.
- Tell the person that his comments or touch make you uncomfortable. If he does not change the way he is acting you should get away from him as soon as possible.

If he has power over you (for example if he is your boss, your doctor, a teacher, or an official):

- The first time he does something that makes you feel uncomfortable, tell him to stop. If he is trying to take advantage of his power, he will look for someone who is easy to frighten. Let him know that you are not frightened. He is less likely to treat you badly (for example to fire you, refuse you medical care, or deny your request) if you can get him to stop bothering you before he has done anything that makes him look foolish.

➤ *Be aware that if a man cannot gain control over a woman through sexual violence, he may try to gain control over her in other ways.*

- Talk to other women about him. You are probably not the only one he has bothered. If you must continue to deal with him, try to bring a friend with you so you are never alone with him. Warn other women to be careful.

HELP CHILDREN AVOID SEXUAL ABUSE

- Teach children about the possibility that they may be touched sexually, and how to tell the difference between touching that is affectionate and touching that is sexual.
- If possible, have girls and boys sleep separately, especially after age 10 or 11 years old.
- Make sure children know who they can talk to if something should happen to them.
- Believe a child who says he or she feels uncomfortable around an adult or older child—no matter who that person is.

➤ *Sometimes sexual abuse of children continues for many years. A girl may be told that she will be harmed or even killed if she tells anyone about it.*

Self Defense for Women

Practice these self defense movements with a friend, so that you will be prepared to fight off an attacker. Hit him as hard as you can. Do not be afraid to hurt him—he is not afraid to hurt you. For more self defense ideas, see page 146.

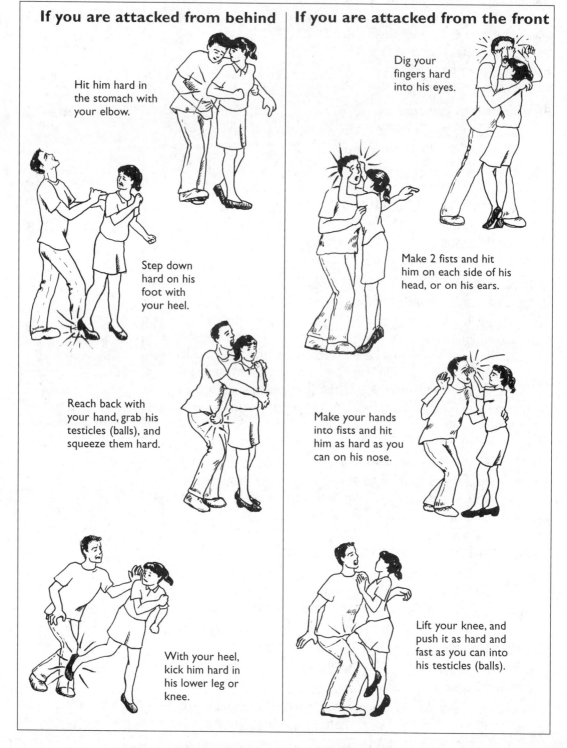

If you are attacked from behind

Hit him hard in the stomach with your elbow.

Step down hard on his foot with your heel.

Reach back with your hand, grab his testicles (balls), and squeeze them hard.

With your heel, kick him hard in his lower leg or knee.

If you are attacked from the front

Dig your fingers hard into his eyes.

Make 2 fists and hit him on each side of his head, or on his ears.

Make your hands into fists and hit him as hard as you can on his nose.

Lift your knee, and push it as hard and fast as you can into his testicles (balls).

If You Are Sexually Assaulted

If a woman is able to resist her attacker, she will usually be able to avoid the rape, even if the rapist has a weapon. The more different ways a woman tries to keep from being raped, the more likely she is to be able to avoid the rape, or to suffer fewer injuries and mental health problems from the rape afterward.

It is impossible to know ahead of time how a woman will react when someone is trying to rape her. Some women are filled with rage and feel strength they did not know they had. Others feel like they cannot move. If this should ever happen to you, know that you will do what you can.

Here are some ideas that may help you during a sexual assault:

• **Do not cry, plead, or give in. It usually does not help**. In fact, women who try this often suffer more injuries than women who fight back.

• **Stay aware**. Watch the rapist carefully. There may be times when he is not watching you, or when he loses his control.

• **Try different things**. Kick, yell, bargain, trick him—do whatever you can think of to make him realize you are not an easy victim. Try to make him realize that you are a person, not an object.

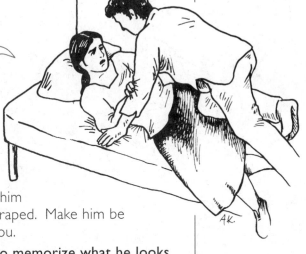

I have 6 brothers and they'll kill you if you hurt me!

• **If you know the rapist, tell him how you feel**. Do not let him believe that women like to be raped. Make him be aware of what he is doing to you.

• **If the rapist is a stranger, try to memorize what he looks like**. How big is he? Does he have scars, marks, or tatoos? What kind of clothes is he wearing? Try to remember them so that you can tell the police and warn the other women in your community.

• **Use your best judgement**. Only you can decide how much to fight back. In some rape situations, for example, during war, the rapist may have no reason to keep you alive if you resist.

➤ *If there are several people trying to rape you, or if the rapist has a weapon, you can still resist, but it is usually better not to fight back physically.*

What to Do if You Have Been Raped

➤ *Do not blame yourself. You did not deserve to be raped. There was nothing you did that made it right for a man to force sex on you.*

Every woman's experience with rape is different. But there are a few things you need to do to help yourself recover.

First, ask yourself these questions:

- **Who can you ask for help?**
- **Do you want to tell the police about the rape?**
- **Where can you go for medical care?**
- **Do you want to try to punish the rapist?**

You need someone to talk to when you feel sad, hurt, scared, or angry, to go with you for medical care, and to help you figure out what to do. Choose someone who cares about you, who you trust will not tell others, and who is strong and dependable. Sometimes a woman's husband or parents are too upset themselves to be able to give much support.

If someone you know has been raped

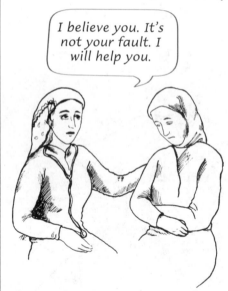

I believe you. It's not your fault. I will help you.

- Reassure her that it is not her fault.
- Be supportive. Listen to her feelings, help her decide what she needs, and reassure her that she can go on with her life (see page 423).
- Respect her wishes for privacy and safety. Do not tell anyone else unless she wants you to.
- Go with her to see a health worker, to report the rape to the police, to talk with someone who is trained to listen and support her, to see a lawyer, and to go to court if she wants to do those things.
- Do not protect the rapist if you know him. He is a danger to every woman in the community.

The decision to use the law must be made carefully.

- Can someone go with you to talk to the police?
- Has the law helped other women in your community who have been raped?
- Do you want the rape to remain private? Can the police keep others from learning about the rape?
- Did the rapist threaten to hurt you more if you reported the rape?
- If the rapist is caught and you can prove that he raped you, how will he be punished?

If you think you may want to report the rape to the police, do it as soon after the rape as possible. Do not wash before you go, and bring the clothes that you were wearing in a bag. These things can help you prove that you were raped. Take a friend with you, and ask to have a female health worker examine you, if possible.

If you do not want to go to the police, or if you cannot go until later, you should see a health worker anyway—even if you are not badly hurt. Tell the health worker that you have been raped. She should then check you for cuts or tears, and give you some medicines to prevent pregnancy and *sexually transmitted diseases (STDs)*. Ask her to write down everything that she finds because it will help prove to the police or to others in the community that you were raped.

➤ *If there is no health worker who can treat you, the information on pages 336 and 337 can help you prevent and treat some of the problems yourself.*

emergency family
planning, 224
STDs, 261

To the health worker

If you see someone who has been raped:

Treat her with kindness and understanding. Do not blame her. Since she may find it difficult for you to see or touch her, explain everything and wait until she is ready to be touched. Remember that her feelings about the rape may last for a long time, even years.

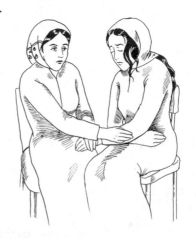

Treat her health problems. Give her medicines to prevent STDs and pregnancy. If she is already pregnant, help her to decide what she wants to do.

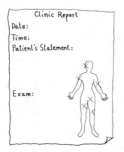

Write down who raped her and exactly what happened. If your clinic does not keep records, make one and keep it somewhere safe. If you can, draw a picture of the front and back of her body and mark the places where she has been hurt. Show or tell her what you have written and that it can be used to support the fact that she was raped if she goes to the law.

Treat her mental health needs. Ask her whether she has someone to talk to. Help her to respect herself again and to gain control of her life.

Help her to make her own decisions. If she wants to go to the law, help her find legal services. Help her find other services in the community for women who have been raped.

Help her to tell her partner or her family. If they do not know already, offer to help her tell them. You can help them find ways to support her until she recovers. Remember that family members usually also need help to overcome their feelings about the rape.

In some countries, women have worked with the police to have specially trained female police officers to help victims of rape and violence.

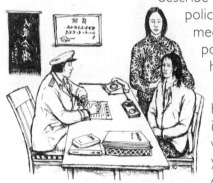

➤ *Always take someone with you to the police.*

Health Problems of Rape

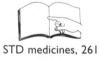

STD medicines, 261
the HIV test, 288

IF YOU GO TO THE POLICE

In most places rape is a crime. But it may take a long time and be very difficult to prove you were raped.

The police will ask you what happened. If you know the rapist, tell them who it is. If you do not, you will need to describe what he looks like. You may have to go with the police to try to find him. You may also be asked to get a medical exam from a legal doctor who works with the police. This is not an exam to help you get well, but to help prove that you were raped.

If the rapist is arrested, you will have to identify him, either in front of the police or in front of a judge in court. If there is a trial, try to find a lawyer who has worked with rape cases before. The lawyer will tell you what to expect and help you prepare for the trial. Always take someone with you.

Going to court for a rape is never easy. Describing what happened may make you have the feelings of being raped all over again. Not everyone will be understanding. Some may try to blame you or say you are lying.

PREGNANCY

Pregnancy can be prevented if you act quickly and use emergency family planning (see page 224). You must use it as soon as possible, but **no later than 3 days (72 hours) after the rape.**

IMPORTANT *In some countries, abortion is safe and legal if a girl or woman has been raped. Ask a health worker or women's organization if this is true in your country.*

SEXUALLY TRANSMITTED DISEASES (STDs)

STDs are passed more easily with violent sex because the skin in the *vagina* is often torn and the *infection* can get into the woman's body easily. If the man who raped you had an STD, he may have passed it to you. Since you cannot know if he was infected, you should be treated just in case, so you can keep from getting the disease and passing it on to others. Take medicines for gonorrhea, syphilis, and chlamydia, and watch for signs of other STDs. **Take the medicines whether or not you think you were infected.** It is better to prevent an STD than to wait for one to start.

You should also try to have an *HIV* test in 6 months. Until then, it is better to use condoms if you have sex to protect your partner from possible infection.

TEARS AND CUTS

Sometimes rape damages the *genitals* by causing tears and cuts. These usually cause pain, but will go away in time. If there is a lot of bleeding, you may need to see a health worker trained to stitch tears. For small cuts and tears:

- Soak your genitals 3 times each day in warm water that has been boiled and cooled. Putting chamomile leaves in the boiling water can help soothe the tears and help with healing. Or you can put gel from an aloe plant on the tears.
- Pour water over your genitals while passing urine so that it will not burn. Drinking a lot of liquid makes the urine weaker so it will burn less.
- Watch for signs of infection: heat, yellow liquid *(pus)* from the torn area, a bad smell, and pain that gets worse.
- After violent sex it is also common for women to have a *bladder* or *kidney* infection.

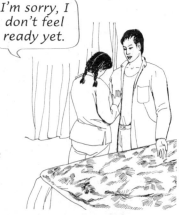

wounds and sores, 306

bladder and kidney infections, 366

SEXUAL RELATIONS AFTER RAPE

You can have normal sexual relations again after rape. You will need to wait until your genitals no longer hurt and any tears have healed. For many women, having sex makes them think about the rape. If this happens to you, talk with your partner about why you need to wait.

I'm sorry, I don't feel ready yet.

Sometimes a woman's partner may reject her after she has been raped. He may feel ashamed or act as though he is angry with her. This can be very hard for a woman who is already dealing with many difficult feelings.

OVERCOMING FEELINGS ABOUT THE RAPE

The rape may still bother you long after your body has healed. Here are some common reactions:

What did I do wrong?

It happened so long ago... Why can't I just forget about it?

If nobody else knows, maybe I can forget what happened.

How DARE he have done that to me!

It is important for a woman who has been raped to talk to someone or to do something to help herself feel better after the rape—every woman needs to find her own way to heal. For some women, this can mean performing a ritual. For others it means trying to punish the rapist, or working to prevent other women from being raped. Whatever you do, be patient with yourself and ask others to be patient, too.

➤ *It may take a long time before you feel better, but talking with someone you trust, or who has also survived rape, can help you to heal. See page 423.*

Working for Change

Rape affects everyone in a community. Women who have been raped can suffer long-lasting problems because of the rape. But almost all women, whether they have been raped or not, learn to be afraid. They learn not to trust men, and they learn to not to do things that attract attention. Women learn not to walk alone, or not to talk to men they do not know.

To create a world in which rape does not happen, we need to work toward having:

- communities where a person's choices and behavior are not limited by whether the person is a man or a woman.

- an equal chance for everyone to participate in the community.

- the chance for men and women to talk openly and honestly with each other about what they each expect from a sexual relationship.

But until we achieve these goals, we need to find ways to help women who have been raped. We can:

- educate elected leaders, clergy, and teachers about rape. Ask for their help and make a plan for change.

- train doctors and health workers to treat women who have been raped. They should be trained to provide STD testing, emergency family planning, and how to listen and be kind to the woman and her family.

- encourage health workers to find out what information their country's laws require in order to punish a rapist, so they can help the woman fill out legal forms.

- teach women and girls how to defend themselves.

- teach boys and girls about sex and sexuality. Teach girls to be clear about their wishes, and teach boys to ask girls about their wishes and then respect them.

- learn about laws in your country that protect women who have been raped, and teach them to others.

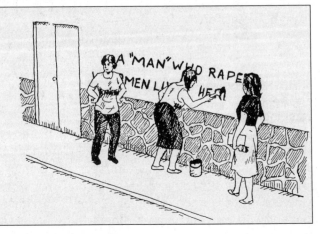

In a small town in El Salvador, the police refused to stop a known rapist because he was the son of a wealthy man. So the women of the town began painting the word 'rapist' outside his house. His family was so ashamed that they forced him to stop.

How a community in South Africa organized against rape

Early one Saturday morning, a 59-year-old woman was raped and stabbed by a man who had raped other women in the past. The victim pointed the rapist out to the police. He was arrested and the woman was taken to the hospital. But the police released the rapist the same afternoon. He was not charged with rape or assault—he was free.

We women of the township were very angry. The police had protected a man who made women afraid to walk alone on the streets. The township's women's organization decided to organize a protest.

Most of us work as domestic servants for rich white women who live in a nearby city. So all of us stayed away from our jobs, demanding that the police charge the rapist with rape and assault, before we would go back to work.

We also asked the women we worked for to come to speak with us. We wanted to show and tell them about our problems. We know that all women, black and white, fear rape. We felt the white women might understand and be sympathetic to us. We also wanted the women whose husbands worked for the police to explain our problems to their husbands and how bad it was for them to release a violent rapist back into the township.

But the white women were not sympathetic—they just got angry. We think they were upset because they had to do their own housework. When the Employers' Federation came to see about the protest, we told the men, "Please do not speak for us. This is a women's problem. Men do not get raped." The Employers' Federation would not meet with us, but after a week, a group of white women came to talk to us. We showed them around the township, and they decided to meet with us again. We called off the protest, even though the rapist was only charged with assault, and not rape. But people in the township were so angry that the rapist could no longer live there.

The police arrested several of us who had organized the protest. They did not believe that women had organized the protest. They think men are behind everything that women do. But we women had become very strong.

It is very important to talk openly about the problem of rape. Most people don't talk about rape—they feel ashamed and shy. Often the family of the raped girl or woman does not want to talk about it.

But here it is different. We started organizing in the community for education, child care, pensions, and so on. We started talking about all the problems and things that we need to change. So we talk about rape, and any sexual assault on a woman. People now see sexual assault as another kind of oppression. Men and women think the same about this; we are united in the struggle.

A raped woman is trusted. If she says she was raped, we support her, no matter who she is. Even if she is a drunkard, a rape is still a crime against her. In fact, it is worse because she was in a weak position. Our women and men do not blame a woman for a rape. We do not say that the rape was the woman's fault. So women can talk about sexual violence openly and they will get community support.

Chapter 20

In this chapter:

Sex Workers

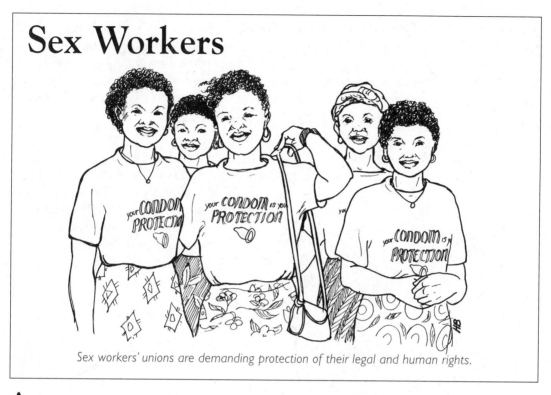

Sex workers' unions are demanding protection of their legal and human rights.

A sex worker is anyone who trades sex for money or other favors. Many people picture sex workers as women who do not wear many clothes, flirt with men, and work in brothels or on the street. But women who sell sex are a diverse group. A sex worker may be a young girl or an older woman with 6 children at home. She may work in a brothel, in a bar or a club, on the street with a *pimp*, or in her own home. What most of these women share in common, though, is that they sell sex because they desperately need money.

In this book we use the term 'sex worker' instead of 'prostitute'. We do this because many people think of a prostitute as a bad woman who should be punished. The term 'sex worker' emphasizes that sex workers, like other women, are working to make a living. For the same reason, we call the men who buy sex 'clients' or 'customers'.

There are also many women who do not think of themselves as sex workers, yet occasionally they trade sex for favors, like a place to live or a job. We call this 'survival sex'. These women face many of the same problems that sex workers face.

The purpose of this chapter is to provide information on the health problems sex workers face, and about ways sex workers can help themselves. It also helps people understand what life is like for women who must trade sex to survive.

➤ *Sex workers, like other women, are working to make a living.*

Why Women Become Sex Workers

➤ *Most women who sell sex would rather have a job that pays well and that gives them dignity and respect.*

Many people think women become sex workers because they are immoral or too lazy to find other work. But most women do so because they need money and have no other way to earn it. These women need money for food and shelter, to support their children and families, to pay debts, or to buy drugs.

This desperate need often arises in situations a woman cannot control: for example, her husband dies, or she gets divorced, or her husband or family abandons her. Or she may be raped or have an unplanned pregnancy and find that no one will marry her. If she has no job skills or ways to get money, she sells the only thing she has—her body—in order to survive.

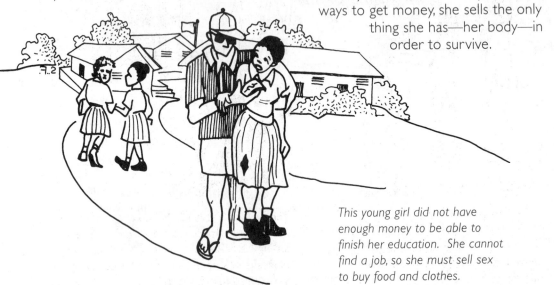

This young girl did not have enough money to be able to finish her education. She cannot find a job, so she must sell sex to buy food and clothes.

STORY OF A POOR WOMAN

Every morning around 9 o'clock, Nawal (not her real name) steps out of the tiny room she shares with her husband, locks her two small children inside, and walks to the wealthy area of town where she 'works'. Wearing a traditional dress with faded colors and a cheap black scarf thrown loosely around her head, she looks just like any other poor woman you see everywhere in Cairo, Egypt. She is not. Nawal is 20 years old and she is a prostitute.

'Working' a certain street until it is time to go home around 2 or 3 in the afternoon, Nawal earns an average of L.E. 20 (US $6) a day. She does not work on Fridays or religious holidays so she can spend time with her family: her husband, who works occasionally as a construction worker, a 4-year-old son, and a 1-year-old daughter.

Nawal's father was blind, and he made money by begging in central Cairo. When she was a young girl, Nawal spent more time in the street guiding her father around than at home. She never saw her mother. At 13, she got married.

Other women are forced into sex work. Often women are tricked into thinking they are going to get jobs or rich husbands in other countries and are sold into sex work instead. Then it is almost impossible to stop selling sex. The woman may be in a new country illegally where she has no rights, no money, and no way to return home. She may have large debts to repay, or her employer may threaten to hurt her if she leaves. She has become a sexual slave.

➤ *Because many men fear they will become infected with HIV/AIDS when they have sex with older sex workers, there is an increasing demand for younger girl children to work in the sex trade.*

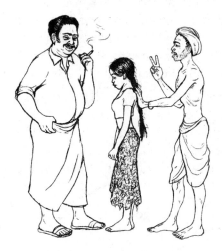

This girl was sold by her family, thinking she would get a job in another country. Instead, she was sold again to a brothel owner who forces her to sell sex.

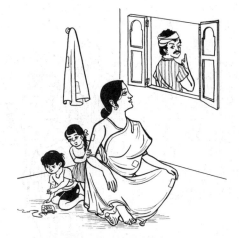

This woman lost her home and land when her husband died, because there were no laws saying his property must be given to his wife. Now she has no money. She started selling sex to feed her children.

Two years later, after giving birth to her son, she had to look for a job. Her husband was getting less and less work. With no education or skills, Nawal tried working as a house cleaner in an apartment building. But she stopped when the building guards refused to introduce her to customers unless she had sex with them.

Nawal does not use the word 'prostitute' to describe herself. She refers to herself as a servant. She knows she has to save money for her children: "I want my children to go to school so that they don't grow up to be criminals."

Because her work is not considered 'real' work, Nawal, and thousands of women like her, get no help from the government or the police. Nawal has been robbed several times, but no one would help her. Officially, she does not exist. And the thing that really puzzles her is that a lot of people think that she enjoys sex work. She does not. She just does not know any better way to survive.

—*from an interview by Ahmed Badawi*

Health Problems of Sex Workers

STDs, INCLUDING **HIV/AIDS**

Because of her work, a sex worker has a greater risk of getting *sexually transmitted diseases (STDs)* and HIV/AIDS than other women. Her risk is increased because sex work does not pay well, and so she must take a large number of clients each day. She may want to protect herself by using condoms and other *safer sex* practices, but the men who pay her can make this difficult. They may demand sex in the *vagina* or *anus* but refuse to use *condoms*. They may even become violent if she refuses unsafe sex practices.

If a sex worker is *addicted* to drugs, her need for drugs may make her more willing to exchange unsafe sex for money or drugs, and less able to take care of herself.

As with any woman, if a sex worker gets an STD, it may lead to *infertility* or *cancer* of the *cervix*. *Infection* with an STD like herpes, syphilis, gonorrhea, or chlamydia greatly increases her chance of also becoming infected with HIV/AIDS. These risks are even more serious for young girls. Since their *genitals* are not fully grown, they can be damaged more easily during sex.

Many sex workers do not have good information about STDs, or about how to treat or prevent them. Information and health services are often not available to sex workers because of people's prejudice against them. When sex workers do go to a health center for help, they may be treated badly or refused services.

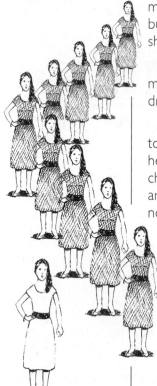

In some communities up to 9 out of 10 sex workers are infected with HIV.

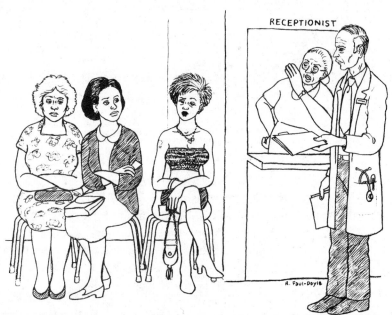

Are sex workers responsible for HIV/AIDS?

Sex workers are blamed for much of the AIDS epidemic. But it is the men who buy sex from them who infect sex workers **and** often their own wives. By blaming sex workers, these men fail to take responsibility for spreading the disease.

Sex workers **want** to practice safer sex. But HIV and AIDS may not seem like the most important problem they face. They often have more immediate, daily problems—such as bad treatment by the police, low wages, dirty and expensive hotels, difficult or violent men, and problems with keeping clean, getting enough to eat, and taking care of their children. If a sex worker does become infected with HIV, she may have no choice but to continue selling sex to survive. As one sex worker says:

> *"Those who blame us do so on full stomachs. I should feed myself and my children adequately. My children should go to school. To say that AIDS kills without giving me a well-paid job is like saying I should die of hunger. To me, that is the only way to survive."*

PREGNANCY

Women who sell sex need safe, effective, and low-cost *family planning* methods to prevent pregnancy. If these methods are not available in her community, a sex worker is likely to have an unwanted pregnancy. If she continues the pregnancy and must also continue selling sex, she puts both herself and her unborn baby at risk for *complications* or STDs. Or she may feel she has no other choice but to have an unsafe *abortion*. All these situations are dangerous.

choosing a family
planning method, 200

unsafe abortion, 241

VIOLENCE

A sex worker may live with others in a house for sex work (brothel) or work on the street. These conditions make it easy for her to be violently attacked, raped, or robbed, especially if she is a child. If a sex worker is 'owned' or controlled by a man who gets part of her money (pimp), he will often use violence to keep her under his control.

self-defense for
women

➤ *In some places, women can be arrested for sex work simply by having condoms for their own protection.*

Because sex work is illegal in most countries, a sex worker is often denied any legal rights, including protection from the police. Or she may have to pay the police a large part of her earnings in exchange for 'protection'. Since most laws are made to protect men from 'immoral' women, a sex worker may be arrested, beaten, harassed, or even *raped* by the police instead.

If you are being mistreated by the law because you are a sex worker, try to learn more about your rights. There may be a prostitutes' rights group in your city or country. Or you can write to one of the organizations listed on page 557 for advice on how to organize a group.

How to Protect Yourself from STDs, Including HIV/AIDS

Many women do not have the choice to stop selling sex. If you must continue, it is important to protect yourself from STDs and HIV/AIDS. For more information, see the section on 'Safer Sex' on page 186, and the chapters on "Sexually Transmitted Diseases and Other Infections of the Genitals" (page 261) and "Family Planning" (page 197).

Here are some other ideas:

- Use *latex* condoms every time you have sex. Make sure you always have condoms when you work.

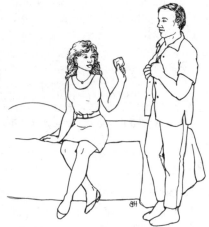

- Hand sex (manual *masturbation*), *oral sex, or sex stories (fantasy),* are safer than sex in your vagina or anus if you cannot get a client to use a condom.

➤ *"If they don't want to use a condom, I ask them if they ever listen to the news. If they have ever heard of AIDS. I tell them I'm not willing to take the chance."*
— Jolanda

- If you are unable to use a male or female condom (see pages 202 to 204), using *spermicide* alone or with a *diaphragm* (pages 205 and 206) will give less protection than a condom, but it is better than no method at all.

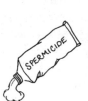

  - Spermicides give some protection against 2 common STDs, gonorrhea and chlamydia. But using spermicides too often can also irritate the skin in your vagina, making it easier for germs to pass through the skin and infect you with an STD, especially HIV. Spermicides used every other day are less likely to cause irritation.

➤ *Protecting yourself and others from STDs means having safer sex with your clients, and also with your husband or boyfriend.*

  - You can put your diaphragm in before you begin work, in case the man refuses to use a condom. Add spermicide between sex acts, but do not remove the diaphragm. It must stay in for 6 hours after you have finished working.

IMPORTANT *Do not use* chemicals *like bleach or detergent to wash our your vagina. They can cause serious injury!*

- Inspect your clients' genitals for sores or *discharge* before you have sex. Refuse to have sex with any man who has signs of an STD. Remember you cannot tell by looking if a person has HIV/AIDS.

TREATMENT FOR STDs WHEN PROTECTION FAILS

It is always best to prevent STDs by practicing safer sex. But sometimes these methods fail. Condoms can break, or clients can refuse to use them.

Get early treatment

If you think you have been exposed to an STD, early treatment can prevent the infection from getting worse. STDs that are not treated quickly can lead to serious illness and even death.

If possible, have regular exams for STDs. If you are having signs of an STD—discharge or bleeding from your vagina, pain or sores on your genitals, or pain in your lower belly—see a health worker trained to treat STDs as soon as possible. Even if you have no signs of infection, go to a health center or clinic at least once a month for treatment if you have unsafe sex often. If you use condoms every time you have sex, you may need to visit a health center less often.

Since you probably do not know what STDs you have been exposed to, you should be treated for as many as possible. Different *antibiotics* can treat different STDs, so you may need to take several medicines at once. Remember, no medicine can cure HIV/AIDS. See the chapter on "Sexually Transmitted Diseases and Other Infections of the Genitals" for information about how to treat STDs.

Testing for AIDS

If you want to be tested for the HIV/AIDS virus, see page 288. Check with your local clinic to see if they have a National AIDS Control Program. They may have special programs for testing sex workers for HIV and for treating their problems if they have AIDS.

➤ *STDs that are not treated quickly can lead to serious illness and even death.*

➤ *If you are at very great risk for getting STDs because of unsafe sex, a medicine called azithromycin can be useful because it treats a number of STDs with only one dose (see page 278).*

IMPORTANT *When you take antibiotics to treat STDs, be sure to take the recommended dose for the full amount of time. If you take too small an amount, or do not take it for the right number of days, your signs may go away, but the infection stays in your body and continues to cause damage. And the next time you try to treat the infection it will be harder to cure. Then you may need to use other, more expensive drugs. Many medicines that once worked for STDs are no longer effecitve because people used them incorrectly.*

Working for Change

➤ *Use role plays to practice negotiating condom use with your clients. Ask other sex workers to practice with you.*

NEGOTIATING CONDOM USE

In order to get more men to use condoms, men must believe that it is in their own interest and that of their sex partners to prevent STDs, including HIV/AIDS. This kind of education is best done at the community level.

As a sex worker, you can help by joining together with other sex workers to make condom use the expected or normal practice. Then clients will begin to want to use condoms.

When you are with clients, your attitude is important. If you believe in yourself and know what you are talking about, you are more likely to convince a man that condom use makes good sense. Here are some ideas:

- Explain that condoms can:
  - protect him as well as you from disease.
  - make him less likely to pass on STDs to his wife.
  - make his pleasure last longer.
- Assure him that you will still make sex good for him.
- If you practice oral sex, learn to put the condom on with your mouth.

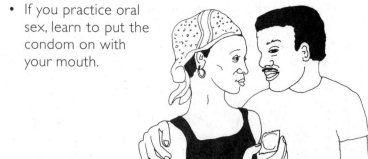

A sex worker in a discotheque in Duala, Cameroon, tells the following story:

Where I work, we understand the risk to our health and our lives from HIV and AIDS, so all the girls are given condoms. We teach our clients that it is in their own interest to protect themselves. Most clients now agree. We make sure that the act will be enjoyable, so they will come back for more.

But there are always those men who think that by not using condoms, they are being 'real men'. That going 'live' is getting the real thing. We almost always find that after a guy has tried without luck to get 4 or 5 of us to have unsafe sex, he will either just leave or agree to see if he can have just as much pleasure with a condom on. If he insists on unsafe sex, we gather together and chase him out!

We do not like to lose clients, but we value our lives and our health. Slowly, things are changing. Where we work, using condoms has become the smart thing.

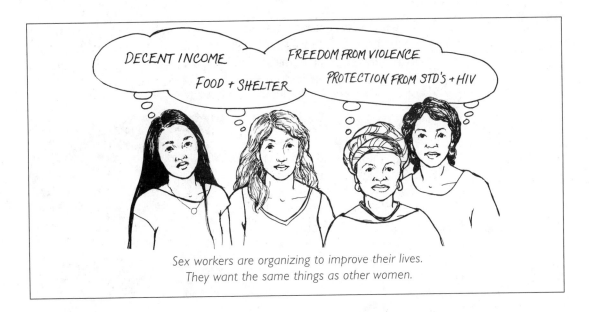

Sex workers are organizing to improve their lives.
They want the same things as other women.

STRENGTH THROUGH ORGANIZING

Because of their low *status* as poor women and as sex workers, women who sell sex sometimes feel unworthy and unable to change their lives. Working alone, it can be very difficult for a sex worker to make her clients use condoms, or to protect herself from violence.

But in many places sex workers have learned that by working together they have more power to make the changes necessary to improve their lives. In some places sex workers are organizing to improve their working conditions, by insisting that their clients use condoms, or organizing against rough treatment from police. In other places, sex workers with the help of others in their community have started programs to get training, or to learn new skills so they will be less dependent on sex work.

Here are some ideas that sex workers from around the world have shared about how they are working together and working with others to make their lives better.

➤ *"I used to work in a club where we didn't always use condoms. There was a lot of pressure NOT to. So I left. Now I work in a house where condoms are the RULE. It saves me a lot of worrying and arguing." —Anita*

Teach each other how to make your work safer. You can get a group of sex workers together to talk about:

- how to use condoms to prevent STDs, including HIVAIDS, and how to get treatment for STDs when necessary.
- family planning methods, how to get them, and how to use them.
- how to choose a customer and avoid dangerous situations.
- how to support each other in handling a client's unwanted demands.
- how to limit the time a sex worker spends with clients.

Organize for greater safety. Working together and supporting each other can help sex workers reduce the threat of violence from clients, police, and pimps. Join with other sex workers to plan how you can support and protect each other.

Learn new skills. You can work to organize programs that teach reading and writing or job skills. Sometimes sex workers can teach each other new skills, or it may be possible to get help from people in your community who can be teachers.

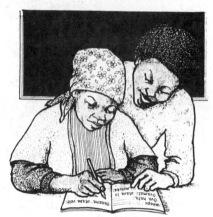

I told him "No condom, no sex" and now that I earn some money doing hair, I can say "no" and still pay my bills.

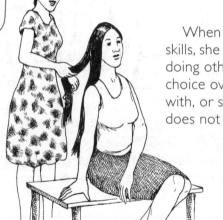

When a sex worker has other skills, she can earn some money doing other jobs. She then has more choice over which man to have sex with, or she can refuse a client if she does not feel safe.

Create a loan fund. A group of sex workers in Nairobi, Kenya, joined their money to create a loan fund for their members. Many use the fund to pay their children's school fees. Other groups have used loan funds to help each other set up small businesses so they can earn money in other ways besides sex work.

Many groups of sex workers are trying to change the negative ways other people think about them. For example, a sex workers' organization in Calabar, Nigeria does not allow members to fight in the streets or in the brothel. Members are also not allowed to use language or wear clothes that may offend the community. By changing the things that had made it easy for the community to criticize sex workers, they hope that people will begin to understand that sex workers are just women doing a job to survive.

The community can help

Community members can help sex workers to organize for safer working conditions. You can:

- demand laws that punish those who exploit sex workers. This includes brothel owners, pimps and middlemen, police, clients, and drug pushers.
- pressure police to stop violent treatment of sex workers.

- work for laws that encourage condom use by clients of sex workers. For example, in Thailand, the Ministry of Health requires sex workers to use condoms. If they do not, the brothel can be shut down or have to pay a fine. This law has helped sex workers to insist upon condoms. This protects the sex workers, the men who pay them, and their wives.

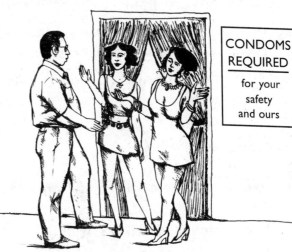

CONDOMS REQUIRED

for your safety and ours

You can also work to prevent children from being sold or forced into sex work:

- Talk with parents in your community about the dangers of selling girls into service in other countries.
- Provide help, such as jobs, *counseling*, and a place to stay, for children who run away from their families. With your help they will not be forced to sell sex to survive.

To the health worker

You can make the biggest difference in the life of a sex worker by helping her to get the care she needs:

- Give the same respectful care to sex workers as you give to others.
- Learn to diagnose and treat STDs. See the chapter on "Sexually Transmitted Diseases and Other Infections of the Genitals," page 261.
- Learn which medicines provide the most up-to-date, affordable treatment, and try to keep a supply available.
- Find a regular and adequate supply of free or cheap condoms for your community. Make them available at health clinics, local shops, bars, cafes, and from outreach workers.
- Make sure health services are available, including family planning, *abortion*, and free or low-cost treatment of STDs and drug *abuse*.

Chapter 21

In this chapter:

How to use this chapter:

1. For sudden, severe pain in the belly or abdomen, see page 354 and follow that advice.

2. Look up the different kinds of pain on pages 354 to 356. Most of these problems are described in other parts of the book. Turn to the page listed for more information.

3. If you are still unsure of the cause of the pain, look at the questions on page 357.

4. For information on how to examine a woman with pain in the abdomen, see page 530.

Pain in the Lower Abdomen

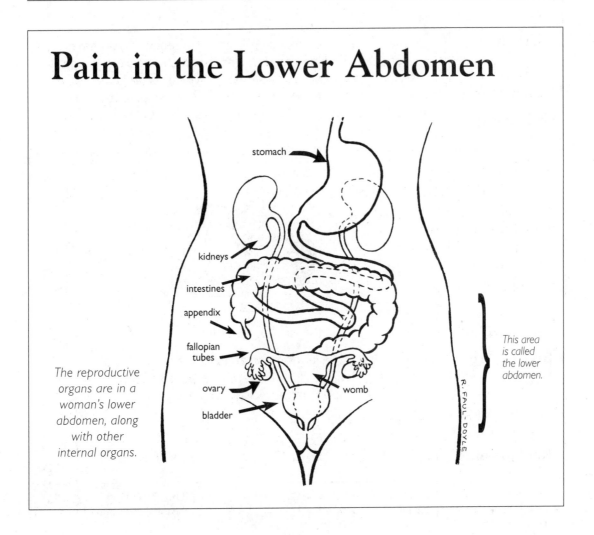

stomach

kidneys

intestines

appendix

fallopian
tubes

ovary

bladder

womb

*The reproductive
organs are in a
woman's lower
abdomen, along
with other
internal organs.*

R · FAUL · DOYLE

*This area
is called
the lower
abdomen.*

Most women have pain in the lower belly or abdomen at some time in their lives. Often women are taught that this pain is normal for them, and that they should endure such pain in silence. Some people think that a woman's pain is not serious until she cannot stand, walk or talk. But when a woman waits that long to seek care for pain, the result could be serious *infection*, *infertility*, loss of a pregnancy, and even death.

This chapter describes different kinds of pain in the lower abdomen (below the *navel*), and what might be causing the pain. Some pain in the lower abdomen spreads above the navel and could have other causes. Some problems of the lower abdomen will also cause pain in the low back. If the pain seems different from what is described in this chapter, see a health worker trained to give an abdominal exam.

➤ *Pain should not be a normal part of a woman's life—it is a sign that something is wrong. Seek care before you are so ill that you cannot stand, walk, or talk.*

Sudden, Severe Pain in the Abdomen

Some lower abdominal pain is an emergency. **If you have any of the following danger signs, go to the nearest hospital.** A trained health worker will need to do an *examination* of your abdomen, a *pelvic exam*, and perhaps special tests. For information about how to do an abdominal exam and a pelvic exam, see page 530.

> *Danger signs:*
> - sudden, severe pain in the abdomen
> - high fever
> - nausea and vomiting
> - swollen abdomen, which is hard like a piece of wood
> - silent abdomen (no noises)

Kinds of Pain in the Lower Abdomen

Pain in the lower abdomen can have many causes. It can be difficult to find the cause because so many organs in the abdomen are close together.

Kind of pain	May be caused by	What to do	See page
Severe, unusual pain during *monthly bleeding* or after a monthly bleeding was missed	*pregnancy in the tube* 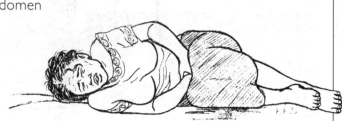	URGENT! Go to a hospital right away.	73
Ongoing pain during monthly bleeding	*fibroids*	See 'pain with monthly bleeding', and 'problems of the womb' Use a mild pain medicine.	50 380 482
Cramps during monthly bleeding	normal squeezing of the womb. Some kinds of *intra uterine devices* (IUDs) may make the pain worse.	See 'pain with monthly bleeding'	50
If the monthly bleeding is late	*miscarriage*	If pain becomes severe, go to a hospital.	234

Kind of pain	May be caused by	What to do	See page
Pain after childbirth, miscarriage, or abortion	infection from pieces of afterbirth (placenta) left in the *womb*, or *germs* that got into the womb during the birth or abortion	See 'womb infection', and 'infection after abortion'.	97 255
Severe pain with fever (infection) with or after having an STD or pelvic infection on one side of the abdomen, with *fever, nausea, vomiting*, and no appetite	another pelvic infection, or a pocket of *pus* in the abdomen (pelvic abcess) *appendicitis* or other *intestinal* infection kidney infection	URGENT! Go to a hospital right away. URGENT! Go to a hospital right away. See 'bladder and kidney infections'	272 366
Pain with *diarrhea*	intestinal infection from bacteria or parasites	See 'diarrhea'.	298
Severe pain in the first 3 months of pregnancy, often with bleeding that comes and goes	pregnancy in the tube	URGENT! Go to a hospital right away.	73
Severe pain in the last 3 months of pregnancy, with or without bleeding	placenta has pulled away from the wall of the womb	URGENT! Go to a hospital right away.	73
Mild, occasional pain during pregnancy	probably normal	No treatment needed.	
Pain with frequent urination Pain with blood in the urine	*bladder* or *kidney* infection kidney stone	See 'bladder and kidney infections', See 'kidney or bladder stones'.	366 369
Pain with discharge or light bleeding from the vagina, sometimes with fever	pelvic infection which may be caused by a *sexually transmitted disease (STD)*, or by infection after miscarriage, *abortion*, or childbirth	See 'pelvic inflammatory disease', 'womb infection', and 'infection after abortion'.	272 97 255

Kind of pain	May be caused by	What to do	See page
Pain during sex	pelvic inflammatory disease (PID), or scars from an old pelvic infection	See 'PID'.	272
	a growth on an ovary (ovarian cyst)	See 'problems of the ovaries'.	383
	fibroids	See 'problems of the womb'.	380
	unwanted sex	See 'if sex is painful'.	193
Pain when moving, walking, or lifting	old pelvic infection, or any of the reasons listed above	Use mild pain medicine if needed.	482
Pain that lasts only a few hours in the middle of your *monthly cycle*	the lining of the abdomen gets irritated when the ovary releases an egg (ovulation) because there is a small amount of blood	Use mild pain medicine if needed.	482
	blood	See the chapter on "Understanding Our Bodies."	43
Pain within 3 weeks of getting an intra uterine device (IUD)	infection with an IUD is most common soon after the IUD is put in	See a health worker right away.	216
Pain without other signs	pelvic infections, which can cause constant or on-and-off pain in the abdomen or lower back that lasts for months or years	See a health worker trained to do a pelvic exam.	272
	intestinal infection from *bacteria* or *parasites*	See a health worker or *Where There Is No Doctor*.	
	tumor or growth on the womb or ovary	See a health worker trained to do a pelvic exam.	375

Questions about Pain in the Abdomen

If your pain does not fit one of the kinds described on the previous pages, these questions may help to learn more about it.

What is the pain like? Is it sharp and severe—or dull, achy, and not so bad? Does it come and go, or is it constant?

- Terrible pain that comes and goes could be from a kidney stone. Severe grabbing, clenching, or cramping pain could be from an intestinal problem.
- Sharp, severe pain, especially just in one place, could be appendicitis or a pregnancy outside the womb in the tube.

How long has the pain lasted?

- Sudden, severe pain that does not get better is probably serious. It could be from a pregnancy in the tube, appendicitis or other gut problems, something wrong with the ovary, or pelvic inflammatory disease (PID).
- Pain that lasts for many days or weeks, especially if it is not severe, may be caused by scars from an old infection, indigestion, or nerves. It may be possible to treat this at home.

Does the pain affect your hunger?

- If you have pain in the abdomen and you DO NOT want to eat anything, you may have a serious infection in your intestines, or appendicitis.
- If you have pain and you DO feel like eating, you probably do not have one of these problems.

For more information on pain in the lower abdomen, see *Where There Is No Doctor* or another general medical book.

Yuni, go to the clinic today to see about this pain you are having. It will only get worse.

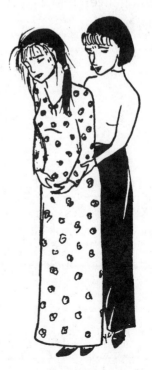

A woman who walks with pain today could die from it tomorrow. Get help early if you are not sure.

Chapter 22

In this chapter:

Problems with Monthly Bleeding

Other Kinds of Bleeding Problems

How to use this chapter:

Most of the causes of the bleeding problems in this chapter are described in other parts of this book. If you have a bleeding problem, look it up here and then turn to the numbered page listed for more information. If the problem is not covered in this book, see a health worker trained to do pelvic exams.

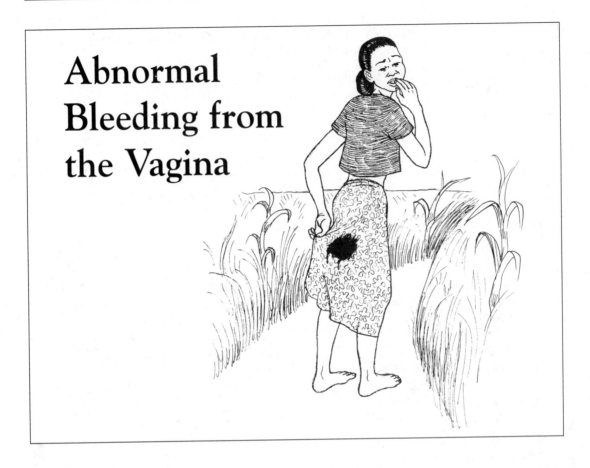

Abnormal Bleeding from the Vagina

It is normal for *monthly bleeding* to change from time to time because of illness, *stress*, pregnancy, breastfeeding, a long journey, overwork, or a change in diet. But if a change in monthly bleeding happens suddenly, lasts more than a few months, or if it comes with other problems, it may be a sign of a more serious problem.

➤ *If monthly bleeding suddenly changes, always think about the possibility of pregnancy—even if a family planning method is being used.*

Danger signs

If a woman has any of these danger signs, she may need medical help right away. Turn to the numbered page listed for more information.

- bleeding and pain in the abdomen when regular monthly bleeding has been missed (page 73)
- bleeding in late pregnancy (page 74)
- heavy bleeding after childbirth, *miscarriage*, or *abortion* (pages 92, 234, and 251)

monthly bleeding

pregnancy

Problems with Monthly Bleeding

HEAVY MONTHLY BLEEDING, OR BLEEDING THAT LASTS A LONG TIME

- Monthly bleeding is heavy if a pad or cloth is soaked through in less than one hour.
- Monthly bleeding is long if it lasts for more than 8 days.
- Blood clots (soft, dark red, shiny lumps in the blood that look like liver) are also a sign of heavy bleeding.
- Heavy bleeding that goes on for many weeks, months or years can cause weak blood (*anemia*, see page 172).

Causes:

- The *hormones* may be out of balance so the *ovary* does not release an egg. This is common for women under 20 and women over 40 years of age (see page 47).

- An *intrauterine device (IUD)* may be making monthly bleeding more heavy (see page 216).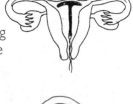

- *Miscarriage*, even if you did not think you were pregnant (see page 234).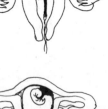

- If you have pain in the abdomen with bleeding, you may have a pregnancy outside the womb in the tube. URGENT. Go to a hospital right away (see page 73).

- You may have a problem with the *thyroid gland.*

- You may have growths (*fibroids* or *polyps*) or *cancer* in your womb (see page 380).

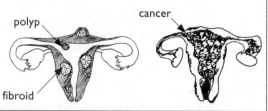

polyp

cancer

fibroid

IMPORTANT *See a health worker trained to do* pelvic exams *if you have heavy bleeding and:*
- *blood gushes from your* vagina.
- *monthly bleeding has been heavy and long for 3 months.*
- *you think you might be pregnant.*
- *you have severe pain with the bleeding.*

LIGHT MONTHLY BLEEDING

Light bleeding each month is not a health problem.

Causes:

208

family planning, changes in bleeding

- Some family planning methods—like injections, *implants*, and the pill—can make you bleed less after you have been using them for some time.
- Your ovary may not have released an egg.

MONTHLY BLEEDING THAT COMES TOO OFTEN, OR BLEEDING AT OTHER TIMES

Something may be wrong if monthly bleeding comes more often than every 3 weeks, or if it comes and goes without a regular pattern.

Causes:

- The ovary may not have released an egg (see page 48).
- There may be growths (fibroids or polyps) or cancer in the womb, especially if monthly bleeding is heavy and not regular (see page 380).

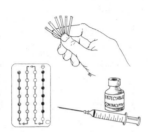

- Taking the medicine called *estrogen* after *menopause* (see page 125).

- Some family planning methods—like the pill, *implants,* and injections—can cause you to bleed more often (see pages 208, 213, and 214).

➤ Hormonal *family planning methods such as pills, implants, or injections, can change monthly bleeding.*

WHEN MONTHLY BLEEDINGS COME TOO FAR APART, OR HAVE STOPPED

Monthly bleeding usually comes about every 21 to 35 days. It may be normal to have an even longer time between bleeding. But something may be wrong, or you may be pregnant, if your monthly bleeding does not come at all.

➤ *If you are over 18 and have never had a monthly period, get medical help.*

Causes:

- You may be pregnant (see page 67).
- You may be pregnant and having a miscarriage (see page 98).
- The ovary may not have released an egg (see page 231).
- You may have a serious illness—like *malaria, tuberculosis,* (see page 387) or *AIDS* (see page 283).
- If you are over 40 or 45, you may be nearing menopause (see page 124).
- Some family planning methods—like the pill, injections, and implants—can make monthly bleedings come far apart (see pages 208, 213, and 214).

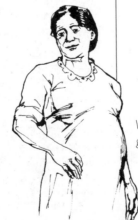

When a woman grows older, her monthly cycle changes.

Other Kinds of Bleeding Problems

BLEEDING DURING PREGNANCY OR AFTER CHILDBIRTH			
Bleeding problem	**May be caused by**	**What to do**	**See page**
Bleeding during the first 3 months with constant pain or pain that comes and goes	*pregnancy in the tube*	URGENT! Go to a hospital right away.	73
Bleeding during the last 3 months of pregnancy	the afterbirth (*placenta*) is coming off the wall of the *womb*. the placenta is covering the *cervix*.	URGENT! Go to a hospital right away.	74
Bleeding during the first 6 months of pregnancy	may be a *miscarriage* (especially if you also have *cramping* pains like birth pains)	Watch and wait. If bleeding becomes heavy, go to a hospital.	98
Heavy bleeding during or just after childbirth	pieces of the placenta are left in the womb the womb is too tired to squeeze or tighten	URGENT! See a midwife or go to a hospital if bleeding is heavy.	92
Light, pink bleeding during the first 3 months of pregnancy without pain	this can be normal, or it may be a sign of early miscarriage	See 'bleeding early in pregnancy'.	74
Spotting or light bleeding instead of your normal monthly bleeding	the developing baby (*fetus*) is attaching to the wall of the womb (*implantation*). This is normal.	See the chapter on "Pregnancy and Childbirth."	67

BLEEDING AFTER AN ABORTION OR MISCARRIAGE

Bleeding problem	May be caused by	What to do	See page
Heavy bleeding, or bleeding that lasts longer than 15 days, or bleeding with pain or fever	pieces of the pregnancy may still be in the womb *infection* in the womb	Go to a hospital or clinic right away.	251 255
Bleeding like a normal monthly bleeding, but lasting 5 to 15 days, getting lighter and lighter	this is normal	See 'what to expect after an abortion'.	249

BLEEDING AFTER SEX

Bleeding problem	May be caused by	What to do	See page
Bleeding during or after sex	*sexually transmitted disease (STD)*	See 'gonorrhea and chlamydia'.	265
	pelvic inflammatory disease	See 'PID'.	272
	forced sex	See Ch. 19, "Rape."	327
	growths or cancer of the cervix or womb	See 'cancer of the cervix' and 'problems of the womb'.	377 380

BLEEDING AFTER MENOPAUSE

Bleeding problem	May be caused by	What to do	See page
Bleeding that begins 12 months or more after menopause	growths or cancer of the womb	See a health worker trained to do a pelvic exam.	380
	growths or cancer of the cervix	You may need to have a Pap test or a *D and C*.	377

Chapter 23

In this chapter:

Problems of the Urine System

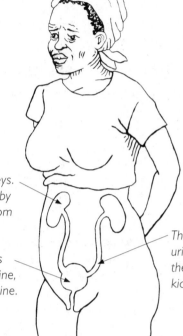

There are 2 kidneys. They make urine by cleaning waste from the blood.

The bladder is a bag. It stretches and gets bigger as it fills with urine, and gets small after you pass urine.

There are 2 upper urine tubes. They carry the urine from the kidneys to the bladder.

When you pass urine, the urine goes down the lower urine tube and comes out a small hole in front of your vagina.

This chapter describes the most common problems that affect the urine system. Sometimes these problems are difficult to tell apart. So if your problem seems different from those described here, get medical help. You may need special tests to find out what the problem is.

If you can identify the problem, it may be possible to treat the problem at home—especially if treatment is started right away. But remember that some serious problems begin with signs that do not seem very bad. These problems can quickly become painful and dangerous. So if you do not feel better within 2 to 3 days, get medical help.

Female circumcision

This can damage the urine system and cause serious health problems for a woman all her life. If you have been circumcised and have problems passing urine, or *infections* that return again and again, talk to a health worker. You may need surgery to correct the problem. For more information, see the chapter on "Female Circumcision," page 459.

Infections of the Urine System

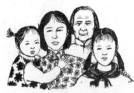

A girl or woman of any age—even a small baby—can get an infection of her urine system.

I hope the truck stops soon so I can pass urine.

➤ *Teach little girls the correct way to wipe after passing stool.*

There are 2 main kinds of urine system infections. A bladder infection is the most common and the easiest to treat. A kidney infection is very serious. It can lead to permanent damage to the kidney and even death.

WHAT CAUSES BLADDER AND KIDNEY INFECTIONS?

Infections of the urine system are caused by *germs* (*bacteria*). They get into the body from the outside through the urinary opening near the *vagina*. Infection is more common in women than in men because a woman's lower urine tube is much shorter. This means germs can more easily climb up the short urine tube into the bladder.

Germs often enter a woman's body or start to multiply when she:

- **has sex**. During sex, germs from the vagina and *anus* can be pushed up through the urinary opening into the lower urine tube. This is one of the most common causes of a bladder infection in women. To prevent infection, pass urine after having sex. This washes out the urine tube (but does not prevent pregnancy).

- **goes for a long time without drinking**, especially if she works outside in hot weather and sweats a lot. Germs will start to multiply in the empty bladder. Try to drink at least 8 glasses or cups of liquid a day. When working in the hot sun, drink even more.

- **goes for a long time without urinating** (for example, when traveling). Germs that stay in the urine system for a long time can cause an infection. Try to pass urine every 3 to 4 hours.

- **does not keep her genitals clean**. Germs from the *genitals*—and especially the anus—can get into the urinary opening and cause infection. Try to wash the genitals every day, and always wipe from front to back after passing *stool* (see page 154). Wiping forward can spread germs from the anus into the urinary opening. Also, try to wash your genitals before having sex. Keep the cloth and pads used for your monthly bleeding very clean.

- **has a** *disability*, especially those from backbone (spinal cord) injuries, or with a loss of feeling in the lower body. For more information, see the books *Where There Is No Doctor* and *Disabled Village Children*.

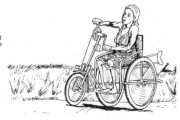

SIGNS AND TREATMENT

Bladder infection signs:

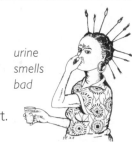
urine smells bad

- need to pass urine very often (It may also feel as though some urine is still left inside.)
- pain or a burning feeling while passing urine
- pain in the lower belly just after passing urine
- urine smells bad, or looks cloudy, or has blood or *pus* in it. (Dark urine can be a sign of *hepatitis*. See page 271.)

Kidney infection signs:

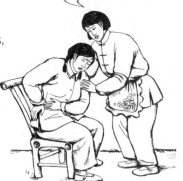

Don't worry Lihua. I will help you get to the health center.

- any bladder infection signs
- *fever* and chills
- lower back pain, often severe, that can go from the front, around the sides, and into the back
- *nausea* and *vomiting*
- feeling very ill and weak

If you have signs of both a bladder and a kidney infection, you probably have a kidney infection.

When a woman has a kidney infection, she may be in great pain and feel very ill. This can be very frightening. If this happens to you, try to get a family member or a neighbor to help you get to a health worker or health post.

IMPORTANT *If your signs are serious, start taking medicine right away. See the next page.*

Treatment for a bladder infection:

Bladder infections can often be treated with home remedies. **Start treatment as soon as you notice the signs.** A bladder infection can sometimes travel quickly up the urine tubes into the kidneys.

- **Drink a lot of water**. Try to drink at least one cup of clean water every 30 minutes. This will make you pass urine often. Sometimes the germs will wash out of your urine system before the infection gets worse.

- **Stop having sex** for a few days, or until the signs have gone away.

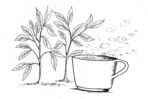

- **Make a tea** from flowers, seeds, and leaves that are known to help cure urine infections. Ask the older women in the community which plants will help.

➤ *STDs, especially chlamydia, can cause a burning feeling when a woman passes urine.*

If you do not feel better in 1 to 2 days, stop taking the home remedies and start taking the medicines in the box below. If you do not feel better in 2 more days, see a health worker. You may have an STD rather than a urine system infection (see page 263).

IMPORTANT *Before taking any of these medicines, especially if you are pregnant or breastfeeding, first read about them in the "Green Pages" of this book.*

Bladder Infection Medicines

Medicine	How much to take	When to take
amoxicillin	3 g (3000 mg)	once only by mouth
or		
co-trimoxazole 480 mg (80 mg trimethoprim and 400 mg sulfamethoxazole)	4 tablets	once only by mouth

Treatment for a kidney infection:

If you have signs of a kidney infection, home remedies are not enough. Start taking these medicines right away. But if you do not start to feel better after 2 days, see a health worker.

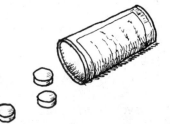

Kidney Infection Medicines

Medicine	How much to take	When to take
amoxicillin	500 mg	3 times a day, by mouth, for 10 days
or		
co-trimoxazole 480 mg (80 mg trimethoprim and 400 mg sulfamethoxazole)	2 tablets	2 times a day, by mouth, for 10 days
<u>If you cannot swallow medicines because you are vomiting, take:</u>		
ampicillin	500 mg	Inject into a muscle 4 times a day.
or		
gentamicin	80 mg the first time only, then 60 mg each other time	Inject into a muscle 3 times a day.

When you can swallow medicine again without vomiting, stop injections and continue with the medicine by mouth for kidney infection for 7 more days.

BLOOD IN THE URINE

If your urine has blood in it, and if there are no other signs of a bladder or kidney infection, you may have bladder or kidney stones (see below). Or you may have one of these diseases, if they are common in your community:

- *Bilharzia* (**blood flukes, schistosomiasis**) can cause permanent damage to the urine system if it is not treated early enough. See a health worker trained in problems of the urine system for treatment, and to learn how to prevent bilharzia from happening again. For more information about bilharzia, see *Where There Is No Doctor* or another general medical book.
- *Tuberculosis (TB)* can damage the bladder and kidneys. For more information, see page 387.

KIDNEY OR BLADDER STONES

These are small hard stones that start to grow in the kidney, and then move through the urine system.

Signs:

- Sudden, very bad pain:

in the back where the kidneys are,

or in the side near the kidneys,

or lower down in the urine tubes or bladder.

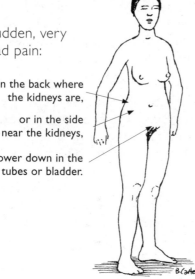

Other signs are:

- Blood in the urine. This can happen if the stones scratch the inside of the urine system.
- Difficulty passing urine. This can happen if a stone blocks the tubes.

Treatment:

- Drink large amounts of liquid (at least 1 or 2 cups every 30 minutes). This will help wash the stone out of the kidney and down the urine tube.
- Take a pain medicine. If the pain is very bad, get medical help.

Sometimes the blocked urine tubes become infected. Treat this problem the same way you would treat a kidney infection.

Other Problems of the Urine System

tuberculosis

medicines for pain

NEED TO PASS URINE OFTEN

This may happen because:

- the muscles around your bladder and *womb* have become weak. The 'squeezing exercise' (page 371) may help strengthen these muscles.
- a growth (like a fibroid) in your abdomen is pushing against the bladder so it cannot hold much urine.
- you have a bladder infection.
- you have *diabetes*.

growths, 380
diabetes, 174

LEAKING URINE

Poor control of urine (incontinence)

This can be caused by weak or damaged muscles around the bladder. It happens mainly to older women or to women after childbirth. The urine leaks out when a woman puts pressure on the weak muscles in her lower belly during sex, or by laughing, coughing, sneezing, or lifting. The 'squeezing exercise' (page 371) may help.

Urine leaking from the vagina (vesico-vaginal fistula, VVF)

When a woman leaks urine all the time, she may have a hole between her vagina and bladder. (Sometimes the hole is between the rectum and the vagina, and stool leaks out.)

This serious problem happens as a result of a blocked birth. It happens to girls who have babies when they are very young, before their bones are fully grown. The problem can also happen to older women who have had many babies, if their muscles are no longer strong enough to push a baby out. In both cases, it is difficult for the baby to get out. Its head presses on the skin between the bladder and the vagina, and damages the skin. This causes an opening (fistula) to form between the bladder and the vagina. Often the baby is born dead.

This girl's husband was embarrassed by the smell of her leaking urine. He made her leave his house.

After the birth, the fistula does not heal and urine leaks from the bladder out through the vagina all the time. The girl or woman has to wear a cloth or pad all day and night to catch the urine.

If she cannot get help (see the next page), fistulas can cause serious problems for a girl or woman in her daily life. Her husband, family, and friends may avoid her because she smells of urine all the time.

Treatment:

After the birth, if you are leaking urine or stool, talk with a health worker as soon as possible to find out if she or he knows of a hospital where the fistula can be repaired. You should **go to the hospital as soon as possible**. If you cannot get to the hospital quickly, the health worker may know how to put in a plastic or rubber tube (catheter) through the urine hole into the bladder (see page 373). This tube will drain the urine and may help the fistula heal. But you must still go to the hospital. When you get there, the doctor will examine you to see if the fistula has healed or if you need an operation to repair the fistula.

Do not despair. The problem can often be made better.

IMPORTANT *To help prevent infection while the tube is in, drink a lot of fluid (at least 10 to 12 cups a day). This will make you pass urine often and flush out germs.*

Prevention:

- Avoid marriage and pregnancy until a girl is fully grown.
- If a girl under 17 is pregnant, she should try to see a trained midwife or health worker as soon as possible to find out how to have the safest birth.
- Do not have babies too close together, so that your muscles can get strong again in between births (see page 197).

➤ *If you have leaking urine after giving birth, seek medical help right away.*

72
pregnancy

The squeezing exercise

This exercise can help strengthen weak muscles that cause you to pass urine often or to leak urine. First practice while you are passing urine. As the urine comes out, stop it by tightly squeezing the muscles in your vagina. Count to 10, then relax the muscles to let the urine come out. Repeat this several times whenever you urinate. Once you know how, practice the squeezing exercise at other times during the day. No one will know. Try to practice at least 4 times a day, squeezing your muscles 5 to 10 times each time.

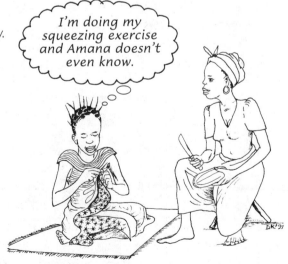

I'm doing my squeezing exercise and Amana doesn't even know.

Some women may need surgery to help control leaking urine. If your urine leaks a lot and this exercise does not help, get advice from a health worker trained in women's health. The squeezing exercise is good for all women to do every day. It helps keep muscles strong and can prevent problems later in life.

When You Have Problems Passing Stool or Urine

Many women (and men) do not have normal control over when they pass stool or urine (especially persons who are near death, or who have a spinal cord injury, or a disability that affects the muscles of the lower body). This can be inconvenient and embarrassing. It can also cause skin problems and dangerous infections, so it is important to stay clean, dry, and healthy.

Bowel control

This information will help those persons who have hard stools (constipation) or who have difficulty passing stool. You can learn to help the stool come out when it is easiest for you. The *bowels* work best when you are sitting rather than lying, so try to remove the stool when you are sitting on a toilet or pot. If you cannot sit, try to do it lying on your left side.

How to remove stool:

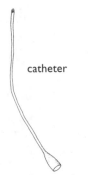

1. Cover your hand with a plastic or rubber glove, or a plastic bag. Put oil on your pointing (index) finger (vegetable or mineral oil both work well).

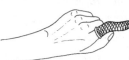

To keep your finger clean, use a thin rubber glove or 'fingercot'.

2. Put your oiled finger into the anus about 2 cm (1 inch). Gently move the finger in circles for about 1 minute, until the muscle relaxes and the stool pushes out.

3. If the stool does not come out by itself, remove as much as you can with your finger.

4. Clean the anus and the skin around it well, and wash your hands.

To prevent hard stools:
- drink lots of water every day.
- keep a regular bowel program.
- eat foods that are high in *fiber*.
- exercise or move your body every day.

Bladder control

catheter

Sometimes it is necessary to remove urine from the bladder by using a rubber or plastic tube called a catheter. **Never use a catheter unless it is absolutely necessary.** Even careful use of a catheter can cause infection of the bladder and kidneys. So it should only be used if someone has a:
- very full, painful bladder and cannot pass urine.
- vesico-vaginal fistula (VVF). See page 370.
- disability or injury, and cannot feel the muscles that control passing urine.

How to put in a catheter

1. Boil the catheter (and any syringe or tool you may be using) for 15 minutes.

2. Wash well with soap and clean water between the folds of the vulva and skin around the genitals.

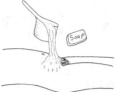

3. Wash your hands. After washing, only touch things that are *sterile* or very clean.

4. Put very clean cloths under and around the genitals.

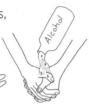

5. Put on sterile gloves, or rub hands well with alcohol or surgical soap.

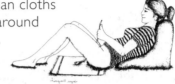

6. Cover the catheter with a sterile lubricant (slippery cream) that dissolves in water (not oil or petroleum gel).

7. Open the folds of the vulva and wipe the opening with a sterile cotton cloth made wet with soap and clean water, or with a solution of 1 teaspoon of povidone iodine to 1 cup of clean water.

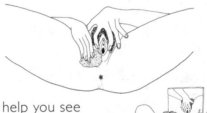

8. If you do this for yourself, use a mirror to help you see where the urinary opening is, and use your pointing (index) finger and third finger to hold the folds of the vulva open. The urinary opening is below the clitoris almost at the opening to the vagina.

9. Then, with your middle finger, touch below your clitoris. You will feel a sort of small dent or dimple, and right below that is the urinary opening. Keep your middle finger on that spot, and with your other hand, take the clean catheter and touch the tip to the end of your middle finger, and gently guide the catheter into the opening until urine starts to come out.

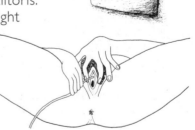

You will know if the catheter goes into the vagina instead of the urinary opening because it will go in easily, but no urine will come out. Also, when you remove it, the catheter will have discharge (mucus from the vagina) in it. Try again with a clean catheter.

IMPORTANT *To avoid infection when using a catheter, it is important for you to be very clean, and to use only a catheter that is sterile, boiled, or very clean (see page 521).*

Chapter 24

In this chapter:

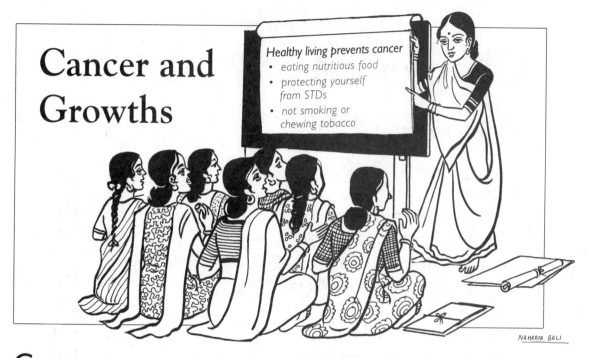

Cancer and Growths

Healthy living prevents cancer
• eating nutritious food
• protecting yourself from STDs
• not smoking or chewing tobacco

NAMRATA BALI

Cancer is a serious sickness that can affect many different parts of the body. If it is treated early it is often curable, but if left too long it can cause death. Many people who get cancer die from it, especially those with little *access* to health care.

Women often do not see a health worker or doctor unless they are very sick. So women who get cancer are more likely to get very sick or die, because the cancer is not found early enough. Also, women who get cancer are sometimes considered 'cursed' and may be shunned by their families or communities. This isolation is not only bad for the women who are sick, but also for the whole community, since it keeps everyone from knowing about how cancer makes people sick.

WHAT IS CANCER?

All living things, like the human body, are made up of tiny *cells* that are too small to see without a *microscope*. Sometimes these cells change and grow in an abnormal way, causing growths (tumors). Some growths go away without treatment. But some growths get larger or spread and may cause health problems. **Most growths do not become cancer**, but some do.

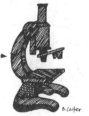

B.Carter

Cancer starts when some cells begin to grow out of control and take over parts of the body. When cancer is found early, it can often be removed by surgery, or treated with medicines or *radiation*, and the chance of it being cured may be good. Once cancer spreads, however, curing it is more difficult and eventually becomes impossible.

➤ *'Tumor' is another word for growth or swelling. Some tumors are cancer and some are not.*

Cancer

Cancer of the *cervix*, breast, and *womb* are the most common 'women's' cancers. Other common cancers that both men and women get are cancer of the *lung*, colon, *liver*, *stomach*, mouth, and skin.

CAUSES OF CANCER

The direct causes of most cancers are not known. But these things may make you more likely to get cancer:

- smoking tobacco, which is known to cause lung cancer, and also increases the risk of getting most other cancers
- certain viral infections, like *hepatitis* B or *genital warts*
- eating foods with too much fat or with harmful chemicals
- using some medicines, like *hormones*, incorrectly
- working with or living around certain *chemicals* (like pesticides, dyes, paints, and solvents)
- living or working near nuclear power plants

Also, if others in a woman's family (blood relatives) have had a certain kind of cancer, this may mean she is more likely to get that same kind of cancer (this is called a hereditary risk).

Healthy living can prevent many cancers. This means eating *nutritious* food and avoiding things that may cause cancer. For example:

- Do not smoke or chew tobacco.
- Try to avoid harmful chemicals in your home or workplace, including foods grown or preserved with them.
- Protect yourself from *sexually transmitted diseases (STDs)*.

FINDING AND TREATING CANCER EARLY

Finding cancer early can often save a woman's life, because she can get early treatment, before the cancer spreads. Some cancers have warning signs that show something may be wrong. But usually, to find out if you have cancer, you must have a test that takes a few cells from the part of your body where the cancer may be. Then the cells must be examined with a microscope, by someone who is trained to recognize cancer.

Cancers that do not have early signs can often be found with screening tests, routine tests given to people to see if everything is normal. A Pap test for cancer of the cervix (see page 378) is one kind of screening test.

If you have warning signs, or a test shows something may be wrong, do not wait. Follow the advice in this chapter for finding and treating the problem as soon as possible.

➤ *Cancer is not an infection. It is not 'catching' and cannot spread from one person to another.*

149

staying healthy

186

safer sex

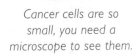

Cancer cells are so small, you need a microscope to see them.

COMMON PROBLEMS OF THE CERVIX

Nabothian cysts are small blisters or bumps on the cervix that are filled with fluid. There are no signs, but they can be seen during a *pelvic exam* (with a *speculum*). These cysts are harmless, so no treatment is needed.

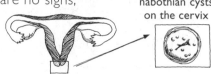

nabothian cysts on the cervix

Polyps are dark red growths, sometimes found at the cervix. They also grow inside the womb. For more about them, see 'Common Growths of the Womb', page 380.

Inflammation of the cervix. Many infections of the vagina— like trichomonas—and some STDs affect the cervix, and can cause growths, sores, or irritation and bleeding after sex. For information about those types of problems, including treatment, see the chapter on "Sexually Transmitted Diseases and Other Infections of the Genitals."

CANCER OF THE CERVIX

Cancer of the cervix is the most common cancer in the less-developed world. The main cause is a virus—human papilloma virus, or HPV—which is the same virus that causes genital warts. This cancer grows slowly for about 10 years, and if it is treated early it can be completely cured. But many women die every year from cancer of the cervix because they never knew they had it.

A woman is at greater risk of getting cancer of the cervix if she:

- is older than 35.
- began to have sex at a young age (within only a few years of starting her *monthly bleeding*).
- has had many sex partners, or has a partner who has had many sex partners.
- has had frequent STDs, especially genital warts.
- has *HIV/AIDS*.
- smokes tobacco.

Warning signs:

There are usually no outward signs of cancer of the cervix until it has spread and is more difficult to treat. (There **are** often early signs on the cervix, which can be seen during a pelvic exam. This is why regular exams are so important.)

Abnormal bleeding from the vagina, including bleeding after sex, or an abnormal *discharge* or bad smell from the vagina can all be signs of a serious problem, including advanced cancer of the cervix. If you have any of those signs, try to get a pelvic exam and a Pap test.

Problems of the Cervix (the Opening of the Womb)

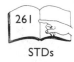

261

STDs

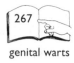

267

genital warts

9

Mira's story

IMPORTANT
If you are treated with medicines for a vaginal discharge and do not get better, you should try to have your cervix examined and get a Pap test to look for cancer.

Finding and treating cancer of the cervix

> If you are a health worker, try to get training in testing for cervical cancer. Encourage your community to offer cancer screening.

Because cancer of the cervix does not have early warning signs, but can be cured if it is found early, it is good to be tested for it regularly, if possible. The tests are designed to look for abnormal tissue on the cervix. Such tissue may be slightly abnormal (mild dysplasia), more abnormal (severe dysplasia), or early cancer (before it has spread).

The Pap test

The most common test is the Pap test. For this test, a health worker scrapes some cells from the cervix (this is not painful) during a pelvic exam and sends them to a *laboratory* to be examined with a microscope. When you have this test, you must return for the results, usually after several weeks.

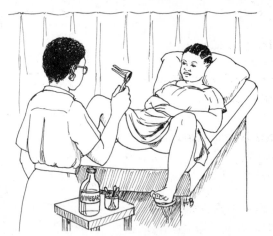

Visual inspection

A new, low-cost method of screening women for cancer of the cervix uses a vinegar solution (acetic acid) which is painted on the cervix, and turns abnormal tissue white. The cervix is examined, sometimes with the aid of a small lens that makes it easier to see. If a woman has abnormal tissue, she may need other tests or treatment.

Regular testing for cancer of the cervix can save many lives.

Other tests used to find cancer

• **Biopsy**. A piece of tissue is taken from the cervix and sent to a laboratory to be examined for cancer cells.

• **Colposcopy**. This tool, available in some hospitals, magnifies the cervix (makes it look bigger) so it is easier to see signs of cancer.

How often women should be tested

To find cancer of the cervix early enough to treat it simply and successfully, women should be tested at least every 3 years. In places where this is not possible, women should try to get tested at least every 5 years, especially women over 35.

You should be tested more often, if possible, when:

• you are more at risk for developing cancer of the cervix (see page 377).

• you have a Pap test that shows some slightly abnormal cells. These cells often do not become cancer, and they return to normal in 2 to 3 years. But since those cells **could** be early signs of cancer, you should have another Pap test in 1 to 2 years to make sure cancer is not growing.

Treatment:

If a test shows that you have severe dysplasia or a more advanced cancer, you will need treatment. You and your doctor should decide together what treatment is best. Treatment in the early stages can be simple, using methods that remove or destroy the cancer tissue.

36

deciding about treatment

In some places a method called *cryotherapy* is available, which freezes the cervix and kills the cancer. Another treatment is to remove part of the cervix (cone biopsy). If it is available, this treatment may be best if you still want to have children and the cancer has not spread, because you can keep your womb. When cancer is found and treated before it spreads, it can be cured.

➤ *You may need to go to a large, special hospital for cancer treatment.*

If the cancer is found after it has grown for a long time, it may have spread beyond the cervix to other parts of the body. In this case you will usually need surgery to remove both the cervix and womb (hysterectomy). Sometimes radiation therapy can help.

381

hysterectomy

Deaths from cancer of the cervix can be prevented

When people do not know about the risks for cancer of the cervix and how finding it early can prevent death, more women die. To change this, we can:

- learn what increases a woman's risk, and work together on finding ways to reduce these risks. It is especially important for girls to be able to wait until they are grown women before having sex. All women also need to be able to protect themselves from STDs.

- learn about cancer screening. Finding cancer of the cervix early can save lives.

In some parts of the world Pap tests are available to women who live near hospitals. Other women are able to get Pap tests from clinics that offer maternal and child health services, family planning, and treatment for STDs.

Developing screening programs may seem too costly but it is cheaper than treatment. Screening programs can help the most women while costing the least if they:

- target older women. Young women can also get cancer of the cervix, but women over 35 are most at risk.

- test as many women as possible, even if this means testing them less often. Testing all women at risk every 5 to 10 years will find many more cancers than testing only some women more often.

- train local health workers in how to give Pap tests and do visual inspection.

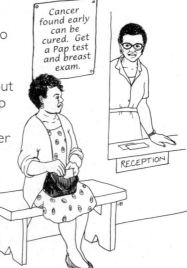

Cancer found early can be cured. Get a Pap test and breast exam.

RECEPTION

Problems of the Womb

COMMON GROWTHS OF THE WOMB

Fibroid tumors

Fibroids are growths of the womb. They can cause abnormal bleeding from the vagina, pain in the lower belly, and repeated miscarriage (losing a pregnancy). They are almost never cancer.

fibroids

womb

Signs:

- heavy monthly bleeding or bleeding at unusual times of the month
- pain or a heavy feeling in the lower belly
- deep pain during sex

Finding and treating fibroids

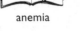

pelvic exam

Fibroids are usually found during a pelvic exam. The womb will feel too large or be the wrong shape. A test called an *ultrasound*, if it is available, can show how large the fibroids are.

If fibroids cause problems, they can be removed with surgery. Sometimes the whole womb is removed. But most of the time, surgery is not necessary because fibroids usually

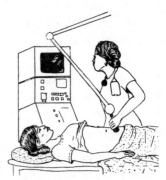

An ultrasound test can show how large fibroids are.

become smaller after menopause and stop causing problems. If *monthly bleeding* is heavy because of fibroids, *anemia* may develop. Try to eat foods rich in iron.

172

anemia

Polyps

Polyps are dark red growths that can grow inside the womb or at the cervix. They are rarely cancer.

polyps

Signs:

- bleeding after sex
- heavy monthly bleeding or bleeding at unusual times of the month

Finding and treating polyps

D and C

Polyps at the cervix can be seen and removed easily and painlessly during a pelvic exam by someone who has been trained. To find polyps inside the womb, the inside of the womb must be scraped out (this is called a D and C). The D and C also removes the polyps. The growth is sent to a laboratory to make sure there is no cancer. Once polyps are removed, they usually do not grow back.

CANCER OF THE WOMB
(CANCER OF THE UTERUS, *ENDOMETRIAL* CANCER)

Cancer of the womb usually starts in the lining inside the womb (the endometrium). If it is not treated it can spread to the womb itself and to other parts of the body. This cancer happens most often to women who:

- are over 40 years old, especially if they have gone through *menopause*.
- are overweight.
- have *diabetes*.
- have taken the hormone estrogen without also taking progesterone.

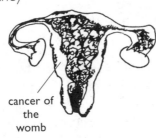

cancer of the womb

125

medicines during menopause

Signs:

- heavy monthly bleeding
- irregular monthly bleeding, or bleeding at unusual times of the month
- bleeding after menopause

IMPORTANT *If you have any bleeding at all, even light spotting, after you have finished menopause (12 months without monthly bleeding), get checked by a health worker to make sure you do not have cancer.*

Finding and treating cancer of the womb

To find out if a woman has cancer of the womb, a trained health worker must scrape out the inside of the womb with a D and C, or do a biopsy, and send the tissue to a laboratory to be checked for cancer. If cancer is found, it must be treated as soon as possible with an operation to remove the womb (hysterectomy). Radiation therapy may also be used.

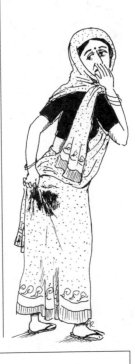

Hysterectomy

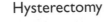

In a hysterectomy, sometimes only the womb is removed and sometimes the tubes and ovaries are also removed (total hysterectomy). Since your ovaries make hormones that help protect you against heart disease and weak bones, it is always better to leave them in, if possible. Talk to a doctor about this.

If cancer of the womb is found early, it can be cured. If it is more advanced, curing it is more difficult.

IMPORTANT *Any woman who is over 40 years old and has unusual bleeding should get checked by a health worker.*

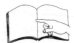

abnormal bleeding, 359

heavy bleeding or bleeding in the middle of the month, 129

Problems of the Breast

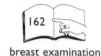

162

breast examination

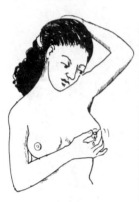

117

breast infections

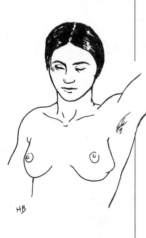

HB

Breast lumps

Breast lumps are very common in most women, especially soft, fluid-filled ones (called cysts). These usually change during a woman's monthly cycle, and sometimes feel sore or painful when pressed. **Few breast lumps are cancer.** But since breast cancer is always a possibility, a woman should try to examine her breasts for lumps once a month (see 'warning signs' below).

Discharge from the nipple

Milky or clear discharge from one or both nipples is usually normal if a woman has breastfed a baby within the last year. Brown, green, or bloody discharge—especially from only one nipple—could be a sign of cancer. Get checked by a health worker who can examine your breasts.

Breast infection

If a woman is breastfeeding a baby and gets a hot, red sore area on the breast, she probably has *mastitis*, or an *abscess*. This is not cancer and is easily cured. If the woman is not breastfeeding, it may be a sign of cancer.

CANCER OF THE BREAST

Breast cancer usually grows slowly. If it is found early, it can sometimes be cured. It is hard to tell who will get breast cancer. The risk might be greater for a woman whose mother or sisters have had breast cancer, or for a woman who has had cancer of the womb. Breast cancer is more common in women over age 50.

Warning signs:

- a hard painless lump with a jagged shape, that is in only one breast and does not move under the skin
- redness, or a sore on the breast that does not heal
- skin on the breast that is pulled in, or looks rough and pitted, like orange or lemon peel
- a nipple that is pulled inward
- abnormal discharge from a nipple
- sometimes, a painful swelling under the arm
- rarely, pain in the breast

If there is one or more of these signs, get help from a trained health worker right away.

Finding and treating breast cancer

If you examine your breasts regularly, you are likely to notice if there are any changes or if a new lump develops. A special X-ray called a mammogram can find a breast lump when it is very small and less dangerous. But mammograms are not available in many places, and they are very expensive. And it cannot tell for sure if a lump is cancer.

The only way to know for sure that a woman has breast cancer is with a biopsy. For this, a surgeon removes all or part of the lump with a needle or a knife and has it tested for cancer in a laboratory.

Treatment depends on how advanced the cancer is and what is available where you live. If a lump is small and found early, just removing the lump may be effective. But for some cases of breast cancer, an operation may be needed to remove the whole breast. Sometimes doctors also use medicines and radiation therapy.

No one knows yet how to prevent breast cancer. But we do know that finding and treating breast cancer early makes a cure more likely. For some women it never comes back. In other women, the cancer may come back years later. It may come back in the other breast or, less often, in other parts of the body.

162

how to examine
your breasts

➤ See a health
worker right away if
you have already had
breast cancer and
find another lump in
the breast or notice
other warning signs
of cancer.

CYSTS ON THE OVARIES

These cysts are fluid-filled sacks that women can get on their ovaries. They happen only during the reproductive years, between *puberty* and menopause. A cyst can cause pain on one side of the lower *abdomen* and irregular monthly bleeding. But most women only find out they have a cyst if a health worker feels one during a pelvic examination.

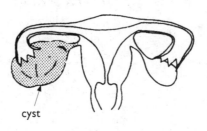

cyst

Most cysts last only a few months and go away on their own. But some can grow very large and must be removed by surgery. If you have severe pain, see a health worker right away.

CANCER OF THE OVARIES

Cancer of the ovaries is not common. There are usually no warning signs, but a health worker might feel an ovary that is very large while doing a pelvic examination. Surgery, medicines, and radiation therapy are all used for treatment, and cure is very difficult.

Problems of the Ovaries

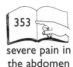

353

severe pain in
the abdomen

Other Common Cancers

Smoking causes cancer.

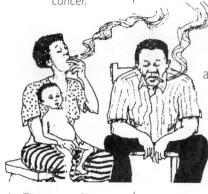

➤ *The signs of lung cancer are the same as tuberculosis (TB). Seek medical help if you have these signs.*

➤ *Try to make hepatitis B vaccine available in your community.*

STDs, 261
hepatitis B, 271

LUNG CANCER

Lung cancer is a growing problem that is often caused by smoking tobacco. It is more common in men because they usually smoke more than women. But because many women now smoke as much as men, they are starting to get more lung cancer. In some countries, more women now die from lung cancer caused by smoking than from any other kind of cancer. And in many places, girls are starting to smoke as early and as much as boys. As more girls and women smoke, even more women will end up getting lung cancer.

Lung cancer does not usually affect people until they are over 40 years old. If a woman stops smoking, her risk of getting lung cancer becomes much less. The signs (coughing up blood, losing weight, difficulty breathing) appear when the cancer is advanced and difficult to cure. Surgery to remove part of the lung, medicines, and radiation therapy are all used to treat lung cancer.

MOUTH AND THROAT CANCER

Mouth and throat cancer can be caused by smoking and chewing tobacco. If you smoke or chew tobacco, and have sores in your mouth that do not heal, get medical advice.

CANCER OF THE LIVER

Some people who become infected with hepatitis B develop cancer of the liver years later. Signs of liver cancer are a swollen abdomen and general weakness. See a health worker if you think you may have liver cancer.

Hepatitis B can be prevented by having *safer* sex and by getting *vaccinated*. Babies can be protected against hepatitis B by vaccination at birth. Adults can be vaccinated at any time.

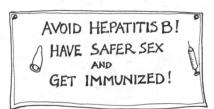

AVOID HEPATITIS B!
HAVE SAFER SEX
AND
GET IMMUNIZED!

Cancer of the liver can be caused by hepatitis B.

CANCER OF THE STOMACH

Cancer of the stomach can occur in women and men over age 40. Usually there are no signs until it is advanced. Surgery is the only treatment and may not be successful.

When Cancer Cannot Be Cured

Many cancers can be cured, but others cannot, especially if the cancer has spread to several parts of the body. Also, hospitals that treat cancer are often far away, in large cities, and treatment is costly.

Sometimes, when cancer is found late, there is no cure. Then it may be best to stay at home in the care of your family. This time can be very difficult. Eat as well as you can and get enough rest. Medicines for pain, anxiety, and sleeping problems can make you more comfortable (see page 482). Talking with someone close to you can help you prepare for death, and help you plan for your family's future after you are gone.

If you are caring for someone who must stay in bed, or who is near death, see the information on the following pages: 142, 143, 306, 308, 309, and 372.

Working for Change

Many unnecessary deaths from cancer could be prevented if more cancers were found and treated earlier. To help make this happen, organize women and men to promote:

- better cancer screening in local health services and rural areas.
- training for local health workers to do visual inspection for cancer of the cervix, Pap tests, and breast exams.
- more labs and trained technicians to read Pap tests.
- better education and more community awareness about how cancer can be prevented, who is at risk, what the warning signs are, and the benefits of cancer screening.
- lower cost care for women who have cancer.

It is also important for women to:

- learn to do breast self-examinations.
- know the signs of cancer, especially cancer of the womb, breast, and cervix.

When people in the community know more about the things that are likely to cause cancer, they may be better able to avoid them. This could prevent many cancers from starting. Help people in your community learn that they can prevent many unnecessary deaths from cancer if they avoid smoking or chewing tobacco, and if women are able to protect themselves from STDs.

Chapter 25

In this chapter:

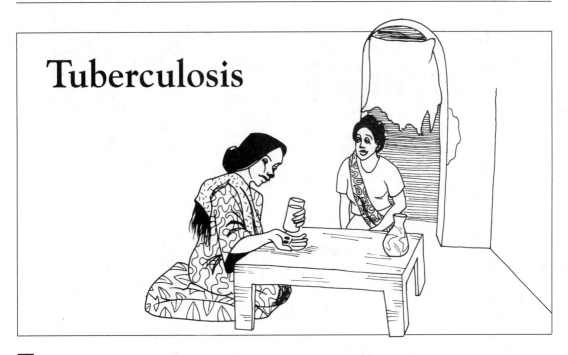

Tuberculosis

Tuberculosis (TB) is a serious disease that usually affects the *lungs*. Every year TB causes more deaths than any other *infectious* disease—more deaths than tropical diseases, *malaria*, and *AIDS* combined. About 2 billion people (1/3 of the world's population) carry the TB *germ* in their bodies. Of these, 10 million people are actually sick with TB right now.

➤ *With proper treatment, TB can almost always be cured.*

As living and work conditions become more crowded, even more people are becoming infected or sick with TB. This is because TB spreads easily in crowded conditions—for example, in cities, slums, refugee camps, factories, and office buildings—especially in indoor areas where the air does not move much. Also, people who are infected with *HIV* and TB can easily get sick with TB because their *immune systems* are weak and unable to fight disease.

WOMEN AND TB

TB affects both men and women, but fewer women than men get treatment. Nearly 3000 women die every day from TB, and at least 1/3 die because they never knew they had the disease or because they did not receive proper treatment. It is often more difficult for a woman to get health care to cure TB because she may not be able to leave her family and work, or does not have the money to travel to a clinic. In some places a woman may not seek treatment for TB because she fears her husband will reject her as 'sickly' or too weak to do her work. A woman who works outside the home is often afraid she will be dismissed because her employer may think she will infect others.

➤ *Caring for sick family members may also put a woman at greater risk of becoming infected with TB.*

What Is TB?

diabetes, 174
AIDS, 283

➤ *Sometimes TB germs attack other body organs, the lymph nodes, or the bones and joints. This is called extrapulmonary TB. When TB germs attack the spine and brain, it is called TB meningitis.*

TB is caused by a small germ, or bacteria. Once this germ enters a woman's body, she is infected with TB and will remain so for many years, probably for life. Healthy people can usually fight off the sickness, and only a small number of people who are infected actually get sick with TB. About 1 out of 10 persons infected becomes sick with TB in his or her lifetime.

But if a person is weak, malnourished, *diabetic*, very young or very old, or infected with HIV, the TB germs may start to attack her body. Usually this happens in the lungs, where germs eat holes in the *tissue* and destroy blood vessels. As the body tries to fight the disease, the holes fill with *pus* and small amounts of blood.

This is what the lungs look like inside the body.

Without treatment, the body starts to waste away, and the person usually dies within 5 years. If a person is infected with HIV and TB, she or he may die in a few months without treatment.

How TB Is Spread

➤ *Women who are sick with TB often infect their children and others they take care of every day.*

TB spreads from one person to another when someone who is sick with TB coughs germs into the air. The TB germs can live in the air for hours.

People who are sick with TB in their lungs can spread the germs to others. People who are infected with TB but not sick with signs of TB, and those who are sick with TB in other parts of the body, are not *contagious*.

If not treated correctly, a person sick with TB will infect about 10 more people with TB each year. But once a person has been taking medicines for about a month, he or she is probably no longer contagious.

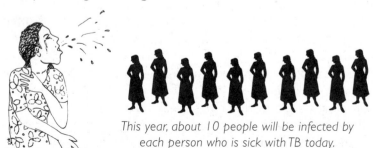

This year, about 10 people will be infected by each person who is sick with TB today.

A person with these signs is likely to have TB in the lungs:

- cough for more than 3 weeks, especially if the cough brings up mucus (sputum) from the lungs
- blood in the sputum
- weight loss

But the only way to know for sure that a person has TB is to have the sputum tested. To get a sample of sputum—and not just saliva (spit)—a person must cough hard to bring up material from deep in her lungs. The sputum is then examined in a *laboratory* to see if it contains TB germs (is positive).

A person should take at least 2 sputum tests, ideally 2 mornings in a row. If both of her sputum tests are positive, the woman should begin treatment. If only one of the 2 tests is positive, she should have her sputum tested again and, if it is positive, begin treatment. If the third test is negative, she should get a chest x-ray, if possible, to be certain that she does not need treatment.

How to Know if a Person Has TB

➤ *If someone with signs of TB in the lungs has negative sputum tests, she should see a health worker trained in treating problems of the lung. She may have pneumonia, asthma, or cancer of the lungs.*

TB can almost always be cured if a woman has TB for the first time, and if she takes the right kinds of medicines in the right amounts for the full length of the treatment.

The treatment has 2 parts. In the first, a woman takes 3 to 4 medicines for 2 months, and then her sputum is tested. If it is negative, she begins part 2, in which she takes 2 drugs for another 4 to 6 months (a total of 6 to 8 months of treatment). When the treatment is finished, her sputum should be checked again to make sure that she has been cured.

The medicines usually given to treat TB include ethambutol, isoniazid, pyrazinamide, rifampicin, streptomycin, and thiacetazone. For information about these medicines see the "Green Pages." But the treatments used to cure TB vary from country to country. A health worker should always follow the recommendations of the TB program in her or his country.

If a woman's sputum is still positive after 2 months of treatment, she should see a health worker for more tests. These can show if her TB germs are *resistant* to the medicines.

How to Treat TB

➤ *TB medicines can make hormonal methods of family planning (like birth control pills) less effective. Women being treated for TB should use a different family planning method. See page 200.*

TB treatment during pregnancy

A pregnant woman should never take streptomycin, because it may cause deafness in her unborn baby. She should also avoid taking pyrazinamide whenever possible, because its effect on the baby is not known. TB medicines may cause pain and numbness in the hands and feet, especially during pregnancy. Taking 50 mg of pyridoxine (vitamin B6) daily will help.

IMPORTANT *Persons infected with HIV must not take thiacetazone, because it can cause their skin to peel off. If there is any possibility that a person is infected with HIV, other medicines should be used instead.*

➤ *After the first 2 months of treatment, it is sometimes possible to take medicines 2 or 3 times a week, instead of every day. Talk to a health worker to see if you can get this kind of treatment.*

Anyone who is being treated for TB should follow these rules:

• Take all the medicine. **Never stop treatment when you feel better. If you do stop, the illness will come back and you can infect others.**

• Learn which side effects are normal and which are serious for the medicines you are taking. If you have serious side effects, you should stop taking the medicines and see a health worker immediately. The health worker may have you start them again one at a time or give you a new medicine.

• Get plenty of rest and eat as well as possible. If you can, stop working until you begin to feel better.

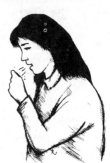

• Keep from spreading TB germs to others. If possible, sleep separately from those who are not sick with TB for one month after starting medicines. Cover your mouth when coughing and spit sputum into a piece of paper. Throw it into a *latrine* or toilet, or burn it.

• If you give birth during treatment, your sputum should be tested. If it is negative, your baby should be given a BCG (Bacille Calmette-Guerin) *vaccine,* but no medicines. If your sputum is positive, your baby will need medicines. You do not need to be separated from your baby or to stop breastfeeding.

RESISTANCE TO TB MEDICINES

If a person does not take enough of the right kinds of medicine, or stops taking medicines before the treatment is finished, not all the TB germs will be killed. The strongest germs will survive and multiply, and then the medicine will be unable to kill them. This called 'resistance'. Anyone whose sputum is still positive after 2 months of treatment may have TB germs that are resistant to the medicines she is taking. She should see a health worker trained in treating TB to get other medicines to take.

➤ *If a woman is infected by someone with drug resistant TB, the germs causing her sickness will also be resistant.*

➤ *Health workers should always ask if a person has been treated for TB before. If she has, she is more likely to have drug-resistant TB.*

Germs that have become resistant to both isoniazid and rifampicin can cause drug-resistant TB, which is very difficult to treat. The treatment takes between 12 to 18 months, and is much less successful and more expensive than treatment for ordinary TB. A person with drug-resistant TB can still spread the disease to others for several months after beginning treatment.

Because the treatment for TB is so long and the effects of stopping treatment are so serious, extra care should be taken to make sure that a person takes all her medicine. A health worker or community volunteer should watch the sick person take every dose and record that it is taken. This is called 'directly observed treatment, short-course', or DOTS. **Health workers should use DOTS whenever possible, but it is most important for the first 2 months of treatment.**

IMPORTANT *The best way to prevent the spread of TB is to cure people who are sick with TB.*

Preventing TB

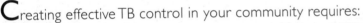

These things can also help:

- Encourage people to get tested for TB if they live with a person who is sick with TB and have any signs, or if they have a cough for 3 weeks or more.
- Try to keep the air moving in enclosed areas. This reduces the number of TB germs in that area.
- Let sunlight in whenever possible. Sunlight helps kill TB germs.
- Immunize healthy babies and children with BCG vaccine to prevent the most deadly forms of TB. But children sick with *AIDS* should not get BCG vaccine.

Working for Change

Creating effective TB control in your community requires:

- community and family education about the signs of TB and how it is spread. Encourage women to seek treatment for the signs of TB.
- trained health workers or community volunteers to participate in the DOTS program, and to find and work with persons sick with TB if they stop treatment early. DOTS programs must be flexible to be able to meet each person's needs.
- a continual supply of medicines so that treatment does not get interrupted, and laboratory equipment and trained workers for testing sputum.
- a good system for keeping track of who has TB, how the treatment is going, and when a person is cured.

A good TB program must give care to all people sick with TB, including women. TB services can help more women by:

- providing care and treatment in women's homes or as near to the home as possible.
- including midwives and traditional birth attendants in TB screening and DOTS programs.
- combining TB screening and treatment with other health services women are more likely to use.

Chapter 26

In this chapter:

Work

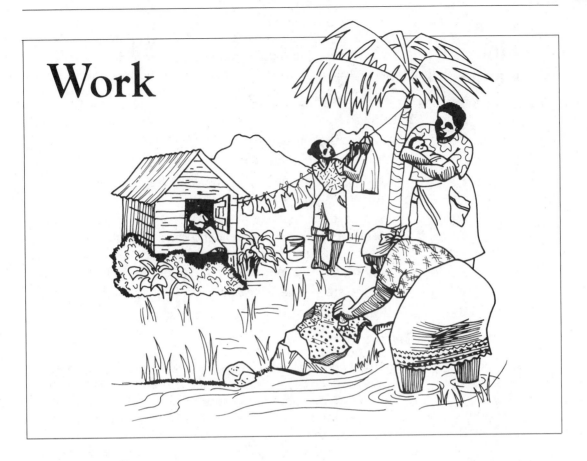

Nearly every woman spends most of her life working. Women farm, prepare food, carry firewood and water, clean, and care for children and other family members. Many women also work to earn money to help support their families. Yet much of women's work goes without notice, because it is not considered as important as men's work.

The work women do, and the conditions in which they work, can create health problems—which often go without notice as well. This chapter describes some of these problems, their causes, and ways to treat them. But unless women's working conditions are changed, these problems cannot really be solved. Women must work together to make these changes happen.

➤ *When a woman works to keep her family clean and fed, and to earn income to support her family, she is actually working two jobs.*

One type of work that some women do—getting paid for sex—involves some specific and serious health risks, so we have devoted a whole chapter to it. "Sex Workers" starts on page 341.

Health workers, and others who care for sick people, are at risk for getting illnesses from the people they treat. Ways of preventing these problems are discussed on pages 521 and 295.

Cooking Fires and Smoke

caring for burns

Most women spend many hours a day preparing food. This puts them at risk for health problems caused by cooking fires and smoke.

FIRES

Kerosene and other liquid and gas fuels can cause explosions, fires, and burns. To use these fuels more safely:

- do not let the fuel touch your skin or drip anywhere. If it does, wash it off right away.
- keep anything that can burn away from the stove. This will prevent fires from spreading and causing great damage. Store extra fuel in a safe place away from where you cook (and do not use matches or cigarettes nearby).
- put the stove where air can move freely around it.
- always be careful when lighting the stove.

SMOKE

Women who cook with fuels that produce a lot of smoke—such as wood, coal, animal dung, or crop remains—often have health problems. These fuels cause more problems when they are burned indoors where the smoke does not move out quickly. And if the fuel has *chemicals* in it—such as pesticides or fertilizers in the crop remains—the smoke is even more harmful.

Breathing smoke from cooking fires can cause *chronic* coughs, colds, *pneumonia*, *bronchitis*, *lung infections*, and lung disease. Breathing coal smoke can also cause *cancer* in the lungs, mouth, and throat.

Pregnant women who breathe cooking smoke can suffer from *dizziness*, weakness, *nausea*, and headaches. And because a woman's body is less able to fight infection when she is pregnant, she is even more likely to get the lung problems mentioned above. Smoke can also make her baby grow more slowly, weigh less at birth, or be born too early.

➤ *Small children who spend much of their day playing near a smoking cookstove are at greater risk for colds, coughs, pneumonia, and lung infections.*

➤ *Women are at greater risk for these health problems than men, because women spend more time breathing smoky air.*

Preventing health problems from smoke

To reduce the amount of smoky air you breathe:

Cook where air can move freely. If you cannot cook outdoors, then make sure there are at least 2 openings for air in the room. This creates a draft, so the smoke will leave the room.

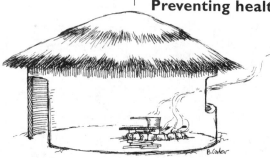

Cook in turns with other women. This way each woman will breathe less smoke.

Find ways to prepare food that require less cooking time (but still cook foods completely). This way you will breathe in less smoke, and you will also use less fuel. Food cooks more quickly and completely if you:

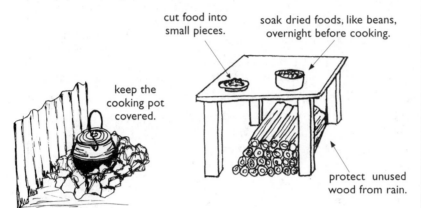

cut food into small pieces.

soak dried foods, like beans, overnight before cooking.

keep the cooking pot covered.

protect unused wood from rain.

protect the fire from wind. A nest of rock, clay, or iron sheets can help keep heat around the pot.

Use stoves that produce less smoke. This is the best way to prevent health problems caused by cooking smoke. Stoves that burn less fuel and produce very little smoke may be available in your area, but they can also be made easily with local materials. See the next page for instructions.

➤ *Smoke is a sign that fuel is being wasted, since it is caused by fuel that does not burn completely. Finding ways to cook with less smoke can save money as well.*

Stoves burn less fuel and produce less smoke when they have:

- protective lining (insulation) between the fire and the outside of the stove. Materials that trap a lot of air—like ash, pumice rock, dead coral, or aluminum foil—keep heat inside, instead of escaping out of the sides of the stove. This keeps the fuel burning hotly, which reduces smoke. Avoid using clay, heavy rock, sand, cement, and brick to prevent heat escaping from your stove because they do not trap enough air.

- chimneys inside the stove (see page 396) that help the air move around the fire. A longer chimney outside can also help cut down the smoke in the cooking area.

- 'skirts' (material around the cooking pot) to reflect the heat coming out of the chimney and direct it back to the pot. The pot then absorbs heat from all sides.

- a small burning chamber (see page 396) that allows you to burn one end of a piece of fuel in the chamber while the rest of the fuel stays outside. As the part inside burns, you can push the fuel further in.

How to make a stove and cooker that reduce smoke

The rocket stove

This is one example of a stove that is easy to make. You may need to adapt it for the fuel you use and the materials available in your area.

You will need:

- a large (5 gallon) can, such as a cooking oil can, soy sauce can, large paint can (well-cleaned), or a can that medical supplies were packed in. This will be the body of the stove. Cinderblocks or bricks may also be used, but a large can is better because it is thin and does not absorb as much heat.

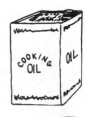

- a 4-inch wide metal stove pipe with a 90-degree bend (elbow) in it. The pipe on one side of the elbow should be longer than the pipe on the other side. You will also need a straight stove pipe to attach to the short end of the elbow. These pipes will be used to create the burning chamber and chimney for your stove. (4 or 5 tin cans with their tops and bottoms cut out can be used instead of stove pipes.)

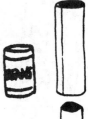

- insulation such as wood ash, pumice rock, vermiculite, dead coral, or aluminum foil.

- tin snips and a can opener for cutting the metal.

- extra metal for creating a 'skirt' around the pot.

- grating or thick fencing for the top of the stove, where the pot rests for cooking.

How to make the stove:

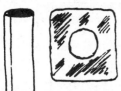

1. Use the can opener or tin snips to take the lid off the big can. Cut a 4-inch round hole in the middle of the lid for the chimney. Cut another 4-inch round hole in the lower front side of the can, about 1 inch up from the bottom of the can, for the burning chamber. The holes you cut should fit around your stove pipe or tin cans.

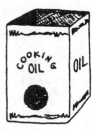

2. Place the stove pipe with the elbow inside the can so that one end sticks out of the front of the can. Make 2 parallel cuts 1/2 inch apart at the long end of the pipe and bend the section back to create a lip. This way the pipe will not slip back into the can. The long section of this pipe will be the burning chamber (where the fuel burns). Attach a straight section of pipe to the short end of the elbow to make a chimney that ends 1 inch below the top of the can. Make a lip on this pipe, too, so the top of the pipe will not fall into the can.

Note: A chimney made from tin cans will only last 1 to 3 months, and then you will need to replace it. To prevent this, try making a fired clay chimney with a mixture of 3 parts sand and 2 parts clay. Put this clay around the chimney of tin cans. When the cans burn through, you will have a clay chimney supported by all the insulation (see the next page) packed around it.

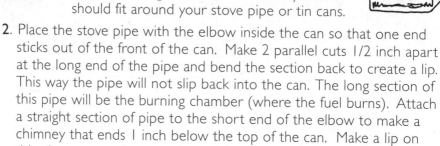

3. Fill the body of the stove, around the chimney, with insulation such as wood ash.

4. Replace the can lid over the insulation and around the chimney.

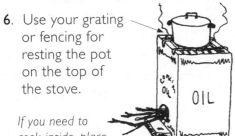

5. Use a tin can to make a shelf inside the burning chamber. Remove the ends of the can and flatten it. Then cut it into a T shape that will fit inside the pipe. The top of the T will stick out and keep the shelf from slipping inside. Place a brick or rock under the outside part of the shelf to support the twigs while they are burning.

6. Use your grating or fencing for resting the pot on the top of the stove.

If you need to cook inside, place the stove near a wall with an opening in it. The smoke can climb along the wall and leave the building.

7. Make a skirt with extra metal. It should surround the pot, leaving a 1/4- inch gap between the skirt and the pot at its base. For an even better skirt, make a double skirt and put insulation between the 2 sheets of metal.

The haybox cooker

To save even more fuel, use a haybox cooker to keep food warm or to simmer it after it has come to a boil on your stove. This cooker can cut fuel use by more than half when cooking beans, meat, rice, or grains. Rice and grains will use 1/3 less water, because not as much water will evaporate.

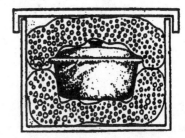

Keep the hay cooker away from an open flame.

Make a haybox by lining a cardboard box with 4 inches of hay (or use straw, sawdust, old clothing, feathers, chaff, cotton, wool, styrofoam, or corrugated cardboard). Leave space inside the box for your cooking pot and for more insulation on top of the pot. The lid of the box should fit tightly.

When using the haybox cooker, remember:
- food cooked in the haybox takes 1½ to 3 times longer to cook than over a fire.
- beans and meat should be simmered on your stove for 15 to 30 minutes before going into the haybox. The foods may need to be reheated after 2 to 4 hours.
- keep the pot closed and **boil meat dishes again before eating**. This prevents *bacteria* from infecting your food.

For more information on stove and oven designs, including easy-to-build solar stoves, contact Aprovecho Research Center. See page 557.

Lifting and Carrying Heavy Loads

HEALTH PROBLEMS

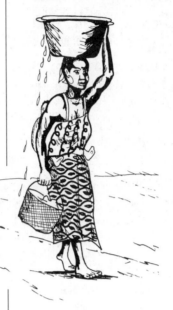

Women everywhere suffer from back and neck problems, usually from heavy lifting during their daily work. Carrying water, wood, and older children for long distances can cause serious strain.

Young girls who carry many heavy loads—especially water—have problems with the back and spine (backbone). Their pelvic bones also develop poorly, which can lead to dangerous pregnancies later on.

Carrying heavy loads can cause young women to suffer more *miscarriages*, and can make older women and those who have recently given birth more likely to have fallen womb (*prolapse*).

Prevention:

How to lift safely:

• Use leg muscles—not back muscles—when lifting. When you lift objects or children from the ground, kneel or squat to pick them up rather than bending over.

> ➤ *It is easier to prevent back problems than to cure them. Whenever possible, let your legs do the work—not your back.*

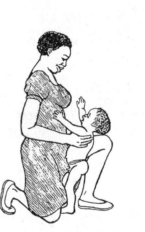 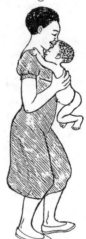

• Keep your back, shoulders, and neck as straight as possible.
• Do not lift or carry heavy objects during pregnancy or right after childbirth.
• Get someone to help you lift heavy objects. It may seem quicker to lift something by yourself. But later on you may lose time because of a back injury.

How to carry safely:

- Carry objects close to your body.
- If possible, carry objects on your back rather than on the side of your body. This way the muscles on one side of your back do not need to do all the work. Carrying loads on your side also makes your spine twist too much. This can cause back strain.
- If you must carry objects on one side, try to switch sides often. This way the muscles on both sides of your back are working the same amount, and your spine twists both ways. Or split the load and carry it on both sides.
- Try to avoid using head straps. They can strain your neck muscles.

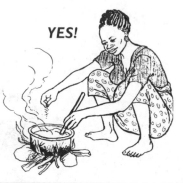

If you already have back problems:

- Sleep on your back with a rolled cloth or pillow under your knees. Or sleep on your side with some rolled cloth behind your back and another between your knees to keep your body straight and support the spine.

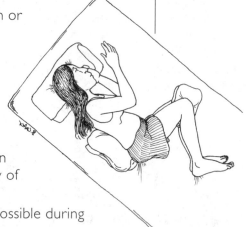

- Do the exercises on the next page every day to strengthen the muscles in your back and lower belly. Stop if any of these exercises cause pain.
- Try to keep your back as straight as possible during the day. Do not slump forward.

Bending

Do not bend over at the waist to reach things on the ground.

Bending forward for long periods of time—which women often do when washing, farming, or with other chores—can cause back strain. If you must work this way, try to stretch often. If you start to feel pain in your back, it can help to try some different positions, like squatting or kneeling. Change positions often.

Instead, squat down by bending your knees and keeping your back straight.

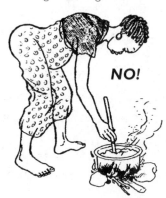

NO!

YES!

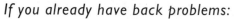

Exercises to relax and strengthen your back and belly muscles:

Try to do these exercises every day, in the order that they are listed:

1. **Stretching your lower back.** Lie on your back and hug your knees. Hold this position for 10-15 seconds as you breathe deeply. As you breathe out, gently rock your knees even closer to your chest to increase the stretch. Repeat 2 times, or until you feel some release in your lower back.

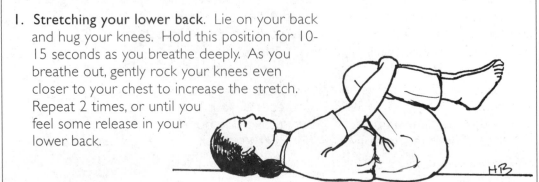

2. **The twist.** Lie on your back with your arms straight out from your sides. Bend your knees, and then move them slowly to one side. At the same time, turn your head to the opposite side, trying to keep your shoulders flat on the ground. Stay in this position as you breathe in and out a few more times. Then raise your knees to the center, and slowly bring them over to the other side. Turn your head the other way. Repeat this exercise 2 times on both sides, or until you feel some release in your lower back.

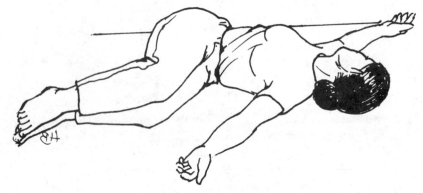

3. **The pelvic tilt.** Lie on your back with your knees bent. Flatten your lower back onto the floor. Slowly tighten your lower abdominal and buttock muscles and hold as you count to 3. Keep breathing as you hold. Then relax. As you do, your back will curve up the way it normally does. Repeat.

For more exercises to relax your back and neck, see page 404.

Tighten your muscles here...

...and here.

omen must often find and carry all the water for their families. Women also do most of the washing and cleaning, and are usually the ones who bathe children. All of these tasks are important for a woman's health and the health of her family.

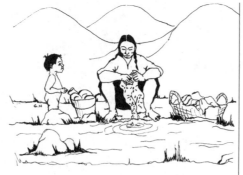

Work with Water

However, these same tasks can cause health problems.

Health problems from work with water:

- Women who spend long hours in contact with contaminated water are exposed to *parasites* and *germs* that live in and near water. These women are more likely to get infected with *bilharzia*, guinea worm, the germs that cause river blindness and *cholera*, and other parasitic diseases.

- Women who live downstream from a factory or large farms may be exposed to chemicals in the water. Chemicals can cause many health problems. For more information, see the next page.

- Water is one of the heaviest things women must carry, so collecting and carrying it can cause back and neck problems, as well as other health problems. See page 398.

➤ *For information about how to treat these infections, see* **Where There Is No Doctor**.

Prevention:

Clean water helps keep everyone healthy. All over the world, people are working together to improve health by organizing community water projects. But women are often left out of the meetings and decisions about these projects, such as where to put community taps, where to dig wells, and what kind of system to use.

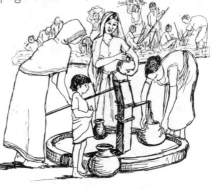

If your community does not have easy access to clean water, work with others to plan and organize a water project. If your community already has a water system, ask for women to be trained in how to fix and take care of the system used for the water supply.

Women should help take care of the system used for the water supply.

➤ *If you live downstream from a factory that dumps chemicals into the water, try to organize your community to work for better conditions. For an example of one community's experience, see page 127.*

Work with Chemicals

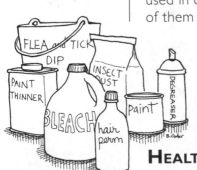

➤ *Avoid all unnecessary contact with chemicals.*

Many women have contact with dangerous chemicals, often without knowing it. This is because many modern products used in daily life and at work contain hidden chemicals. Some of them can be very harmful, such as:

- pesticides, fertilizers, weed killers, and animal dips.
- paints, paint thinners, paint remover and solvents.
- fuels and pottery glazes with lead in them.
- cleaning products containing bleach and lye.
- hair dressing products.

HEALTH PROBLEMS

Some chemicals cause harm to your body right away. Others cause harm that shows up later on, even after you have stopped using the chemicals. Some damage lasts only a short time. Other damage is permanent.

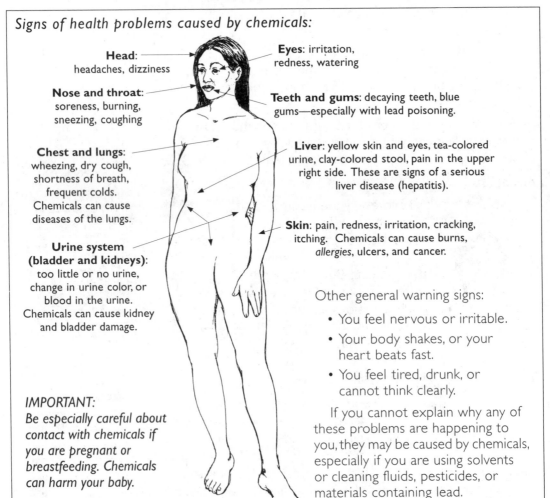

Signs of health problems caused by chemicals:

Head: headaches, dizziness

Nose and throat: soreness, burning, sneezing, coughing

Chest and lungs: wheezing, dry cough, shortness of breath, frequent colds. Chemicals can cause diseases of the lungs.

Urine system (bladder and kidneys): too little or no urine, change in urine color, or blood in the urine. Chemicals can cause kidney and bladder damage.

IMPORTANT: Be especially careful about contact with chemicals if you are pregnant or breastfeeding. Chemicals can harm your baby.

Eyes: irritation, redness, watering

Teeth and gums: decaying teeth, blue gums—especially with lead poisoning.

Liver: yellow skin and eyes, tea-colored urine, clay-colored stool, pain in the upper right side. These are signs of a serious liver disease (hepatitis).

Skin: pain, redness, irritation, cracking, itching. Chemicals can cause burns, *allergies*, ulcers, and cancer.

Other general warning signs:

- You feel nervous or irritable.
- Your body shakes, or your heart beats fast.
- You feel tired, drunk, or cannot think clearly.

If you cannot explain why any of these problems are happening to you, they may be caused by chemicals, especially if you are using solvents or cleaning fluids, pesticides, or materials containing lead.

Prevention:

To reduce the health risks from working with harmful chemicals, try to:

- avoid getting chemicals on your skin. When using chemicals at home, use rubber kitchen gloves (or plastic bags). When farming with pesticides and other chemicals, use thicker gloves and wear shoes. Otherwise, chemicals in the soil can get into your body.
- wash your hands after touching chemicals. If you have been using strong chemicals, like pesticides, change your clothes and wash yourself before eating or coming into the house. Use rubber gloves when you wash these clothes.
- avoid breathing in fumes (vapors) from chemicals. Work where fresh air flows freely. Wear a mask or a cloth over your nose and mouth.
- keep chemicals away from food. **Never use chemical storage containers for food or water**, even after they have been washed. A container that looks very clean can still have enough chemical to poison the food or water. Do not use sprays near food or on a windy day.

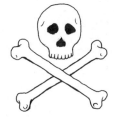

Keep chemicals away from children. Always look for poison warnings, or this picture, on the label.

If a chemical gets in your eye, flush it immediately with water. Keep flushing 30 times. Do not let the water get into the other eye. If your eye is burned, see a health worker.

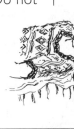

Lead poisoning

Lead is a poisonous part of some common materials—like pottery, paint, fuel, and batteries. Lead poisoning happens when people eat from pots with glazes containing lead or when they eat even a tiny amount of lead dust. It can also happen from breathing in lead dust or from breathing fumes from fuel containing lead.

Lead is especially harmful for babies and children. It can cause low birth weight, poor development, damage to the brain (which can be permanent), and death. So it is important to avoid working with lead during pregnancy.

If you work with lead, try to protect yourself and your family by:

- not getting powdered glaze on your hands or in your mouth.
- keeping children away from your work area.
- cleaning up with damp cloths rather than sweeping, so that less lead dust gets into the air.
- washing your hands well after working.
- eating foods that contain a lot of *calcium* and *iron* (see pages 167 and 168). These foods help keep lead from getting into your blood.

Sitting or Standing for a Long Time

If you must sit or stand for many hours at work, you may suffer health problems. Sometimes they only show up after months or years. Most of these problems can be prevented.

HEALTH PROBLEMS

Back and neck problems. These come from sitting a long time with your back bent or from standing in one place.

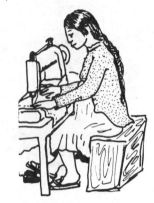

Varicose veins, **swollen feet, and blood clots in the legs.** When you sit or stand for a long time, it is hard for blood to flow easily through your legs, especially with your legs crossed.

Prevention:

• Take short, fast walks during your break. Also try to walk around the room or at least stretch every hour.

• If possible, wear socks or hose with support. They should go above the knee.

• Do each of the exercises described below whenever you feel stiffness or pain, or slump forward. Repeat them 2 or 3 times, taking slow, deep breaths.

Head:

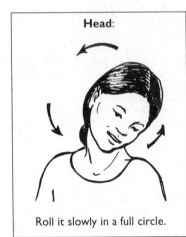

Roll it slowly in a full circle.

Shoulders:

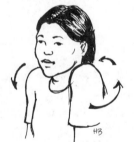

Move them up and down, roll them forward and backward, and pull your shoulder blades together behind your back.

Waist and upper body:

With your back straight, turn from the hip to face the side. You should feel relief in the upper and lower back.

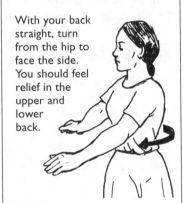

If you sit at work:

• Use a chair with a straight back—with your head, neck, and shoulders straight. If it feels better, put some rolled cloth or pillows behind you to support your lower back.

• If necessary, adjust the height of your chair or table to allow you to work in a better position. You can try sitting on a pillow, or putting a desk or table up on blocks.

• Do not cross your legs at the knees.

• Avoid wearing tight clothing.

Joints are places in the body where bones come together. At these joints tendons connect the bones to muscle. If you repeat the same movement over and over while working, the tendon can be damaged. Injuries to the wrists and elbows are common with farming and factory work. Injuries to the knees are common among domestic workers ('house-maid's knee'), miners, and other workers who kneel for a long time.

Repeating the Same Movement Over and Over

Signs:

- Pain and tingling in the part of your body that repeats the movement.

- For wrists, you will feel pain in your hand or here when your wrist is gently tapped.

- A grating feeling when you place your hand over the joint and move it.

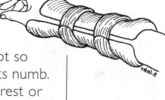

Treatment:

- Rest the joint in a comfortable position as much as possible. If you must continue to use that joint as you work, wear a splint to keep it as still as possible. Try some of the ideas below in the prevention section.

- Make a soft splint by wrapping the joint with cloths so it does not move. Wrapping the cloth around a thin piece of wood first can help keep the joint straight. The cloths should be wrapped tightly enough to keep the joint from moving, but not so tightly that the blood flow is blocked or the area gets numb. Wear the splint while you work, and also while you rest or sleep.

- If the joint is painful or swollen, take aspirin or use one of the pain medicines that reduce inflammation. Hot, moist cloth compresses can also help decrease pain and swelling.

482

medicines for pain

- If the joint does not get better after 6 months, get medical help. You may need to have medicine carefully injected into the joint, or you may need an operation.

Prevention:

- If it is safe, switch hands or body positions as you work. Try to work in a way that bends the joint less and puts less pressure on it.

- Try to exercise the joint every hour, by moving it through all of the motions it can make. This will stretch and strengthen the tendons and muscles. If exercise causes pain, move the joint slowly and gently.

➤ *If a joint is red or hot, it might be infected. See a health worker right away.*

Crafts

Many types of crafts are done in the home, where women work alone. This makes them less likely to know of common health problems caused by work and how to prevent them.

COMMON HEALTH PROBLEMS FROM WORK WITH CRAFTS		
Craft or skill	**Problem**	**What to do**
Pottery making	Lung diseases similar to those miners get (fibrosis, silicosis)	Open windows and doors for better air flow. Blow air out with a fan if there is electricity. Wear a protective mask that keeps dust out.
Pottery painting	Lead poisoning	See 'Lead poisoning', page 403.
Sewing, embroidery, knitting, lace making, weaving	Eye strain, headaches, low back and neck pain, joint pain	If possible, increase the amount of light on your work and rest often. See 'Sitting or Standing for a Long Time' and 'Repeating the Same Movement'.
Work with wool and cotton	Asthma and lung problems from dust and fibers	Improve air flow (see above), and wear a mask that will not let fibers through.
Use of paints and dyes	See 'Work with Chemicals'	See the prevention information in 'Work with Chemicals', page 403.
Soap making	Skin irritation and burns	Use protective gloves and avoid contact with lye.

Unsafe Working Conditions

Many factories have unsafe working conditions, such as:
• closed and locked doors and windows, which make it impossible for workers to get out during emergencies, and which keep air from flowing freely.

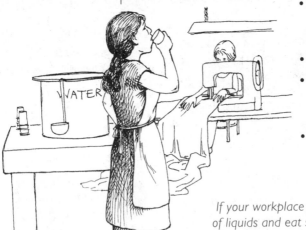

• exposure to toxins, such as chemicals and *radiation*, without protective barriers or clothing.

• unsafe equipment.

• fire hazards, like loose electrical wires, or chemicals or vapors that burn easily.

• no safe water, toilets or *latrines*, or rest breaks.

If your workplace is hot, drink plenty of liquids and eat salted foods— especially if you are pregnant. Women are more likely to get heat stroke than men.

Many of these conditions cannot be changed unless workers get together and demand change. But here are some things you can do yourself to prevent problems:

- When you begin a new task, get instructions about how to safely use all equipment and chemicals. Always ask for advice from women with experience using the same equipment or the same chemicals.

- Whenever possible, wear protective clothing—like hats, masks, gloves, or earplugs for loud noises. When working with machines, avoid wearing loose clothing. Keep long hair tied up and covered.

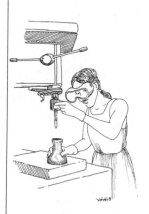

Sexual Harassment

Sexual harassment is unwanted sexual attention from an employer, manager, or any man with power over a woman. This includes saying something sexual that makes a woman uncomfortable, touching her in a sexual way, or making her have sex. Every woman is in danger of sexual harassment. It does not matter if she works for her family in the country or in a factory in the city.

There are many reasons why it is hard for a woman to say 'no' to sexual harassment:

- She may be afraid she will lose her job, which she needs to support herself and her family.

- She may have been raised to obey and respect the wishes of older men and men in power.

- The man may be a relative, and she may be afraid if she says no or complains he will be made to look bad.

But no matter what situation a woman is in, sexual harassment is wrong. It is also against the law in many countries. If you have been sexually harassed, try to find someone to confide in and to give you support. You can also share your experience with other women. Although you may not be able to end the harassment, sharing your story with others can help them avoid being harassed.

327

rape and sexual assualt

➤ *In some countries sexual harassment is called the "lay down or lay off" policy. This is because women are often fired if they do not have sex with the man who is harassing them.*

What you can do to avoid and stop sexual harassment:

- Try to avoid the men who have harassed other women where you work.
- Do not go anywhere alone with male employers.
- Find out if there are laws to protect you from harassment.

Migration

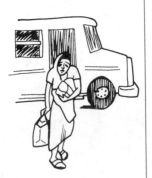

Remember that everyone feels alone at first. This is natural.

Many women work away from their homes. Some women travel daily from home to work, while others have moved many miles to live near work. This is called 'migration'.

Most often women move from rural areas to cities where big factories offer jobs, or where they can get jobs as domestic workers. Some women choose to move, but others are forced to move because there is no food or work at home, or because factories offer more money. Often the money these women make is very important for supporting their families back home.

When women migrate, they may be alone for the first time. This can be very frightening because they are away from the family and friends who gave them support.

Here are a few things you can do to make yourself feel more comfortable in a new home:

- Make friends with other women at work. These women can become a new source of support.
- Find a safe place to live. Many companies run their own hostels. Some are safe, but many are not. Sometimes they are places where women live in poor conditions and pay too much money for rent. The company may also take advantage of these women because they do not have control over where they live.

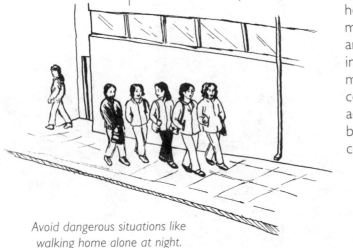

Avoid dangerous situations like walking home alone at night.

Sometimes the only way to get safe housing is to find it yourself. Here is an example of a woman's group that organized for safe housing:

Women who work making clothes in factories in Dhaka, Bangladesh, became tired of their poor, unhealthy living conditions, where they were often sexually harassed and *abused*. With help from a woman with management experience, they set up 2 hostels. Now the workers pay part of their wages to the hostel. In return, the staff, who are all women, provide food, cooking utensils, blankets, clothing, and other help. The workers are safe and close to work, and are able to save more of their wages.

—*Bangladesh*

Many women earn money working at tasks—like selling in the marketplace, making home crafts, and domestic work— that are not considered formal jobs. These jobs have very few protections, so women who do them are at risk for being exploited and abused.

Forgotten Workers

Domestic workers

A domestic worker faces many of the same health problems already described in this chapter. Because she works in someone else's home, she has few rights and little protection. She faces:

- *exhaustion* and poor *nutrition* from long hours and poor pay. Even though she may cook for her employer, she is often given little to eat.

- constant fear of losing her job and of being mistrusted by her employer. She may lose her job if she becomes pregnant. These fears, and the separation from her family, can cause mental health problems.

- sexual harassment, especially if she lives in her employer's house. Because he has power over her job, she may be forced to have sex.

- painful bone and muscle problems from working on her knees for long periods ('house-maid's knee').

- skin and nail problems ('washer-woman's hands') from working with chemical cleaners without using gloves.

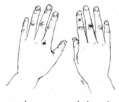

washer-woman's hands

Washer-woman's hands

When a woman uses a lot of cleaning chemicals without using gloves, her skin may become red, cracked, and painful, and develop open sores. The nails often get thick and damaged, and separate from the skin underneath.

What to do:

- If possible, use rubber or plastic gloves to protect your hands.

- Keep your hands as dry as you can. Use lotion or the thick juice from an aloe plant after you finish working. If your nails begin to look thick or damaged, try painting them right away with Gentian Violet.

- Try keeping a bowl of cool black tea or vinegar water (one capful of vinegar in one quart of water) next to the sink. Each time you use soapy water, soak your hands in the tea or vinegar for one minute.

- Use the juices of fresh plants that are known in your area for helping skin problems like rashes, burns, or itching. Gather and wash fresh plants, and grind them into a watery paste. Put your hands in this mixture as often as you can.

Working for Change

In South Africa, domestic workers have a Domestic Workers' Union to help them demand laws to protect themselves. They began by knocking on doors, and by educating people through pamphlets and radio announcements. Now they are a national union. They work with domestic workers' unions in other countries to help workers get fair working hours, fair pay, social security benefits, and other basic protections.

Unions like the South African Domestic Workers' Union are a very good way to organize and protect workers' rights. But it is often difficult to start a local union because there are no larger unions for support or because the company does not allow them. In this case there are other ways women can work together to help themselves.

When women start to work together for better conditions, they sometimes fear that they may lose their jobs or that they will be treated badly if their employers find out. In these cases it is important that women trust those they are organizing with. If it is not possible to talk at work, it may be best to meet in secret in private homes or in the community.

To begin organizing your workplace:

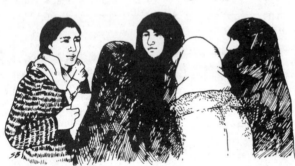

- **Talk** with the women you work with to identify common problems and possible ways to solve them.
- **Meet together** regularly as a group to build trust and help support one another. Be sure to include women who are new at work and make them feel welcome. Remember, there is strength in numbers.

Once you are organized as a group or a workers' association, you may feel strong enough to join a union or start your own. The company may be less likely to challenge you if you are already organized.

WHAT YOUR ORGANIZATION CAN DO

When your group has identifed common problems and possible solutions, decide which problems can be changed and what you need to do to make change happen. Even if the company is not willing to change anything, you can do a lot for yourselves. The next page gives some examples.

Teach each other about safety.
Women who have been doing the job
for a long time will have learned the
safest way to do things. Ask them to
share ideas about how to make the job
easier and safer.

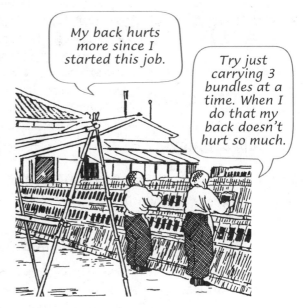

My back hurts more since I started this job.

Try just carrying 3 bundles at a time. When I do that my back doesn't hurt so much.

Help new women. New women
may be afraid to join your group,
especially if the employers do not
support you. But it is still important to
share your knowledge about safety,
because the safer every women is, the
safer you are.

Support each other. Many women
experience conflict at home when
they start working, because their role
in the family changes. Share advice on
solving family problems, and on
balancing housework and child care with paid work. Some
women even help take care of each other's children. They may
organize a child care center, where one woman is paid to care
for young children so that others can work. Or the women
may take turns minding the children.

423

helping relationships

You might also try meeting together with men to discuss
women's workload. For example:

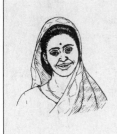

In workshops at the Center for Health Education, Training,
and Nutrition Awareness (CHETNA) in India, men and women
are asked to list their daily tasks. Many are surprised to learn that
a woman's work day starts before a man's does and ends long
after his, and that she rarely gets a chance to rest. This helped
men to see how work is distributed unfairly between men and
women. Then they were able to talk about dividing work fairly,
based on the needs of the family and not only by gender roles.

**If you can, negotiate with your employer for better
working conditions,** such as:

- child care at work.
- bathroom breaks.
- a private place to remove breast milk by hand
  (for mothers with babies).
- higher wages.
- maternity leave (time off when a woman has a baby, with
  the right to return to the same job).

111

when the mother
works ouside the
home

Chapter 27

In this chapter:

Mental Health

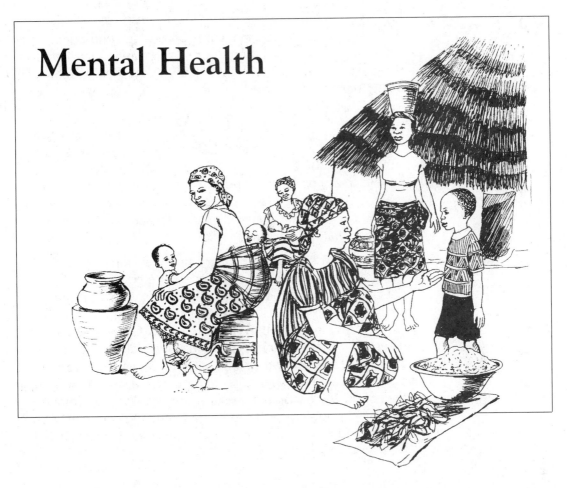

➤ *Good mental health is just as important as good physical health.*

Just as a woman's body can be healthy or unhealthy, so can her mind and spirit. When her mind and spirit are healthy, she has the emotional strength to take care of her physical needs and those of her family, to identify her problems and attempt to solve them, to plan for the future, and to form satisfying relationships with others.

Almost everyone has difficulty doing these things at times. But if the difficulty continues and keeps a woman from carrying out her daily activities—for example, if she becomes so tense and nervous that she cannot care for her family—she may have a mental health problem. These problems are harder to identify than problems in the body, which we can often see or touch. Yet mental health problems need attention and treatment, just as physical problems do.

This chapter describes the most common mental health problems and their causes. It also offers suggestions for how a woman can help herself or others with these problems.

Self-Esteem

When a woman feels she makes a valuable contribution to her family and community, she is said to have good self-esteem. A woman with good self-esteem knows that she is worthy of being treated with respect.

Self-esteem begins to develop in childhood. The amount of self-esteem a woman develops depends on how she is treated by the important people in her life—like her parents, brothers and sisters, neighbors, teachers, and spiritual guides. If these people treat her as someone who deserves their attention, if they praise her when she does something well, and if they encourage her to try things that are difficult, she will begin to feel she is valued.

In some cases, girls have a hard time developing good self-esteem. For example, if their brothers are given more education or more food, girls may feel less valued simply because they are girls. If they are criticized a lot or their hard work goes unnoticed, they are more likely to grow up feeling unworthy. Then, as women, they may not believe they deserve to be treated well by their husbands, to eat as much good food as others, to have health care when they are sick, or to develop their skills. When women feel this way, they may even think that their lack of importance in the family and community is natural and right—when, in fact, it is unfair and unjust.

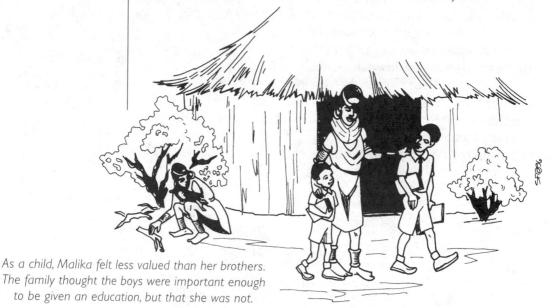

As a child, Malika felt less valued than her brothers. The family thought the boys were important enough to be given an education, but that she was not.

Self-esteem is an important part of good mental health. A woman with good self-esteem will feel more able to cope with (manage) daily problems and better able to work for changes that can improve her life and her community.

Building self-esteem

Building self-esteem is not an easy task. This is because a woman cannot just decide to value herself more. Rather, she must change deeply held beliefs that she may not know she has.

Often these changes must happen indirectly, through experiences that allow a woman to see herself in a new way. Change can come through building on strengths a woman already has, like her ability to form close, supportive relationships with others, or from learning new skills. For example:

➤ *A woman's self-esteem will influence the choices she makes about her health.*

As a child Malika was expected to be quiet and follow orders. When she was 18, her mother forced her to marry a military man. Malika was in love with someone else, but her mother did not care. The military man was an important man.

After they had been married for a number of years and Malika had given birth to 4 children, her husband stopped coming home at night. Friends would report that he had been with other women. Malika complained to her mother, and her mother told her to just live with it—this was how her life would be. Eventually Malika's husband moved out to live with his girlfriend. Malika felt very sad and worthless.

One day Malika was given the opportunity to enter a program where she would learn to take care of children at the community school. She decided to try, even though she had never worked away from home before. Learning new skills and being with the children and other women in training changed Malika. She began to see she had some worth outside of her marriage and that she could be a productive worker. Malika then began to think about what she could do for her family and what she hoped to accomplish in her lifetime.

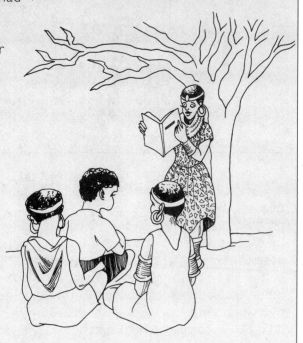

As an adult, Malika learned new skills and began to value herself more.

Common Causes of Mental Health Problems in Women

➤ *To have better mental health, women need to have more control and power over their lives.*

➤ *It is easy not to notice the stress in daily life because it is always there. But it takes a lot of a woman's energy to cope with this kind of stress.*

Not everyone who has to cope with the problems listed below will develop a mental health problem. Rather, a woman usually develops a mental health problem when these pressures are stronger than her ability to cope. Also, not all mental health problems have causes that can be identified. Sometimes we just do not know why someone develops a mental health problem.

STRESS IN DAILY LIFE

Daily activities and events often put pressure on a woman, causing tension in her body and mind (stress). Stress can come from physical problems, like illness or overwork. Or it can come from emotional events, like conflict in the family or being blamed for problems that a woman has no control over. Even events that often bring pleasure—like a new baby or getting a job—can be stressful because they create changes in a woman's life.

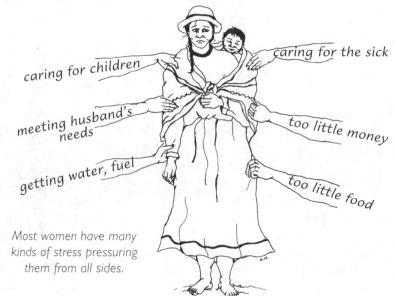

caring for children

caring for the sick

meeting husband's needs

too little money

getting water, fuel

too little food

Most women have many kinds of stress pressuring them from all sides.

When a woman faces a lot of stress every day and for a long time, she may begin to feel overwhelmed and unable to cope. The problem may be made worse if she has been taught to take care of others first and neglects her own needs. With little time to rest or to enjoy things that could help reduce her stress, she may ignore signs of illness or overwork. And as a woman, she may have little power to change her situation.

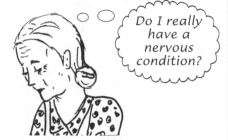

Do I really have a nervous condition?

Often a woman is made to feel that she is weak or ill. But the real problem may be something that is not fair or not right in life.

Other kinds of stress happen less often, but can also contribute to mental health problems:

LOSS AND DEATH

When a woman loses someone or something important—a loved one, her work, her home, or a close friendship—she may feel overwhelmed with grief. This can also happen if she becomes ill or develops a disability.

Grieving is a natural response that helps a person adjust to loss and death. But if a woman faces many losses at once, or if she already has a lot of daily stress, she may begin to develop mental health problems. This can also happen if a woman is unable to grieve in traditional ways—for example, if she has been forced to move to a new community where her traditions are not practiced.

454

difficulty mourning
or grieving

CHANGES IN A WOMAN'S LIFE AND COMMUNITY

In many parts of the world, communities are being forced to change rapidly—because of changes in the economy or because of political conflict. Many of these changes require families and communities to alter their entire way of life. For example:

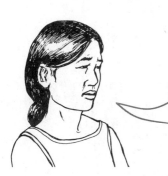

My name is Edhina. When the war started, soldiers came and forced the men in our village to fight. Some of the women were raped. We fled into the mountains, but it was hard to find food. Now we live as refugees in a camp just across the border. We usually have enough to eat, but many people are sick. The camp is crowded with strangers. Every day I wonder—will I ever see my home again?

My name is Jurema. Every year our land produced less. We had to borrow money to buy seeds, and even tried buying fertilizer, but we could never grow enough to pay back the bank. We were finally forced to leave our land. Now we live in a shack at the edge of the city. Every morning when I wake up, I listen for the birds that had always greeted the morning. But then I remember—there are no birds here. There is only another day of scrubbing other people's floors.

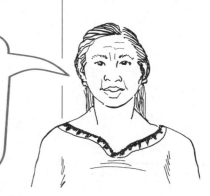

When families and communities break apart, or when life changes so much that old ways of coping do not work any more, people may begin to have mental health problems.

TRAUMA

When something horrible has happened to a woman or to someone close to her, she has suffered a *trauma*. Some of the most common kinds of trauma are violence in the home, rape, war, torture, and natural disasters.

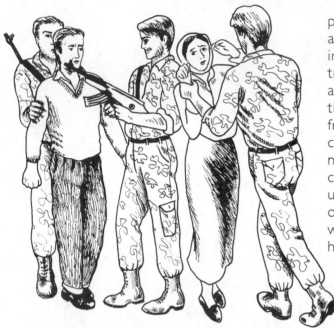

Trauma threatens a person's physical or mental well-being. As a result, a person feels unsafe, insecure, helpless, and unable to trust the world or the people around her. It usually takes a long time for a woman to recover from trauma, especially if it was caused by another person, not by nature. Trauma suffered as a child, before she could understand what was happening or talk about it, can affect a woman for many years without her even knowing it.

PHYSICAL PROBLEMS

Some mental health problems are caused by physical problems, such as:

- *hormones* and other changes in the body.
- *malnutrition.*
- *infections,* such as *HIV.*
- *pesticides, herbicides,* and industrial solvents.
- *liver* or *kidney* disease.
- too much medicine in the body, or the side effects of some medicines.
- drug and alcohol misuse.
- *strokes, dementia,* and head injuries.

Always consider the possibility of a physical cause when treating mental health problems. Remember, too, that physical problems can be the sign of a mental health problem (see page 421).

Although there are many kinds of mental health problems, the most common ones are anxiety, depression, and misuse of alcohol or drugs. In most communities, women suffer from these problems more than men do. But men are more likely than women to have a problem misusing alcohol or drugs.

To decide whether someone has a mental health problem, keep the following things in mind:

- There is no clear line between normal responses to life's events and mental health problems.
- Most people have some of the signs below at different times in their lives, because everyone faces problems at one time or another.
- Signs of mental health problems can vary from community to community. Behavior that looks strange to an outsider may be a normal part of a community's traditions or values.

Common Mental Health Problems for Women

436

misusing alcohol and drugs

➤ *For information about treating mental health problems, see page 422.*

DEPRESSION (EXTREME SADNESS OR FEELING NOTHING AT ALL)

It is natural for a person to feel depressed when she experiences a loss or death. But she may have a mental health problem if the signs below last for a long time.

➤ *Some people call depression 'heaviness of heart' or 'loss of spirit or soul'.*

Signs:

- feeling sad most of the time
- difficulty sleeping or sleeping too much
- difficulty thinking clearly
- loss of interest in pleasurable activities, eating, or sex
- physical problems, such as headaches or intestinal problems, that are not caused by illness
- slow speech and movement
- lack of energy for daily activities
- thinking about death or suicide

Suicide

Serious depression can lead to suicide (killing oneself). Almost everyone has thoughts of suicide once in a while. But if these thoughts come more and more often or get very strong, a woman needs help right away. See page 431 for how to identify people who are most at risk for suicide and how to help them.

Anxiety (feeling nervous or worried)

Everyone feels nervous or worried from time to time. When these feelings are caused by a specific situation, they usually go away soon afterwards. But if the anxiety continues or becomes more severe, or if it comes without any reason, then it may be a mental health problem.

Signs:

- feeling tense and nervous without reason
- shaking hands
- sweating
- feeling the heart pound (when there is no heart disease)
- difficulty thinking clearly
- frequent physical complaints that are not caused by physical illness and that increase when a woman is upset

Panic attacks are a severe kind of anxiety. They happen suddenly and can last from several minutes to several hours. In addition to the signs above, a person feels terror or dread, and fears that she may lose consciousness (faint) or die. She may also have chest pain, difficulty breathing, and feel that something terrible is about to happen.

Reactions to trauma

After a person has experienced trauma, she may have many different reactions, such as:

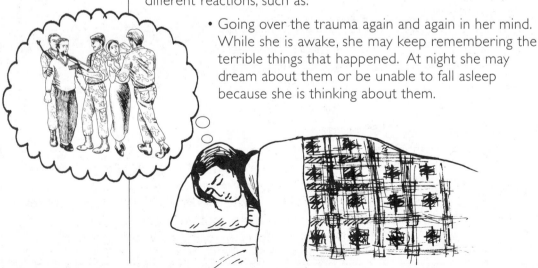

- Going over the trauma again and again in her mind. While she is awake, she may keep remembering the terrible things that happened. At night she may dream about them or be unable to fall asleep because she is thinking about them.

➤ *Other common names for anxiety are 'nerves', 'nervous attacks', and 'heart distress'.*

➤ *When a woman has severe chest pain or difficulty breathing, she should get medical help. These may be a sign of serious physical illness.*

- Feeling numb or feeling emotions less strongly than before. She may avoid people or places that remind her of the trauma.
- Becoming very watchful. If she is constantly looking out for danger, she may have difficulty relaxing and sleeping. She may overreact when startled.
- Feeling very angry or full of shame about what happened. If a person has survived a trauma where others died or were seriously injured, she may feel guilty that others suffered more than she did.
- Feeling separate and distant from other people.
- Having outbursts of strange or violent behavior, in which she is confused about where she is.

Many of these signs are normal responses to a difficult situation. For example, it is normal to feel angry that a trauma has happened, or to be watchful if the situation is still dangerous. But if the signs are so severe that a person cannot carry out daily activities, or if the signs start months after the trauma has happened, the person may have a mental health problem.

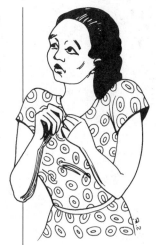

➤ *People suffering from reactions to trauma may also feel anxious or depressed, or misuse alcohol or drugs.*

PHYSICAL CHANGES AND DISEASE CAUSED BY STRESS

When a person experiences stress, the body gets ready to react quickly and fight off the stress. Some of the changes that occur are:

- The heart starts beating faster.
- The *blood pressure* goes up.
- A person breathes faster.
- *Digestion* slows down.

If the stress is sudden and severe, a woman may feel these changes in her body. Then, once the stress is gone, her body returns to normal. But if the stress is less severe or happens slowly, she may not notice how the stress is affecting her body, even though the signs are still there.

Stress that goes on for a long time can lead to the physical signs common in anxiety and depression, like headache, intestinal problems, and lack of energy. Over time, stress can also cause illness, like high blood pressure.

In many places, emotional problems are not considered as important as physical problems. When this happens, people may be more likely to have physical signs of anxiety and depression than other signs. While it is important not to ignore physical signs, it is important to also be sensitive to the emotional causes of illness.

Helping Yourself and Helping Others

A person suffering from mental health problems can begin to feel better with treatment. Although most communities lack mental health services, there are things a woman can do on her own, with very few resources (personal coping skills). Or she can form a 'helping relationship' with another person or group.

The suggestions that follow are just a few of the many ways a person can work toward better mental health. These suggestions will be most effective if they are adapted to a community's needs and traditions.

➤ *For severe problems, medicines may be necessary. Try to talk to a health worker who knows about medicines for mental health problems.*

PERSONAL COPING SKILLS

Women do not often take time out of their busy day to do something for themselves. But every woman needs to put her problems aside sometimes and do what she likes. Simple things that you may not do very often—like spending time alone, or shopping, gardening, or cooking with a friend—can all be helpful.

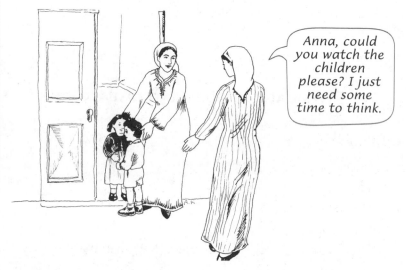

Anna, could you watch the children please? I just need some time to think.

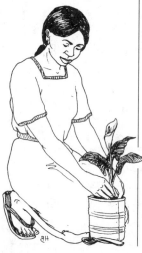

Activities to let your feelings out. Making up poems, songs, and stories can be helpful when you have trouble saying things to others. Or you can draw your feelings without using words—you do not have to be an artist.

Creating pleasing surroundings. Try to fix your living space so that it feels right to you. No matter how small it is, you will feel more order and control when it is arranged the way you like. Try to have as much light and fresh air as possible.

Try to have some beauty around you. This could mean putting some flowers in the room, playing music, or going where there is a nice view.

Practice traditions that build inner strength. Many communities have developed beliefs and traditions that help calm the body and mind, as well as build inner strength. For example:

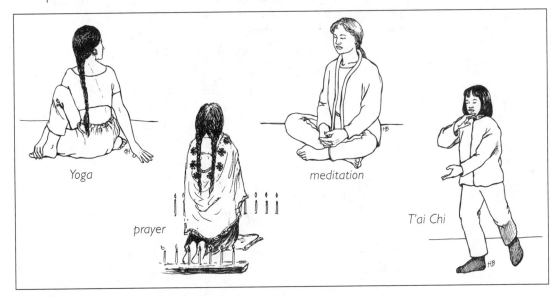

Yoga

prayer

meditation

T'ai Chi

Practicing these traditions regularly can help a person cope better with stress and other difficulties in her life.

HELPING RELATIONSHIPS

In a helping relationship, two or more people make a commitment to get to know and understand each other. This can happen in any relationship—between friends, family members, or women who work together, or in a group that already meets for another purpose. Or a new group may form because the people share a common problem. These are often called 'support groups'.

➤ It is often easier to turn an existing group into a support group than to create a new one. But be careful when choosing helping relationships. Form relationships only with people who will respect your feelings and your privacy.

These women agreed to listen to each other's problems as they worked.

Building a helping relationship

Even when two people know each other well, helping relationships develop slowly, because people usually hesitate to share their problems. It takes time to get over these worries and begin to trust one another. Here are some ways to build trust between people or members of a group:

➤ *No two people have exactly the same life experiences. There is always more to understand about another person.*

- Try to be open to hearing everything another person says, without judging it.
- Try to understand how the other person feels. If you have had a similar experience, think about how you felt. But avoid seeing someone else's experience as exactly like your own. If you do not understand her, do not pretend that you do.
- Do not tell another person what to do. You can help her understand how the pressures of her family, community, and work responsibilities affect her feelings, but she must make her own decisions.
- Never think of a woman as beyond help.
- Respect the woman's privacy. Never tell others what she has told you unless it is necessary to protect her life. Always tell her if you plan to speak with someone else for her protection.

Starting a support group

1. Find 2 or more women who want to start a group.
2. Plan when and where to meet. It helps to find a quiet place, such as a school, health post, cooperative, or place of worship. Or you can plan to talk while doing your daily work.
3. At the first meeting, discuss what you hope to accomplish. If you are in a group, decide how the group will be led and whether new members can join later.

Although the person who began the group will probably need to take the lead at the first meetings, she should not make decisions for the group. Her job is to make sure everyone has a chance to talk and to bring the discussion back to the main point if it wanders off. After the first few meetings members may want to take turns leading the group. Having more than 1 leader can also help shy women lead.

Meeting together with others can help a woman:

- **get support.** Mental health problems often drain a woman's energy and make her discouraged. Meeting together can give a woman more energy, which then helps her cope with daily problems.

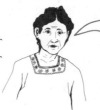

> Sometimes we would arrive at the meeting in a bad way. We didn't have any wish to speak. We felt without energy. Then a hug from someone or the spirits of others would be catching. And all of us would feel more strength.

- **recognize feelings**. Sometimes women hide their feelings (or do not even realize they have them) because they think the feelings are bad, dangerous, or shameful. Hearing others talk about feelings can help a woman notice her own.

> Some of us had been sexually abused in the past, but we had never been able to share it with others. It was only in the group that we could talk about these terrible things.

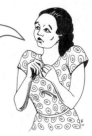

- **control impulsive reactions.** Group members can help a woman think through a problem, so that she will not act on her first impulse, without thinking.

> The group helped me to see others' points of view and to not get carried away by my feelings. This has helped me understand why other people react the way they do.

- **understand underlying causes.** By talking together, women begin to realize that many of them suffer from the same kinds of problems. This helps them identify root causes of the problem.

> I often think poorly of myself and feel as if I am to blame for my family's situation. But it is not our fault that we are poor. Talking about this with others has helped me to understand why we women suffer the way we do.

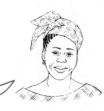

- **put forth solutions.** Solutions that are discussed in a group are often more easily accepted and used than those that a woman thinks of by herself.

> There are things from our past that we have never discussed with our partners. In the group we talked about how to deal better with these things. We get strength from each other.

- **develop collective power.** Women acting together are more powerful than a woman acting alone.

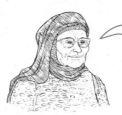

> We all decided to have a ceremony and then accompany one of our members to get a death certificate for her partner and arrange the title for her land. If she had to do these things alone it would be very difficult.

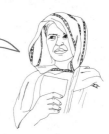

EXERCISES FOR LEARNING HOW TO HELP

Most members of a group need to understand what a helping relationship is and what makes it work before they can really help one another with a mental health problem. These exercises can help:

➤ *These exercises are most often done in groups, but they can also be used by just 2 people.*

1. **Sharing experiences of support.** To become more aware of what support is, the leader can ask members to tell a personal story in which they have received or given support. Then the leader asks questions like: What kind of help was it? How did it help? What are the similarities and differences between the stories? This can help the group come up with general ideas about what it means to support and help another person.

    Or the leader can pose a story of someone with a problem—for example, a woman whose husband drinks too much and beats her. She becomes withdrawn and pretends nothing is wrong, but no longer participates in the community. Then the group can discuss: How could we as a group help her? How can she help herself?

➤ *Some women may feel more comfortable listening as they work with their hands—for example, as they weave or sew.*

2. **Practicing active listening.** In this exercise the group divides into pairs. One partner talks about a topic for about

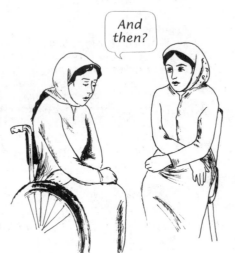

And then?

5 to 10 minutes. The other partner listens, without interrupting or saying anything, except to encourage the speaker to say more. The listener shows that she is listening by her attitude and by the way she moves her body. Then the partners switch roles.

When the partners are finished, they think about how well it worked. They ask each other questions like: Did you feel listened to? What difficulties did you have? Then the leader begins a general discussion among everyone about the attitudes that best show listening and concern. The leader can also emphasize that listening sometimes means talking: asking questions, sharing experiences, or saying something that makes the other person feel understood. It may also mean admitting that you have tried but still do not understand.

EXERCISES FOR HEALING MENTAL HEALTH PROBLEMS

Once the group has learned how to help and support one another, they are ready to begin working on their mental health problems. Here are some ways for the group to help healing begin:

1. **Share experiences and feelings in the group.** People who have mental health problems often feel very alone. Just being able to talk about a problem can be helpful. After one person has told her story, the leader can ask for other similar experiences. When everyone has listened to these, the group can discuss what the stories have in common, whether the problem was partly caused by social conditions, and if so, what the group might do to change these conditions.
2. **Learn to relax.** This exercise is particularly helpful for people who are suffering from stress. In a quiet place where everyone can sit down, the leader asks the group to follow these instructions:

    • Close your eyes and imagine a safe, peaceful place where you would like to be. This might be on a mountain, by a lake or ocean, or in a field.

    • Keep thinking about this place as you breathe deeply in through your nose and then out through your mouth.

    • If it helps, think of a positive thought, such as "I am at peace," or "I am safe."

    • Keep breathing, focusing either on the safe place or the thought. Do this for about 20 minutes (as long as it takes to boil rice).

➤ *If you start to feel uncomfortable or frightened at any time during this relaxation exercise, open your eyes and breathe deeply.*

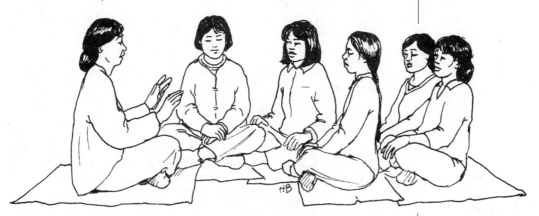

A woman can also practice this exercise at home whenever she has difficulty sleeping, or feels tense and afraid. Breathing deeply helps calm nervous feelings.

➤ *If you tell a story about a problem, it is important to also talk as a group about ways to overcome the problem.*

➤ *If a group has lived through a trauma and enough time has passed, they can analyze their own experiences rather than creating a story.*

3. **Creating a story, drama, or painting.** The group can make up a story about a situation similar to those experienced by members of the group. The leader starts the story, and then another member continues to tell another part—and so on until everyone has contributed something and the story is complete. (The group can also act out the story as it is told or paint a picture of the story.)

Then the group analyzes the different ideas that have been developed. These questions can help people begin to talk:

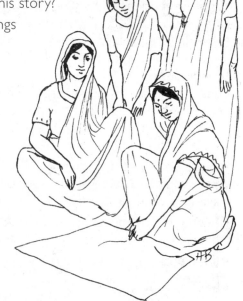

- What feelings or experiences are most important in this story?
- Why did these feelings occur?
- How is the person coping with these feelings?
- What can help her develop a new balance in her life?
- What can the community do to help?

4. **Creating a picture of your community.** This exercise works best after the group has been meeting together for awhile. The leader first asks the group to draw a picture of their community. (It may help for the leader to draw a simple picture to get things started.) Then the group adds to the picture, drawing in those parts of the community that contribute to good mental health, and those that cause mental health problems.

Then the group studies the picture and starts to think about ways to improve the community's mental health. The leader can ask questions like these:

- How can we strengthen those parts of the community that now contribute to good mental health?
- What new things need to be done?
- How can the group help bring about these changes?

28

organizing to solve community health problems

In El Salvador, a group of women from an urban squatters community decided to form a support group. They had lived through the civil war and now worked with victims of the war through their church. One member tells how the group began and how it has helped her:

"One day, all of us felt sad without knowing why. It wasn't as though anything special had happened that day, but all of us were feeling this way. Then one of us realized that it was the anniversary of the war that all of us had lived through. That was when we decided to form this group. We needed to feel close, to understand the things we had experienced, and to cope with how we felt about losing our sons, daughters, husbands, and neighbors to the war—and for what?

In the group we spoke of many experiences we had never been able to share with anyone else. This way we slowly left behind the silence and the feelings of helplessness each of us had. We learned that fears become smaller when we can give them a name. We discovered that we all had the same fears: the fear that others wouldn't understand, of not finding an answer, and that in speaking of our memories they would become more painful.

We spoke, cried, and laughed, but this time we did it together. The group supported us, helped us to change, and helped us see new directions for our lives. We were able to bring new energy and strength to our work. Now we help victims of the war—not just to rebuild their homes and health, but also to overcome their fears and hopelessness. This way they can create a new future for themselves and for their community.

Even though we all lost so much to the war—and peace has not delivered on its promises— we feel as though we have given birth to something new. And like a new baby, this group brings new spirit into the world and gives us the strength to go on."

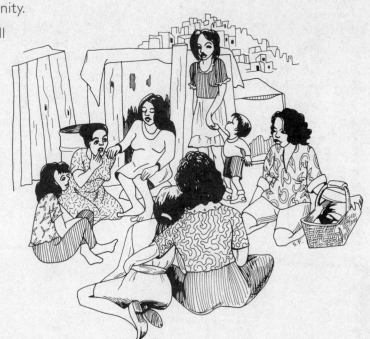

HELPING WOMEN WITH REACTIONS TO TRAUMA

- The most important way to help someone suffering from trauma is to help her learn to trust others again. Let her control how fast the relationship between you develops. She needs to know you are willing to listen, but that she can wait until she feels ready to talk. Doing everyday activities together may be best at first.

➤ *Once a woman understands her reactions, the feelings usually have less control over her.*

- It may help a woman to talk about her life before the trauma as well as her current experiences. This may help her realize that although life has changed a lot, in many ways she is the same person as before. If it seems right, encourage her to do some of the same activities she enjoyed before or that were part of her daily routine.

- Some painful things may be too difficult to talk about, or may be 'buried' away where they cannot be remembered. Exercises like drawing or painting, or a physical activity like *massage,* can help a person express or relieve these painful feelings.

- If a woman dreams of the trauma, she can put an object from her new life next to her as she sleeps. This helps her remember, when she wakes from a bad dream, that she is safe now.

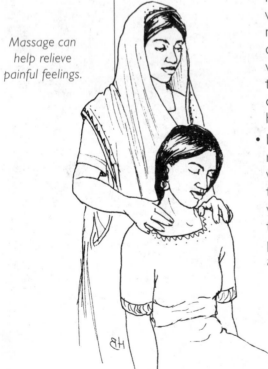

Massage can help relieve painful feelings.

- If reminders of the trauma make a woman react in fearful ways, help her make a plan for those reminders that cannot be avoided. For example, a woman might tell herself: "His face is like the man who attacked me, but he is a different person and does not wish to hurt me."

- If a person was tortured or raped, remind her that she is not responsible for what she said or did while being tortured. All responsibility lies with those who tortured her. Help her understand that one aim of torture is to make a person feel she can never feel whole again, but that this is not true.

HELPING SOMEONE WHO WANTS TO KILL HERSELF

Anyone who suffers from serious depression is at risk for suicide. A woman may not readily talk about thoughts of suicide, but she will often admit them if asked. If she does, then try to find out:

- Does she have a plan about how to kill herself?
- Does she have a way to carry out the plan? Is she planning to kill others as well (for example, her children)?
- Has she ever tried suicide before?
- Is her judgment affected by alcohol or drugs?
- Is she isolated from family or friends?
- Has she lost the desire to live?
- Does she have a serious health problem?
- Is she young and going through a serious life problem?

If a woman has made a plan for killing herself, she needs help right away.

If the answer to any of these questions is 'yes', she is at a greater risk for attempting suicide than other people. To help, first try talking with her. Some people may begin to feel better simply by telling you about their problems. If so, or if she still

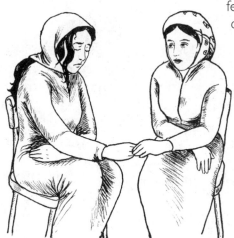

feels bad but is more in control of her feelings than before, ask her to promise that she will not hurt herself without talking to you first.

If talking about her problems does not help, or if she cannot promise to talk to you, then she needs to be watched closely. Always tell the person considering suicide that you plan to talk with others to help protect her. Talk to her family and friends, encouraging someone to be with her at all times. Ask them to remove dangerous objects from her surroundings.

If there are mental health services in her community, find out if someone can talk with her regularly. Medicine for depression may also be helpful.

Mental Illness (Psychosis)

➤ *Similar signs can be caused by illness, poisoning, medicines, drug abuse, or damage to the brain.*

➤ *No matter what treatment is given, a person with a mental illness should be treated with kindness, respect, and dignity.*

A person may be mentally ill if she has any of these signs:

- She hears voices or sees unusual things that others do not hear or see (hallucinations).
- She has strange beliefs that interfere with daily life (delusions)—for example, she thinks that loved ones are trying to rob her.
- She no longer cares for herself—for example, she does not get dressed, clean herself, or eat.
- She behaves in a strange way, like saying things that make no sense.

People who are not mentally ill sometimes act this way, particularly if these behaviors are part of their community's beliefs or traditions. For example, if a woman says that she received guidance in a dream, she may be drawing upon traditional sources of knowledge and guidance—not suffering from mental illness. These signs are more likely to be signs of mental illness if they come so often and are so strong that a person has difficulty carrying out daily activities.

Getting care for mental illness

Although in most places family members care for those who are mentally ill, it is best if the person can also be treated by a trained mental health worker. In some situations medicines are necessary, but they should never be the only treatment.

Traditional healers can also play an important role in treating mental illness. If they come from the same community as the person with the problem, they may know and understand her. Some healers also have treatments or rituals that can help a woman overcome her problem.

Ask these questions before deciding on a treatment:

- What is the purpose of each step in the treatment? What should be expected to happen?
- If the person is not a danger to herself or others, can she get mental health care while living at home, or living together with others in her community?
- Will the family be involved in the treatment?
- Is the person providing treatment respected in the community?
- Do any of the treatments cause physical harm or shame?

If someone must be treated in a hospital, always ask to see it before leaving her there. Make sure that the hospital is clean, that patients are safe and can have visitors, and that they will get regular treatment with trained mental health workers. Patients should be free to move about, unless they are a danger to themselves or others. Also, make sure you find out what must be done to have the person let out of the hospital later.

Ways to Improve Your Community's Mental Health

Identify those who are at risk for mental health problems. Women are at risk if they have:

- had mental health problems in the past.
- lost family members or are separated from their families.
- witnessed violence or have violent partners.
- little social support.

Look for other behaviors that may indicate mental health problems. If you suspect that someone has a mental health problem, get to know her better. Listen to what other people are saying about her behavior and the ways she has changed. Since mental health problems often have roots in the family or community, think about how these may contribute to the problem.

Build on a woman's strengths. Every woman has developed ways of coping with everyday problems. Help a woman identify the positive ways she has dealt with problems in the past and how she might use these strengths in her present situation.

Work within a woman's traditions and culture. Every community has traditional ways of dealing with mental health problems, such as prayer and ritual. These practices are not always helpful, but they should always be considered and used as much as possible. Try to learn as much as you can about a woman's traditions and how they may be a source of strength for her. Anything that helps a woman recognize or give meaning to her experience can help her mental health.

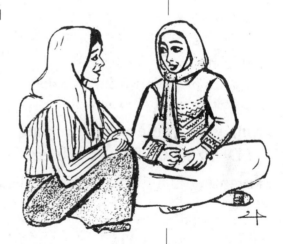

Remember that there are no quick solutions to mental health problems. Beware of anyone who promises this.

Ask for help when you need it. If you do not have experience with a mental health problem, try to talk to a trained mental health worker who does. Listening to other people's mental health problems can make you feel burdened, especially if you listen to a lot of people. Watch yourself to see if you are feeling pressured, if you are losing interest in helping others, or if you get irritable or angry easily. These are signs that you are making other people's problems your own. Ask for help, and try to get more rest and relaxation so you can work effectively.

➤ *The most important part of any treatment is to make the woman feel supported and cared for. Try to involve her family and friends in the treatment.*

Chapter 28

In this chapter:

Alcohol and Other Drugs

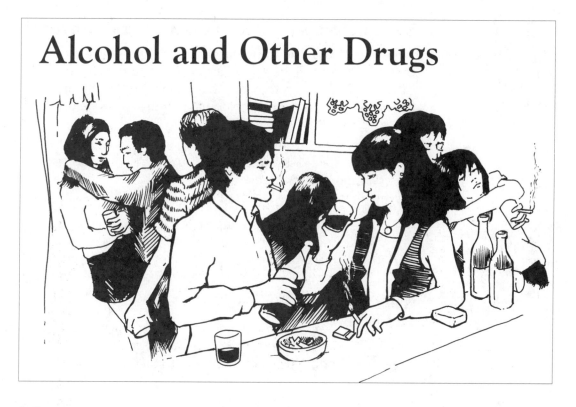

Many kinds of *drugs* are used in everyday life. In some places, drugs or brewed drinks have a sacred role in traditions. In other places, alcoholic drinks like wine or beer are commonly served with meals. Drugs and alcohol are often part of festive or social events. And some drugs are used as medicines.

Some drugs that are often used in harmful ways are:

➤ *Many people do not realize that alcohol and tobacco are harmful drugs.*

- alcohol: drinks such as brew, beer, spirits, liquor, wine.

- cocaine, heroin, opium.

- betel, khat, tobacco leaf.

- marijuana and hashish

- glue, fuels, and solvents.

- pills that help a person lose weight or stay awake.
- medicines, especially those for severe pain, or that help a person sleep or relax.

In this chapter we talk about the health problems these drugs can cause, their effects upon women, and ways to stop using drugs, especially alcohol and tobacco, the most commonly misused drugs in many communities.

Use and Misuse of Alcohol and Drugs

WHY DO PEOPLE BEGIN TO USE ALCOHOL OR DRUGS?

People often begin to use alcohol or drugs because of social pressure. Boys and men may face pressure to drink or use other common drugs to prove their manhood. A man may believe that the more he drinks, or the more drugs he uses, the more manly he is.

Many girls and women are also beginning to face social pressure to start drinking or using drugs. They may feel that they will appear more grown-up or more modern. Or they may think they will be accepted more easily by others.

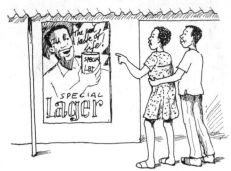

Some advertisements, music, and movies encourage young people to drink and use drugs.

Companies that make and sell alcohol and drugs use social pressure, too. Advertisements that make using drugs and alcohol look glamorous, especially to young people, encourage people to buy them. And when companies that make alcohol, or places that sell alcohol, make it seem easy and even fun to buy, people want to buy more. This kind of pressure is especially harmful, because often people are not aware it is affecting them.

WHEN DOES USE BECOME MISUSE?

Whatever the reason for starting, **alcohol and drugs can easily become misused**. A person is misusing drugs or alcohol if she loses control over **when** she uses alcohol or drugs, over **the amount** she uses, or over **the way she acts** when using alcohol or drugs.

Here are some common signs that people are misusing drugs or alcohol. They:

➤ *If using a drug is changing your life, it is time to stop or to use less. It is better to stop before the drug harms you, your family, or your friendships.*

- feel they need a drink or a drug to get through the day or night. They may use it at unusual times or places, such as in the morning, or when they are alone.
- lie about how much they or others use, or hide it.
- have money problems because of how much they spend on buying drugs or alcohol. Some people commit crimes to get money for drugs or alcohol.
- ruin celebrations because of how much they drink alcohol or use drugs.
- are ashamed of their behavior while using drugs or alcohol.
- are not working as well as before or are not going to work as often because of using alcohol or drugs.
- have problems with violent behavior. A man may become more violent towards his wife, children, or friends.

WHY PEOPLE MISUSE DRUGS AND ALCOHOL

Many people end up misusing drugs and alcohol in order to escape from problems in their lives.

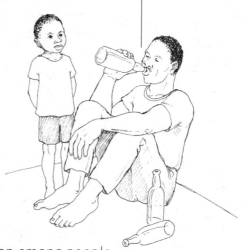

All types of people do this. But people whose parents misused alcohol or drugs are much more likely to try and solve their problems in the same way. This is because a 'weakness' to misuse drugs or alcohol may be passed from parents to children. And as children watch their parents use alcohol or drugs to escape problems, they learn this same behavior.

Alcohol and drug misuse is also common among people who do not feel any hope about changing the miserable conditions of their lives. People who are displaced from their homes or facing desperate problems—like losing their jobs or way of earning a living, losing family members, or being abandoned by a partner—are also more at risk for misusing drugs and alcohol.

Women often begin to misuse drugs or alcohol because they do not feel that they have any control over—or power to change—their lives. They may feel dependent upon, or at the mercy of, their partner or male family members. And if women have low *status* in the community, it may be hard for them to value themselves.

Unfortunately, drugs and alcohol usually make all these problems worse, and people feel even less able to improve their lives. Instead of looking for ways to improve their situations, most people who misuse drugs or alcohol spend their time, money, and health on trying to avoid and forget their problems.

Dependence and addiction

When a person misuses drugs or alcohol, both the mind and the body can begin to feel an overpowering need for the drug. When the mind feels this need, it is called **dependence**. When a person's body feels such a strong need for the drug that she gets sick without it, it is called physical **addiction**.

Alcohol and some drugs can cause addiction. Once a person becomes addicted, she will need more and more alcohol or drugs to feel their effects. (For information about overcoming the physical addition caused by alcohol, see page 441.)

Problems from Alcohol and Other Drugs

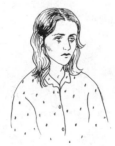

Using drugs and alcohol can permanently damage your health.

➤ *People who chew tobacco are at risk for most of the same health problems as those who smoke tobacco.*

COMMON HEALTH PROBLEMS

People who use alcohol and drugs a lot get sick more often and more severely than others. They are more likely to have:

- poor *nutrition*, which causes more sickness.
- *cancer*, and problems of the heart, *liver*, stomach, skin, lungs and *urine* system—including ones that cause permanent damage.
- brain damage or fits *(seizures)*.
- memory loss—waking up not knowing what happened.
- mental health problems, such as seeing strange things or hearing voices (hallucinations), being suspicious of others, having *flashbacks,* or feeling severe *depression* or *anxiety*.
- death from using too much at one time *(overdose)*.

In addition, injuries or death from accidents happen more often to these people (and often to their families). This is because they make bad decisions or take unnecessary risks, or because they can lose control of their bodies while using alcohol or drugs. If they have unprotected sex, share needles used to *inject* drugs, or trade sex for drugs, they are at risk for *hepatitis* and *sexually transmitted diseases.*

Drugs that are chewed. Chewing tobacco and betel nut often ruin a person's teeth and gums, and cause sores in the mouth, cancer of the mouth and throat, and other harm throughout the body. Khat can cause stomach problems and *constipation.* Many chewed drugs can cause dependence.

Sniffing glues and solvents. Many poor people, and particularly children who live on the streets, sniff glue and solvents to forget their hunger. This is very addicting and causes serious health problems, such as problems with seeing, trouble thinking and remembering, violent behavior, loss of judgement and body control, severe weight loss, and even heart failure and sudden death.

Any use of drugs and alcohol is dangerous if a person:
- is driving, using a machine, or dangerous tool.
- is pregnant or breastfeeding.
- is caring for small children.
- is taking medicine, especially medicines for pain, sleep, fits (seizures), or mental health problems.
- has liver or *kidney* disease.

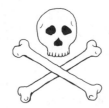

It can be dangerous to use drugs or medicines together with alcohol.

DRUGS AND ALCOHOL CAN BE WORSE FOR WOMEN

In addition to the problems that anyone who misuses drugs or alcohol may suffer, women face some special health problems:

- Women who drink large amounts of alcohol or use a lot of drugs are more likely to get liver disease than men.

- Many women and girls are pushed into sex they do not want when they drink alcohol or use drugs. This may result in unwanted pregnancy, STDs, and even *HIV/AIDS*.

- If used during pregnancy, drugs and alcohol can cause children to be born with *birth defects* and mental disabilities, such as:

    - problems of the heart, bones, *genitals*, and head and face.
    - low birth weight.
    - slow growth.
    - learning difficulties.

NO!

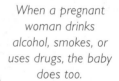

When a pregnant woman drinks alcohol, smokes, or uses drugs, the baby does too.

A baby can also be born dependent on drugs and suffer the same signs of withdrawal (see page 441) as an adult.

Women feel more shame

In most communities, women's behavior in public is more strictly controlled than men's behavior. Often it is considered normal for men to use alcohol or drugs, but not for women to do so. If a woman loses control of her behavior because of using too much alcohol or drugs, she is thought to be a 'loose woman', even if she is not having sex with others.

To avoid the shame that comes from making her drug or alcohol misuse public, a woman is more likely to drink steadily over a long period of time, rather than drinking a lot at one time. This kind of drinking makes it easier for her to control her behavior. She is also more likely to keep her misuse a secret and to put off getting treatment. All these behaviors increase the harm that comes from alcohol or drug misuse.

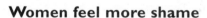

Misuse and violence in the home

Misusing alcohol and drugs makes violent situations worse, especially in the home. Women who have partners who misuse drugs and alcohol often suffer injuries and even death. For more information, see the chapter on "Violence."

Overcoming Problems with Alcohol and Drugs

Although it may seem difficult to overcome a dependence or addiction to alcohol and drugs, it can be done. There are 2 stages: quitting and then learning ways to stay free of drugs and alcohol.

QUITTING

If you think you have a drinking or drug problem and want to quit:

1. Admit you have a problem.

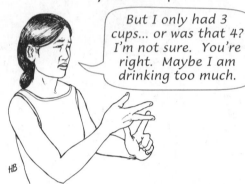

But I only had 3 cups... or was that 4? I'm not sure. You're right. Maybe I am drinking too much.

2. Decide to do something TODAY.

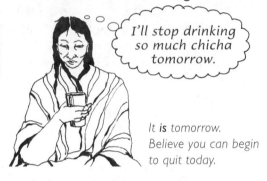

I'll stop drinking so much chicha tomorrow.

*It **is** tomorrow. Believe you can begin to quit today.*

➤ *Stopping is often easier with the help and support of others.*

424

starting a support group

3. Stop. Or use less and then stop. Many people can stop drinking or using drugs all at once. All it takes for them is the will to stop and the belief they can do it. Others need help from a group or treatment program like Alcoholics Anonymous (AA) that helps people with drinking or drug problems. There are AA groups in many countries. There may also be other groups or treatment programs in your area. Most women feel more comfortable in a group with women only. If there are no groups in your area, try starting your own group with someone who has been successful in helping people to stop drinking or using drugs.

4. If you start drinking or using drugs again, do not blame yourself. But try to stop again right away.

Alcoholics Anonymous (AA)

To become a member of AA, a person needs only one thing: a desire to stop drinking. As a member, you will regularly meet with others who have quit drinking, in order to share your experience, strength, and hope. You will also have a sponsor—a person who has stopped drinking for a period of time, and who can give you individual support and guidance.

AA does not charge any money. It does not support or oppose any causes, or have connections to any religious or political groups. Instead, AA tries to stay free of conflict with other groups in order to fulfill its main purpose: to carry its message to the drinking person who still suffers.

Physical addiction and withdrawal

When a person is physically addicted to alcohol or a drug and quits using it, she will go through a period of withdrawal. During this time her body must get used to being without the drug.

Alcohol addiction and withdrawal. After quitting drinking, it can take about 3 days for most signs of withdrawal to stop. Many people get through these days without problems. But since some people have very serious signs, it is important to have someone watch over the person and give help when needed.

Early signs of withdrawal:

- slight shaking
- nervous and irritable feelings
- sweating
- trouble eating and sleeping
- aches all over the body
- *nausea, vomiting,* stomach pain

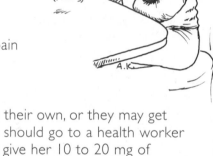

➤ *Some herbal teas can help the liver cleanse the body of poisonous effects of alcohol or drugs. A traditional healer may be able to suggest good local herbs.*

These signs may go away on their own, or they may get stronger. If they do, the woman should go to a health worker immediately. If help is far away, give her 10 to 20 mg of diazepam by mouth to prevent seizures. Give another 10 mg an hour later if the signs are not getting better. If you are still traveling, you can repeat the dose every 4 to 5 hours.

The following signs are an emergency. Any person with these signs must get medical help immediately:

- mental confusion
- seeing strange things or hearing voices
- very fast heartbeat
- seizures

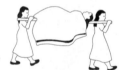

TRANSPORT!

➤ *When someone is addicted to alcohol, lack of alcohol in the body can cause seizures.*

After you have quit drinking

As soon as possible, start eating foods (or drinks) with a lot of *protein, vitamins,* and *minerals* (see page 166). These foods help the body heal itself: liver, yeast, breads made from whole wheat, other whole grains, beans, and dark green vegetables. If you cannot eat, vitamins may be helpful. Take a multi-vitamin or B-complex vitamin that contains *folic acid.*

422

personal coping
skills

LEARNING TO STAY FREE OF DRUGS AND ALCOHOL

Once a person has overcome physical addiction, it is important to learn how to stay free of drugs and alcohol to prevent the problem from developing again. The best way to do this is to learn better skills for coping with life. This is not easy to do and will take time.

A woman who has misused alcohol or drugs often feels powerless and full of shame. She needs to learn that she is able to make changes to improve her life. One way to begin is to make small changes that help prove to herself and to others that she can cope with problems.

Here are some ideas that have helped women build coping skills:

➤ *If you are trying to stay free of drink or drugs, avoid places where you will feel pressure to use them. Work with others to organize social events where drugs and alcohol are not used.*

- Develop a network of support among those close to you and ask for help when you need it. It is much easier to think about problems and begin to solve them when you can talk and work with others.

- Try to solve one problem at a time. That way, problems will not seem so large that you cannot cope with them.

- Try to tell a friend or someone you trust about things that worry or upset you, or that make you sad or angry. You may begin to understand why you feel the way you do and what you can do to feel better.

424

helping
relationships

- Work with other people on a project to improve your community. This proves to you and to others that you know how to work for change. You may also find that doing this helps you make personal changes, too.

- Meet together regularly with other people who are working to stay free of alcohol or drugs.

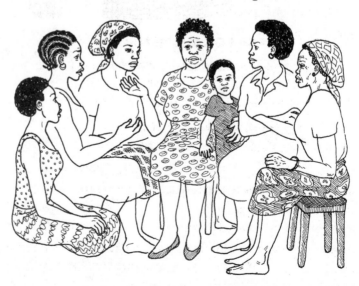

HEALTH PROBLEMS FROM SMOKING

Persons who smoke become addicted to a drug in tobacco called nicotine. Without a cigarette, they may feel sick or nervous. It is very hard to stop smoking, because nicotine is a very addictive drug.

Since more men than women smoke, smoking has mainly been seen as a men's health problem. But smoking is a growing cause of poor health among women. It is also a growing cause of health problems in poor countries. One reason for this is that tobacco companies are trying harder to sell cigarettes in these countries, as more people in rich countries stop smoking.

In both men and women, smoking can cause:

- serious diseases of the lungs, including chronic *bronchitis* and *emphysema*.
- severe colds and coughs.
- *cancer* of the lung, mouth, throat and neck, and *bladder*.
- heart attack, *stroke*, and *high blood pressure*.

Some of these problems can cause death. In fact, I out of 4 people who smoke will die from a health problem connected to smoking.

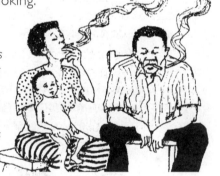

Children whose parents smoke have more lung infections and other lung and breathing health problems than children whose parents do not smoke.

➤ *Smoking can cause disease in those around you who do not smoke.*

SMOKING IS WORSE FOR WOMEN

In addition to the problems above, women who smoke have a greater risk of:

- difficulty getting pregnant *(infertility)*.
- *miscarriage*, and babies born too small or too soon.
- problems when using *birth control pills*.
- monthly bleeding that ends earlier in life *(menopause)*.
- weaker bones that break more easily during mid-life and old age (osteoporosis).
- cancer of the *cervix* and *womb*.

A woman who is pregnant should try to avoid other people who are smoking, so that the smoke will not harm her baby.

Living with Someone Who Has a Drinking or Drug Problem

Often women must care for someone, like a partner or a male relative, who has a drinking or drug problem. Living with someone with these problems is very difficult, especially if the person does not want to change. You can help yourself and your family if you:

- do not blame yourself. It is not always possible to help another person control his or her drug or alcohol use.

- try not to rely on the person's opinion of you to feel good about yourself.

- try to find a *support group* for you and your family. Sometimes this is the only way a family can cope with the problem.

I found out I was a people gatherer... What got me to move forward was other people around me. I did not think of myself as a leader, but there I was, getting people together to talk about this.

Bonnie, from the USA, talks of her struggle with her husband's drinking. She now works with Al Anon.

➤ *Al Anon is an organization like AA, that provides support and help for family members of alcoholics.*

How to help someone with a drinking or drug problem:

- Help him admit he has a problem. This may be all that is needed for him to use less or stop, unless he is addicted.

- Talk to him about stopping when he is not drunk or on drugs.

- Try not to blame him.

- Help him to avoid situations where he may feel pressured to drink or take drugs. This means not being with people with the same problem, even if they are friends.

- Help him to find other ways to cope with life's problems and to have better mental health.

- Help him make a plan for stopping and follow that plan.

423

helping relationships

To successfully prevent drug and alcohol misuse, you must consider the social forces that contribute to drug use.

Try meeting with others to discuss why alcohol or drugs have become important in community life. How did the problem start? What makes people use more? Are there new pressures on men or women that make it harder for them to control their use of alcohol and drugs? How can the drugs or alcohol be made less important in your community?

Once you understand the reasons for the problem, your group might want to work on ways to reduce social pressures to drink or use drugs.

Preventing Drug and Alcohol Misuse

A group of men and women in Chiapas, Mexico organized against alcoholism as part of their movement for democracy and social justice. They realized that people who drink heavily sometimes impose their will on others, in the same way as the police had used force to control the community. The group gave warnings to individuals whose misuse of alcohol was hurting other people, and intervened in cases where drunk men abused their wives. Alcohol played both negative and positive roles in the community. Shamans often drink rum, a sacred symbol, as part of their healing rituals. The group found ways to combat alcoholism and keep the spirit of their tradition by substituting non-alcoholic drinks in these rituals.

Helping young people resist alcohol and drugs

Many people who have drug and alcohol problems as adults began using them when they were young. Drugs or alcohol can seem like an easy way to have fun or escape from problems, especially if others are using them. Young people often feel confused and powerless about the many changes they must cope with—their growing bodies and new responsibilities.
Young people are also influenced by many pressures, especially their friends, older people they admire, and advertising.

One way to reduce drug and alcohol misuse is to help young people learn to resist harmful pressures. Here are some ideas that have worked in many communities:

- Encourage the schools in your community to teach young people about the problems of using drugs and alcohol.
- Make it harder for people to sell drugs to young people.
- Organize to remove advertisements that make cigarettes and alcohol look glamorous and modern.
- Become a good role model. If you drink a lot or use drugs, chances are your children will too.
- Teach your own children about the problems drug and alcohol use can cause. They can then influence their friends.
- Help young people have fun without drugs and alcohol.
- Help your children develop skills and *self-esteem* to resist the social pressure to use drugs and alcohol.

Find popular role models who speak out against drugs. Your children may find the message more powerful if it comes from a person they admire.

Chapter 29

In this chapter:

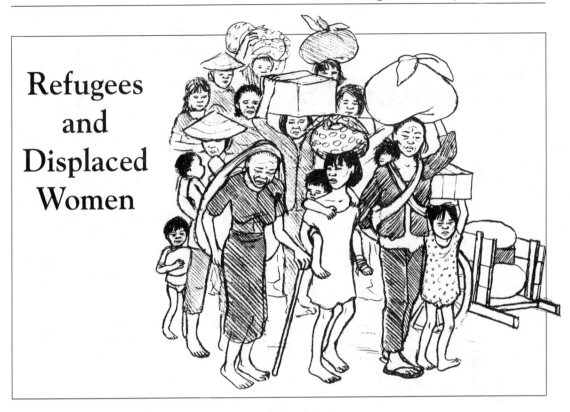

Refugees and Displaced Women

Refugees are people who cross the border of their country into another country, because they fear for their safety at home. Displaced people are people who are forced to leave their homes but remain in their own country. Many refugees and displaced people are victims of a group that has gained power and is prejudiced against the ethnic group, religion, nationality, or political views of others. If this group controls basic resources like food and water, people must leave their homes to survive.

Women and children make up more than 80% of refugees and displaced people. This is because men have often died fighting or been forced to leave their families. Like all refugees and displaced people, women need to be protected from forced return to their homes. They also need laws that give them economic and social rights, so they can get basic resources like food, shelter, clothing, and health care. As women, they need special protection from armed attacks, and from sexual and physical abuse.

This chapter will focus on some of the health problems that refugee and displaced women face. Most importantly, this chapter looks at the role these women can play in their new communities.

➤ *Out of every 10 refugees and displaced persons in the world, 8 are women and children.*

Flight and Arrival

The route to a new place to settle is often very difficult. Families may be separated during their travel (flight). Younger children or older relatives may die of hunger or disease on the way. Women and girls may be attacked by pirates, border guards, army units, and male refugees. All these losses and dangers can make a woman emotionally and physically exhausted even before she arrives at a new home.

Once settled, a woman may face a situation very different from her old home. Often women from small communities find themselves in large, crowded camps that are organized differently from a traditional village or town. Or they may live in cities, often trying to avoid capture by government authorities. Some refugees are thousands of miles away in countries that have allowed refugees to enter and settle there permanently.

In addition, a woman often faces some of these difficulties:

- living among people who do not like her being there or do not speak her language.
- not knowing whether she can return home soon or must stay away for years.
- needing papers showing her refugee status.
- adjusting to new family relationships.
- living in danger if a war is nearby.

Living in a refugee camp and being recognized as a refugee by a new government or the United Nations may give women some protection. But displaced women do not have these protections and are even more at risk.

> ➤ *Having identity documents from either the United Nations or the authorities in the country of refuge can give refugees some protection against being forced to leave (deported).*

Basic Needs

In many communities, women are responsible for providing most of their families' basic needs: they grow most of the food, prepare it, collect water, manage the home, keep the living space clean, and try to maintain the family's health. Away from the home, refugee and displaced women must suddenly depend on outside help to meet basic needs. Often this help is not adequate. Some displaced women may not have any outside help, so meeting basic needs is even more of a problem.

FOOD

Many refugees and displaced women do not have enough food to eat before they flee or during their journey. When they arrive at a new settlement, there still may not be enough food. Or there may not be enough different kinds of food to provide a *nutritious* diet.

> ➤ *Malnutrition is one of the leading causes of death for refugee and displaced women.*

You may be able to improve your diet if you:

- get involved in food distribution. Food should be given directly to women, because men may not be as familiar with the family's needs. Also, women are more likely to feed their families with the food they receive than trade it for weapons or alcohol.

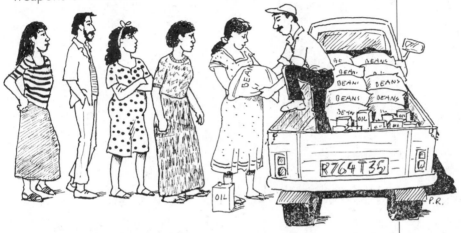

- demand that women get the same amount of food as men and eat at the same time.
- fight for extra food for pregnant women, women who are breastfeeding, and women who are malnourished or sick.
- make sure that women have cooking pots and utensils.
- share cooking tasks with other women. Even if food is prepared in a central place, women can stay involved. This will give them some control over their family's diet.

Emergency Food Distribution

Even in emergency situations, food distribution should involve women. This honors the important role women have had in food management. In Kenya, for example, Oxfam has tried to strengthen traditional social roles by distributing food directly to women. Food is distributed in an open place, overseen by an elected committee of elders. Women are encouraged to give their opinions about what is being done. This kind of food distribution will continue until the local food supply improves.

WATER AND FUEL

Refugee and displaced women often have limited water and cooking fuel. Sometimes water and fuel must be collected away from the camp in an unsafe area. Or the water may be unclean and will make people sick if they drink it. All these problems make women's lives more difficult, because they are responsible for washing and cooking for themselves and their families.

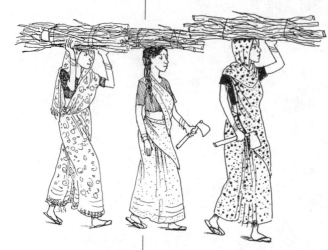

These things can help:

- Learn how to *purify* your water (see page 155).

- Ask organizations that provide support and aid for containers that are not too heavy to carry water.

- Ask those in charge to patrol places where water and fuel are collected, to make sure they remain safe and women can get to them. When you go for water or fuel, go with other people.

PROTECTION FROM SEXUAL VIOLENCE

➤ *Sexual violence is a violation of human rights.*

Rape and sexual violence are common when people are displaced. This happens because:

- guards, government authorities, and workers may demand sexual favors in exchange for food, protection, legal papers, and other help.

- if the area is too crowded, women may be forced to stay with strangers, or even with people who have been enemies. Women who are forced to stay among strangers are in greater danger.

- male refugees, who have lost opportunities they had at home, often become angry and bored. These problems are made worse when men see women taking on new responsibilities. Since men may have weapons with them, they may act violently toward women. This is more common if the men use alcohol or *drugs*.

- people in a nearby community may attack.

There are many ways to prevent attacks:

- Women should try to stay with family and friends. Single women and girls without adults looking after them should stay in a safe place that is separate from men.

rape and sexual
assault, 327

violence against
women, 313

- Men without much to do should be encouraged to begin activities like skills training, sports, or cultural activities.

- Women should be directly in charge of distributing basic resources, like food, water, and fuel, so they do not have to negotiate for their basic needs.

- The camp should be arranged so that *latrines* and other facilities for basic needs are close by and well lit. Women should also demand more protection at night, including women guards.

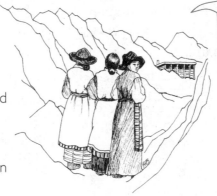

I wish the latrines were closer to the camp. It isn't safe to go here alone or after dark.

➤ *You may risk attack if you have to go a long distance for food, water, fuel, or to use sanitation facilities.*

- Try to arrange meetings for men and women to discuss preventing sexual violence. Make sure everyone understands the dangers. Protection against violence can be included in other programs, such as health and nutrition meetings.

- Ask for education about alcohol and drug misuse.

If you are attacked:

- Request a physical exam right away from a woman health worker. You may be able to prevent pregnancy and *sexually transmitted diseases (STDs)* by taking medicine. If you might be pregnant, be sure to discuss ALL your options—*abortion*, adoption, or keeping the baby—with a health worker.

- If it seems safe to do so, report the attack. Officials will be required to investigate. Remember that you do not have to answer any questions you do not want to, especially about your past sexual history.

- Talk over what happened with a trained mental health worker. This will help you realize you are not to blame for the attack and that many other people have overcome such experiences. If no mental health worker is available, see the chapter on "Mental Health."

- In some cultures, rape is seen as a woman's failure to guard her virginity or her dignity in marriage. If your family is angry at you or ashamed that this happened, they may need *counseling* also.

- If you can, you may want to move to a safer place, away from your attacker. Request that your family or friends come also, if you want them with you.

what to do if you have been raped, 334

emergency family planning, 224

medicine if you are at risk for an STD, 266

mental health, 413

Reproductive Health

Refugee and displaced women often find it very difficult to get proper health care. Health workers may have difficulty reaching displaced persons in dangerous or faraway areas. Or, if services are available, health workers may not know the language of the women they help or the cultural beliefs and practices that affect health care.

In addition to these general problems, women's specific health needs are often overlooked. These needs include:

- **care during pregnancy and birth.** Women need regular care before giving birth (*prenatal care*) and traditional birth attendants (TBAs) who understand a woman's traditional birthing practices.

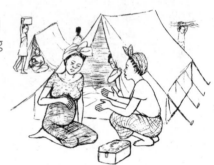

There are no family planning services available here. This is a clinic for emergencies.

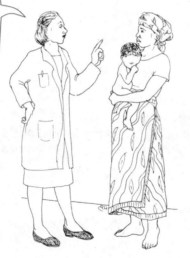

- **family planning.** In many refugee communities, the birth rate is very high. Part of the reason for this is that agencies often do not provide *family planning* information or supplies. Also, crowded refugee camps offer little privacy to use these methods, or secure, personal space to keep things.

- **supplies for *monthly bleeding*.**
- **information about and treatment for STDs.**
- **health workers trained to detect serious health problems of women,** like *pelvic infections* and cervical *cancer*.
- **safe abortion.** This is often unavailable, especially if the agencies providing health care are against it.
- **extra *calcium*, *iron*, *folic acid*, iodine, and vitamin C** in the diet, especially for pregnant or breastfeeding women.
- **being cared for by women health workers.** Some women cannot be examined by men because cultural beliefs forbid it.

Ways to improve women's health

You may be able to improve health services by becoming a link between health services and your refugee community. Help staff understand the traditions and needs of your people. You can also request some of the following changes:

- If the clinic is far away, ask for it to be open more hours at least one day a week. Ask for women health workers to be available on that day, especially if the women in your community cannot be examined by men.

- If the health workers do not speak your language or understand your birthing practices, ask to have a birth attendant or midwife from your community explain these practices to those at the health center.

- Ask for classes for adolescent girls and women on family planning, STDs, prenatal care and birth, and nutrition. Remind health center staff that women need a private area for discussing STDs.

- Request extra feedings for pregnant and breastfeeding women. If there is not enough food available for a healthy diet, these women should receive *vitamin* pills.

- Request that health workers receive training in treating the special health needs of women.

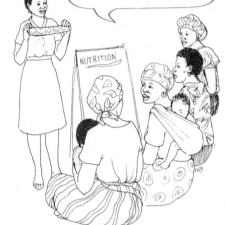

I'm glad they are also teaching us about family planning at these nutrition classes!

Becoming a health worker

Many camps train refugee women to be health workers, *community health workers* (CHWs), TBAs, and health educators, since they can speak the language of the other women and help improve the health of the whole camp.

In Camp Kakuma in northern Kenya, for example, southern Sudanese refugee women are very involved in health care. Many TBAs have been given more training and birthing kits, and other women are now CHWs and health educators.

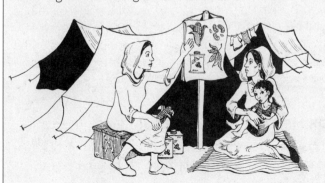

They are being trained in a way that will allow them to work in both the southern Sudan and in Kenya when they leave the camp. Sara Elija, a refugee from the Sudan, says that her new role as a TBA trainer has given her hope for work when she is no longer a refugee.

Mental Health

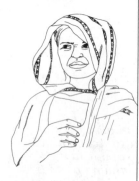

➤ *A woman must be able to cope with sudden and forced change in order to help her family survive.*

CAUSES OF MENTAL HEALTH PROBLEMS

Refugee and displaced women face many of the difficulties listed below, which can cause mental health problems or make them worse. Mental health problems include feeling extreme sadness or not feeling anything at all (depression), feeling nervous or worried (anxiety), or feeling unable to get over horrible things that happened in the past (severe reactions to trauma).

- **Loss of home.** Because home is the one place where a woman often has some authority, losing her home may be especially painful.

- **Loss of support from family and community.** As her family's caregiver, a woman must provide security for her children, and support her partner and parents. If her husband and older sons have died in fighting or joined military forces, she must also become head of the family. All these responsibilities can make her feel afraid and alone. This can happen even when other adults in the family are with her, because often they cannot support her as they did before.

- **Witnessing or being a victim of violence.**

- **Loss of independence and useful work.** Although a woman still has the important job of caring for her family, in other ways her life may be more limited now. For example, before leaving her home, a woman might have been responsible for growing crops, weaving, sewing, and baking bread. If she can no longer do these things, she may feel useless and sad.

- **Crowded living.** Without space, it is much harder for a woman to cope with the extra demands of caring for her family.

- **Difficulty mourning or grieving.** Refugee and displaced women may have lost family members before reaching their new home, but have been unable to carry out traditional burial or mourning ceremonies. Once in a place of refuge, it may still be impossible to bury or mourn in traditional ways. In many places, women are responsible for carrying out these ceremonies, which are important in order to grieve and accept the death of a loved one.

SIGNS OF MENTAL HEALTH PROBLEMS

For information about the signs of mental health problems like depression, anxiety, and severe reactions to trauma, see the chapter on "Mental Health."

413
mental health

WORKING FOR BETTER MENTAL HEALTH

The best way to help overcome mental health problems and to prevent them from becoming worse is to **talk with other women about feelings, worries, and concerns.** Here are some suggestions for encouraging the women you know to listen to and support each other:

helping relationships

- **Organize activities that let women spend time together,** such as nutrition or *literacy* classes, or child care and religious activities. Make extra efforts to include women who seem afraid or uninterested in getting involved. Often these women are the ones who most need to participate and talk with others.

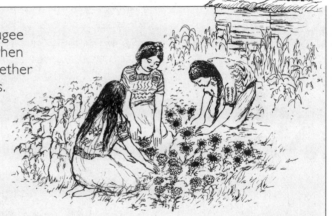

A group of Guatemalan refugee women who felt a deep loss when they left their land worked together to plant vegetables and flowers. This helped them feel close to the earth, to begin to feel like a community again, and to provide some food for their families.

- **Organize a support group.**
- **Work with other women to find ways to grieve and mourn.** You may be able to adapt some of your traditional rituals to your new situation. If you cannot, at least plan some time to grieve as a group.

starting a support group

- **Become a mental health worker.** You can organize a group of friends to talk with women who may not ask for help but who are suffering from mental health problems. Find out if your community has trained mental health workers or religious workers trained in counseling who can also help.

The destruction of homes, families, and communities is very traumatic. Sometimes refugees and displaced women become so affected by these terrible experiences that they cannot work, eat, and sleep in a normal way for a long time. Women need special support and understanding to help them recover and to begin to trust other people again. For more information on how to help people recovering from trauma, see page 430. For more information on helping a woman who has been raped, see page 334.

Women as Leaders

self-esteem

➤ *When programs are developed without consulting the women who will be affected by them, the programs are less effective.*

Women should be involved whenever plans or decisions are made that affect refugees and displaced people. Women should also be encouraged to become leaders in their new communities. This builds *self-esteem*, reduces feelings of loneliness and depression, encourages self-sufficiency, promotes safety for women, and helps those providing services to avoid mistakes.

Here are some ways women can take leadership:

- Participate in planning the way your settlement is arranged—for example, where the latrines, gardens, and water are located.

- Organize separate meetings for women and men about safety, basic needs, nutrition, and community involvement.

- Encourage women to talk about how they feel about their situation. Elect a leader who can talk to those who run the camp.

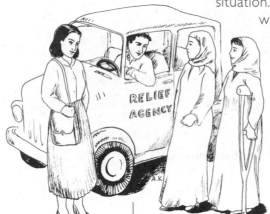

- Help with public information campaigns.

- Organize nutrition and health worker training programs.

- Organize child care centers. Child care is an important way to help women participate in activities where they can talk with others.

- Organize schools for children. Women are concerned about their children even in difficult times. The United Nations says that all refugee children have the right to an education, but few programs are available. Classes are sometimes overcrowded or there may be a shortage of teachers.

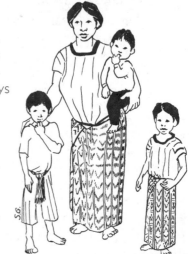

- Help organize reading classes, skills training, music, and sports for women and men.

When we arrived in Honduras we were weak from hiding in the hills and walking long distances to reach safety. There were many sick and malnourished children and old people with us. There was nothing here for us, so the women all worked together to organize nutrition centers. Then we got the local parish to bring us some extra food for the centers and we began to plant vegetables and raise chickens, goats, and rabbits to add to the food we prepared at the centers. Our projects have grown and now we are also able to give every family in the refugee camp a few eggs, a little bit of meat, and some vegetables at least once a month.

We needed to repair our clothing and shoes, so we organized workshops and convinced the agencies to bring us a few sewing machines and tools. Some of the women had worked as seamstresses and an older man knew how to make shoes and they taught others their skills. We are proud of what we have achieved here—we have shown that women can do more than cook.

The agencies trained us to become health and nutrition workers and to raise livestock. We have learned to add, subtract, and plan our expenses so that we can manage these projects ourselves. Because of our experience with these projects, many women are now leaders in the camp and when we return to our country we will be able to run community projects and businesses.

—*Aleyda, a Salvadoran refugee in Colomoncagua, Honduras*

WAYS TO EARN A LIVING

Refugee and displaced women often find it hard to get enough work to support their families. They may lack skills needed to work in their new home or find it difficult to get a work permit. But even in these situations there is often some work women can do.

For example, some refugee women do domestic work in people's homes or work as health workers in organizations that provide aid. Sometimes these organizations also give women money to start projects in traditional women's activities, like handicrafts. But since it can be hard to support a family with these activities, women should also try to find out about larger projects—like planting trees or building shelters—that pay more. Or, if women are given plots of land, they can grow food for their families or to sell. And if a woman has training, she may be able to work in a trade or small business.

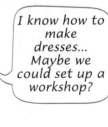

I'm glad they give us food, but there are other things that I need to buy for my family.

I know how to make dresses... Maybe we could set up a workshop?

▶ *Refugee and displaced women need choices, so they will not be forced to sell sex to survive and support their families.*

Chapter 30

In this chapter:

This chapter was written by women who are living and working in communities where female circumcision is practiced.

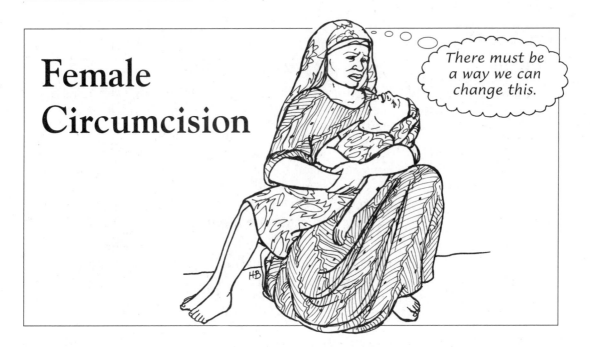

Female Circumcision

There must be a way we can change this.

Throughout history, customs harmful to women's health have been practiced in order to make women seem more attractive or likely to marry. For example, in some European communities, a woman was thought to be more beautiful if she had a very small waist. So starting when they were girls, women were forced to wear a band of stiff cloth called a 'corset' tied so tightly around the waist and hips it sometimes broke their rib bones, and kept them from breathing or eating properly. It was very difficult for them to do anything but sit still or walk slowly.

And in parts of China, a woman had higher status if she had very tiny feet. So the bones of some girls' feet were broken and their feet tightly wrapped in cloth so that when they became women, their feet were deformed and they were unable to do more than walk slowly.

These customs have been stopped, but in some parts of the world, other customs continue. Female circumcision is one them. It is practiced in many communities of Africa, in some communities in the Middle East, and in a small number of communities in Southeast Asia. It involves cutting part of a girl's or woman's *genitals*. Female circumcision is practiced for a variety of reasons, most of them based on culture and tradition. It is often a cause for great celebration in the community.

Female circumcision does not stop a woman's need for love and companionship or affect her moral behavior. But it does interfere with her normal body functions, and can harm her relationship with her husband or partner. Circumcision also causes many health problems, and some of these problems can lead to lasting harm or death.

➤ *Sometimes this practice is called excision.*

➤ *In some communities, a girl must be circumcised before she can become a wife and mother and, in some cases, to own property.*

Types of Female Circumcision

There are 3 types of female circumcision:

1. The *clitoris* is partly or completely removed.

2. The clitoris is removed along with the small skin folds of the outer genitals.

3. The outside genitals are cut away, and the opening to the *vagina* is sewn almost closed. This is called 'infibulation'. A small hole is left for *urine* and *monthly bleeding* to flow out. This type of circumcision is the most dangerous and causes the most serious health problems. **But all types of female circumcision can cause bleeding, infection and death.**

The way that a girl is cut is different in different places, but it is almost always done as part of a ceremony in which a girl moves from childhood into adulthood.

Health Problems Caused by Female Circumcision

These problems may happen right away, or in the first week:

- heavy bleeding
- *infection*
- *shock* from severe pain, bleeding, or infection
- problems with passing urine

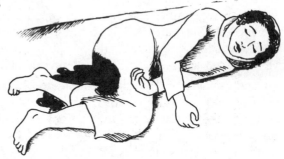

All these problems are extremely dangerous. Get help right away.

254

shock

These problems may happen later, and can last for many years:

- problems with monthly bleeding
- problems with sex
- problems during and after childbirth
- leaking urine and *stool*
- being unable to get pregnant (*infertility*)
- lasting pain
- mental health problems

Heavy bleeding and shock

Heavy bleeding from a deep cut or tear can happen quickly and is very dangerous. If a girl loses too much blood, she can go into shock and die.

Warning signs of shock (one or more of the following):

- severe thirst
- pale, cold, and damp skin
- weak and fast *pulse* (more than 110 beats per minute)
- fast breathing (more than 30 breaths per minute)
- confusion or *loss of consciousness (fainting)*

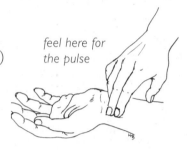

feel here for the pulse

What to do:

- Get help immediately. **Shock is an emergency.**
- Press firmly on the bleeding spot right away. Use a clean, small cloth that will not soak up a lot of blood. Keep her lying down while you take her to medical help.
- Help her drink as much as she can.
- If she is unconscious and you live far from health services, you may need to give her rectal fluids before taking her for help.

Infection

If the cutting tool is not cleaned properly *(disinfected)* before and after each use, *germs* can cause a wound infection, *tetanus*, *HIV/AIDS*, or *hepatitis*.

Signs:

- **of wound infection:** fever, swelling in the genitals, *pus* or a bad smell from the wound, pain that gets worse.
- **of tetanus:** tight jaw, stiff neck and body muscles, difficulty swallowing and *convulsions*.
- **of shock** (see the list above).
- **of an infection in the blood** (sepsis): *fever* and other signs of infection, confusion and shock.

For signs of HIV/AIDS or hepatitis, see the chapters on "AIDS," page 283, and "Sexually Transmitted Diseases and Other Infections of the Genitals," page 266.

IMPORTANT *If a girl begins to show signs of tetanus, shock, or sepsis, take her for medical help right away.*

What to Do for Health Problems

254

shock

TRANSPORT!

537

rectal fluids

522

cleaning and disinfecting

➤ *Signs of infection can begin any time during the first 2 weeks after the circumcision*

255

sepsis

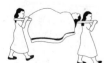

TRANSPORT!

amoxicillin, 490
erythromycin, 501

What to do for infection:

- Give an *antibiotic,* such as amoxicillin or erythromycin.
- Keep watching for warning signs of tetanus, sepsis, and shock. **If she has not yet had a tetanus *vaccination,* she should get one immediately.**
- Give modern or plant medicines for pain.
- Keep the genitals very clean. Wash them with water that has been boiled and cooled and has a little salt in it.

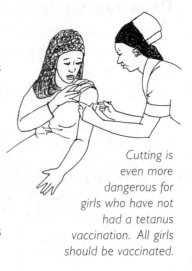

Cutting is even more dangerous for girls who have not had a tetanus vaccination. All girls should be vaccinated.

URINE PROBLEMS

Since circumcision often causes severe pain when a girl passes urine, some girls try to hold their urine back. This can cause infection and damage to the urine tubes, *bladder*, and *kidneys*. Holding back urine frequently can cause stones to form in the bladder.

What to do:

- Run clean water over the genitals when passing urine. This makes the urine less acid, so it causes less pain. Drinking more liquids will also help.
- Pour water into a bucket or pan. The sound of the running water sometimes helps the person start to pass urine.
- Apply a damp towel soaked in warm water to the genitals. This may help relieve the pain.
- Watch for signs of bladder and kidney infection.

367

bladder and kidney infection

372

how to put in a catheter

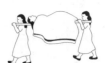

TRANSPORT!

If a girl has not been able to pass urine for more than a day or night, and her lower belly feels tight and full over the bladder, it is an emergency. She must see a trained health worker immediately who can put a tube in the bladder to drain the urine. Do not give her more liquid to drink, because this will add pressure on her bladder and kidneys.

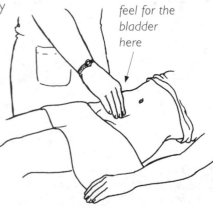

feel for the bladder here

PROBLEMS WITH MONTHLY BLEEDING

If the vaginal hole that is left after infibulation is too small, or if it is blocked by scarring inside the body, the flow of a girl's monthly bleeding can be blocked. This can cause:

- very painful monthly bleeding.
- long monthly bleeding, lasting 10 to 15 days.
- no monthly bleeding because the vaginal opening is blocked and the blood cannot get out.
- trapped blood that can lead to serious *pelvic inflammatory disease (PID)* and scarring in the womb and tubes. This can cause infertility.

What to do:

- Apply a towel soaked in hot water to the lower *abdomen* to relieve pain. (Be careful not to burn the skin.)
- It may help to walk around and do light work or exercise.

If the problems are severe, the vaginal opening may need to be made larger. This should be done by a skilled health worker to prevent harm to the *reproductive parts* inside.

PROBLEMS WITH SEXUAL RELATIONS AND SEXUAL HEALTH

If a circumcised woman has none of the health problems described in this chapter, she may be able to enjoy sex. But many women who have been circumcised, especially those who have been infibulated, find sex difficult.

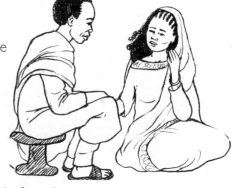

In some communities, young women are circumcised and married on the same day. Or a woman who was circumcised at a young age may have her vaginal opening made larger just before first sex in marriage. If she is expected to have sex before the wound has healed, sex will be very painful and dangerous, and the wound may take longer to heal. Open wounds also increase her risk of catching HIV/AIDS or *sexually transmitted diseases (STDs).*

➤ *All wounds must be completely healed before having sex.*

During sex, a woman may find it difficult to become aroused, since the clitoris has been cut off.

If you live where infibulation is practiced, help men to understand that the vaginal opening should be safely and gently made larger. Opening should be done long before the first time a woman has sex, to allow time for complete healing. Opening should be done by a health worker who uses properly cleaned cutting tools, and who cares for the wound afterward to prevent infection.

➤ *If you can encourage married couples to talk to one another, it will be easier for them to talk about how circumcision affects their sexual relations.*

safer sex

What to do for problems with sex:

A woman can talk with her partner about finding ways to become more sexually aroused, and explain that she may need more time to feel aroused.

She can also talk about ways to make sex less painful. Having enough wetness *(lubrication)* can make sex safer and hurt less.

Getting reproductive health care

If an infibulated woman's vaginal opening is not large enough, she cannot get a *pelvic exam* or a *Pap test* for *cancer* (see page 378). This means she has fewer choices for protecting herself against pregnancy, cancer, and STDs.

PROBLEMS WITH CHILDBIRTH

➤ *Blocked births are more common in young girls whose bodies are not fully grown.*

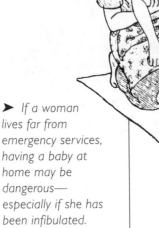

With some types of circumcision, there is a greater risk that the baby will have difficulty getting out of the vagina (blocked birth). If the hole left after infibulation is very small, it must be opened so the baby's head can pass through. This is called 'deinfibulation' (see the box on the next page). If the person who does the opening is not skilled, it can cause other complications.

Scarring from circumcision can also cause the genitals to tear more during childbirth, since scarred skin does not stretch easily. Heavy bleeding may result.

➤ *If a woman lives far from emergency services, having a baby at home may be dangerous— especially if she has been infibulated.*

➤ *Some traditional midwives have had special training for helping circumcised women have safe births, and for problems from infibulation.*

What to do:

Plan in advance for childbirth. During the second half of pregnancy, a pregnant woman should try to see a trained midwife or other health worker trained in helping circumcised women give birth. The midwife can tell her if there is a risk of complications, or if the vaginal opening should be made larger. If there are risks, a woman can make plans for getting medical care ahead of time.

Emergency: If an infibulated girl or woman is giving birth and the baby will not come out (a blocked birth) the *scars* must be cut so the baby can be born. If possible, this should be done by a trained health worker. But if there is no health worker nearby, wash your hands well with soap and clean water before you begin, and wear clean rubber or plastic gloves or bags on your hands. The cutting tool must be cleaned and disinfected first (see page 522). **If you have to cut someone, get her to a health worker who knows how to repair the cut right after the birth.**

To cut the scars open (deinfibulation):

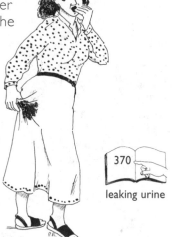

urine hole

(use 1 or 2 fingers)

1. Put 1 or 2 fingers under the band of scar tissue.

2. Inject local *anesthesia* if you know how.

3. Cut the old scar open by snipping the bands of scar tissue until you can see the woman's urine hole. The vagina will probably now stretch enough to let the baby come out.

4. After birth the opening will need repair. This might be a good time to explain to the woman or girl that it would be safer not to be infibulated again—it will cause more scarring and can block the urine tube and vagina. A trained health worker can repair the genitals without closing the opening.

5. To prevent infection, give *antibiotics*: amoxicillin, 3 grams all at once, or erythromycin, 500 mg 4 times a day for 7 days.

LEAKING URINE AND STOOL

During a blocked birth, the lining of the vagina, bladder or *rectum* can tear, causing urine or stool to leak out of the vagina.

If a couple has *anal sex* because the woman's vaginal opening is too small, the anus may become stretched or torn. Stool may leak out of the anus.

Leaking urine and stool are terrible problems to live with. Many young women have been rejected by their partners because of the smell and because they cannot control the leaking. Seek medical help as soon as the problem is discovered.

370

leaking urine

INFERTILITY

Infection can cause scarring of the womb and tubes, which make it difficult for a woman to get pregnant. If you think there may be an infection caused by a sexually transmitted disease, see the chapter on "STDs and Other Infections of the Genitals," page 26. If you think there are problems with scarring in the womb or tubes from blocked flow of monthly bleeding, see a trained health worker about making the opening larger.

229

infertility

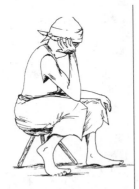

MENTAL HEALTH PROBLEMS

A girl who has been circumcised can become overwhelmed with fear, worry (anxiety), or sadness. When circumcision is done in front of women that a girl knows and trusts to protect her from harm, she may feel that she can no longer trust anyone. It is worse if the girl did not wish to be circumcised.

Chronic pain and suffering can cause other lasting mental health problems, such as deep sadness (depression), and feelings of helplessness and worthlessness. Sexual problems can also cause severe strain between a woman and her partner. A woman may feel she is unable to please him because the pain makes her afraid of sex.

What to do:

mental health

- Encourage her to talk about her feelings.
- If she seems withdrawn, distant, and unable to do daily activities, see pages 418 and 430.

Working for Change

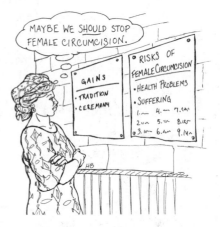

If you are not sure how you feel about female circumcision, weigh the risks to help you decide. Are the benefits of being circumcised worth the health problems? Culture is always changing to meet new community needs. Can this practice also be changed?

What you can do:

If you do not agree with this practice, there are many ways you can help girls in your community:

- If you are a mother, help your daughters feel valued and loved, whether they are circumcised or not.
- Encourage your daughters to continue with their education and to learn enough to make their own decisions about their lives and their futures. Every child has a right to good health and an education.
- Share the information about the health problems caused by female circumcision with other women and men in your community. Work with them for change.
- Find out what women's organizations in your community or region are doing.

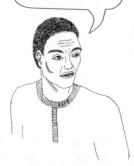

After all the problems my wife and I had with sex and childbirth, I will not let my 2 daughters be circumcised.

- If you are a health worker who does circumcisions, explain the risks to those who ask you.
- Get training on what to do for health problems of female circumcision.
- Work for change with traditional and religious leaders. Religion does not support female circumcision, but this has not been well understood. Try to discuss this with your religious leaders.
- Find ways to discourage circumcision ceremonies in your community. Find other rituals that can mark a girl's passage from childhood to adulthood. These rituals could include prayers to the ancestors, or sacrifices that are not harmful to women. In many places there are coming-of-age rituals for girls that do not harm their health.
- Recognize the important role traditional birth attendants (TBAs) play in the health of the community. Since TBAs often perform circumcision, they need to be trained about its harmful effects. Find ways to replace the gifts they are given after circumcision ceremonies, and look for other ways their help is needed in the community. If other rituals are used to replace circumcision, include TBAs as an important part of the giving and receiving of any gifts.

➤ *For real change to happen in your community, people must work together to end this harmful practice.*

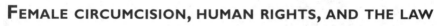

FEMALE CIRCUMCISION, HUMAN RIGHTS, AND THE LAW

This chapter has mainly described the health problems that female circumcision often causes. But even if no health problems occur, a circumcised girl has still been harmed and her human rights to bodily integrity, safety, and health have been violated in the name of tradition. Many believe that circumcision also violates the right to privacy and choice because it is done mainly to girl children who are not old enough to agree to the practice.

Some groups are calling for new laws to make female circumcision illegal and punish those who practice it. These laws need to be written carefully so that in communities where circumcision is practiced, it will not continue in secrecy, which would be even more dangerous. Also, girls and women who have been circumcised should not feel afraid to seek medical help if they have problems.

Chapter 31

In this chapter:

In this book we recommend many medicines. This chapter explains how to use them safely. For more information on *side effects*, warning signs, medicines that need special instructions, and *antibiotics*, see the "Green Pages," page 485.

Use of Medicines in Women's Health

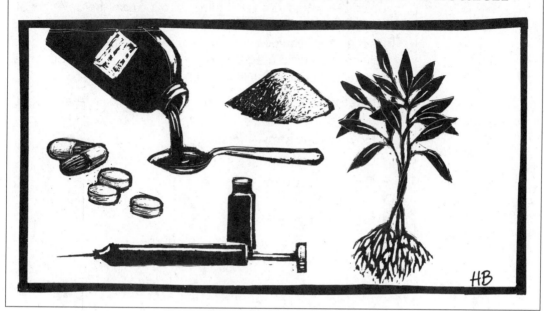

Medicines are drugs that can be used to help the body fight disease or feel better when sick. Medicines can be either modern or traditional. In this book, we mostly talk about how to use modern medicines. This is because traditional remedies vary greatly from one region to another. A remedy that works in one community may not exist or may not work in another community. Ask *traditional healers* where you live to help you find remedies that may work for your problem. (For more information about using traditional remedies, see page 22.)

It is important to use medicines safely. Used properly, medicines can save lives. But used improperly, medicines can hurt and even kill you. For example, some medicines can cause health problems for a pregnant or breastfeeding woman and her baby. And some medicines may cause other problems *(side effects)* that can be annoying, worrisome, or even dangerous to a person's health. If you take too much of a medicine at once, or if you take it too often, it may harm you.

This chapter talks about how to safely use the medicines mentioned in this book to treat women's health problems. It also provides information to help you decide when to use medicines to improve women's health.

➤ *Medicines can be useful, but they cannot replace healthy living, good food, or good health care.*

Deciding to Use Medicine

➤ See the chapters called "Solving Health Problems," (page 18) and "The Medical System" (page 32) for more information to help you decide if you need to take medicine.

Some people think that you always need medicine to get good health care. But medicines can only treat health problems—not solve the conditions that cause them. And not all health problems are best treated with medicine. For some, drinking lots of liquids and resting are most important. A medicine should be used only if you know what the problem is and that the medicine will work for that problem.

To decide whether or not you need a medicine, think about these things:

- How serious is my illness?
- Can I get better without this medicine?
- Can I get better by changing my living or eating habits?
- Is there a traditional remedy that works?
- Are the benefits of using this medicine greater than the risks and costs?

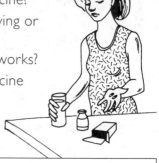

To the health worker:

When giving medicine, remember these guidelines:

1. **Medicine is not a substitute for good health care.** Good health care means explaining why people have a health problem, what they can do to get better, and how they can *prevent* that problem in the future.

2. **Medicine is safe and helpful only if you give good instructions about how to take it** (see pages 474 to 476 in this chapter). Be sure the woman understands your instructions.

3. **Medicine will be used correctly only if you understand a woman's beliefs and fears.** If a person believes that taking more medicine will make her heal faster, she may take extra and harm herself. If she is afraid that a medicine will harm her body, she may not take it at all. But if she understands how the medicine works, she will be more eager to take it correctly.

4. **Help find the cheapest and best treatment for the people you see.** Most people worry about the cost, since buying a medicine can take all the money a family has for a week or month.

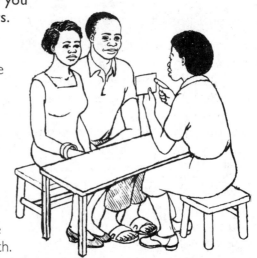

HARMFUL USES OF MEDICINES

Medicines are used to fight dangerous illnesses, but medicines have their own dangers. Used improperly, medicines can hurt or even kill you. These are some common examples of ways medicines can be misused in women's health:

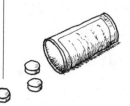

- Oxytocin and ergometrine are sometimes misused to hurry the birth of the baby or the afterbirth (*placenta*). This is dangerous. These medicines can kill the woman and her baby. Unless you are a trained health worker, use these medicines only to stop heavy bleeding AFTER childbirth. Also, do not use them to cause *abortion*. They may burst (rupture) the *womb* and kill the woman before they cause an abortion.

- Women and girls sometimes try using dangerous medicines—such as aspirin, malaria medicines, and ergometrine—to cause abortion. These medicines almost never work. Instead of ending the pregnancy, some medicines can cause serious problems, such as poisoning and death from too much medicine. For more information on new medicines that can be used for safe abortion, read the chapter on "Abortion," page 239.

- Some women have died from using bromocriptine to stop the flow of breast milk. Never take it. Your breast milk will dry up naturally when your baby stops suckling.

- In many places, women are encouraged to take medicines to calm their fears, to improve their mood, or to help them sleep. But these problems are usually caused by life's difficulties. Most of the time, medicines will not make these difficulties go away, and the cost can quickly use up a family's money. If you have difficulty getting through each day, see a trained mental health worker before using a medicine for your nerves or mood.

- DES (diethylstilbestrol), a *hormone*, was used by women in Western Europe and North America from 1941 to 1981 to prevent *miscarriage*. It is no longer used because it can cause *cancer* of the *cervix* and *vagina* in girls and *testicles* in boys whose mothers used it while pregnant. This medicine may still be used in other places, such as parts of Africa and Latin America, to prevent miscarriage and stop the flow of breast milk. Do not take this medicine.

- Some doctors prescribe hormone replacement therapy (HRT) for problems that can happen when your monthly bleeding stops forever (menopause). Sometimes these medicines are helpful. But most women can have a normal and healthy menopause without taking medicines.

- Buying *vitamins* and *minerals* can be a waste of money, unless you have an illness that will be helped by them. Nutritious food is cheaper and healthier for the whole family. If possible, women who have weak blood (*anemia*) and who are pregnant should take iron pills and *folic acid*. But injections of vitamin B12 and liver extract do not help anemia—iron pills and good nutrition will do more good.

How to Use Medicine Safely

Any time you use a medicine, follow these guidelines:

- **Be sure it is necessary.**
- **Get good instructions from the person who told you to take it.** You should know:
    - how much to take (the *dose*).
    - how often to take it each day and for how many days.
- **Take the full amount.** If you stop taking the medicine too soon, the problem may come back.
- **Know the warning signs** for any problems (side effects) the medicine can cause (see page 478).
- **Know if the medicine reacts badly with particular foods** and if you should take it on a full or empty stomach.
- **Avoid taking many medicines at the same time.** Some medicines can stop other medicines from working. Some medicines can combine with other medicines to cause problems that neither would cause by itself.
- **Be careful when buying combination medicines (2 or more medicines in 1 tablet).** Some combination medicines are necessary, but they usually cost more, and you may be putting medicine in your body that you do not need. For example, some eye drops and eye ointments contain both *antibiotics* and *steroids*. The steroids can be harmful. Combination medicines can also cause more side effects.
- **Make sure the package is labeled.** If there is no label, ask the person to show you the bottle or box the medicine came in, and to write down the name and dose for you.

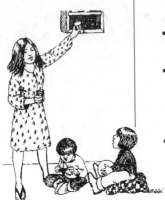

Keep all medicines in a cool, dry place or they may lose their usefulness before the expiration date. Make sure children cannot reach them. They can be deadly to a child.

Avoid medicines that are too old

It is best to use a medicine before its expiration date. This date is written in small print on the package or bottle. For example: If you see 'exp. 10/29/98' or 'exp. 29/10/98' or 'exp. Oct. 29, 1998', this means the medicine should be used before the 29th day of October, 1998. Sometimes expired medicine is better than no medicine. But do not use expired medicines if they are:

- pills that are starting to fall apart or change color.
- capsules that are stuck together or have changed shape.
- clear liquids that are cloudy or have anything floating in them.
- *injections*.
- eye drops.
- medicines that require mixing. If the powder looks old or caked, or if the medicine does not pour evenly after shaking, do not use it. (These must be used soon after they are mixed.)

IMPORTANT *Do not use doxycycline or tetracycline after the expiration date has passed. They may be harmful.*

Throughout this book, we have given the names and doses of medicines that can be used to treat some common women's health problems. But to be able to buy and then use a medicine safely you must also know:

- what the medicine is called where you live (see below).
- in what forms the medicine comes (see page 474).
- how to take the medicine correctly (see page 474).
- whether the medicine is safe for you to take (see page 477).
- if the medicine causes side effects (see page 478).
- what happens if you take too much (or not enough) of the medicine (see page 479).
- what to do if you cannot find (or afford) the medicine, or if you should take another medicine because you are pregnant or breastfeeding or have an *allergy* (see page 480).

This information for each medicine is presented at the end of this chapter in the "Green Pages" (see page 485). The rest of this chapter explains more about how to buy and safely use all of the medicines mentioned in this book.

GENERIC NAMES AND BRAND NAMES

Most medicines have 2 names—a generic or scientific name, and a brand name. The generic name is the same everywhere in the world. The brand name is given by the company that makes the medicine. When several companies make the same medicine, it will have several brand names but only one generic name. As long as the medicine has the same generic name, it is the same medicine.

In this book, we use the generic or scientific name for medicines. For a few medicines, such as those used in *family planning*, we also use the most widely available brand name. If you cannot find the first medicine we recommend, try to buy one of the others listed in the same treatment box.

For example: Your health worker has told you to take **Flagyl**. But when you go to the pharmacy, they do

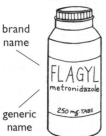

not have any. Ask the pharmacist or health worker what the generic name is for Flagyl (metronidazole) and ask for another brand that has the same generic name. The generic name is usually printed on the label, box, or package. If you ask for the medicine by its generic name, you can often buy it more cheaply.

brand name

FLAGYL
metronidazole
250 mg TABS

generic name

Using the Medicines in this Book

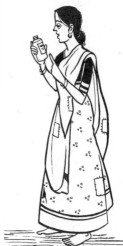

Read the label carefully before you take any medicine.

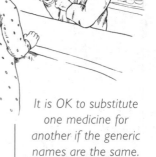

We don't sell that medicine. This one is just as good.

It is OK to substitute one medicine for another if the generic names are the same. Always take the same dose.

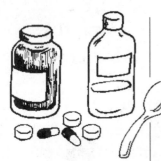

how to give an
injection

MEDICINE COMES IN DIFFERENT FORMS

Medicines come in many different forms:
- Tablets, capsules and liquids are usually taken by mouth. In some cases (rarely) they may need to be used in the *vagina* or *rectum*.
- Inserts (suppositories, pessaries) are made so they can be put into the vagina or the rectum.
- Injections are given with a needle directly into a person's muscle, under the skin, or into the blood.
- Creams, ointments, or salves that contain medicine are applied directly to the skin or in the vagina. They can be very useful for mild skin *infections*, sores, rashes, and itching.

Which kind of medicine, and how much of it you take depends on what is available and on the disease you are trying to treat.

HOW MUCH MEDICINE TO TAKE

How to measure medicine

Many medicines, especially antibiotics, come in different weights and sizes. To be sure you are taking the right amount, check how many grams, milligrams, micrograms, or Units each pill or capsule contains. If the pharmacy does not have the weight or size you need, you may have to take part of a pill, or more than one.

Here are some helpful symbols to know:

= means **equal to** or the **same as**

+ means **and** or **plus**

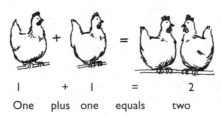

One	plus	one	equals	two
I	+	I	=	2

Fractions. Doses that are less than one whole tablet or pill are sometimes written as *fractions*:

I tablet = one whole tablet =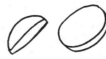

½ tablet = half of a tablet =

I ½ tablet = one and one-half tablets =

1/4 tablet = one quarter or one-fourth of a tablet =

If you are not sure you have the right dose, ask someone who is good at numbers to help you.

Kinds of measurements

Grams and milligrams. Medicine is usually weighed in grams (g) and milligrams (mg):

> 1000 mg = 1 g (one thousand milligrams makes one gram)
> 1 mg = .001 g (one milligram is one-thousandth part of a gram)

For example:

One aspirin tablet has 325 milligrams of aspirin.   .325 g 0.325 g 325 mg   All of these are different ways to say 325 milligrams.

Micrograms. Some medicines, such as family planning pills, are weighed in milligrams or even smaller amounts called micrograms (mcg or μcg):

> 1 μcg = 1 mcg = 1/1000 mg (0.001 mg)   This means there are 1000 micrograms in a milligram.

Units. Some medicines are measured in units (U) or international units (IU).

For liquid medicine: Sometimes instructions for syrups or suspensions tell you to take a specific amount, for example, 10 ml or 10 milliliters or 10 cc (cubic centimeters). A cubic centimeter is the same as a milliliter. If the medicine does not come with a special spoon or dropper to measure liquid, you can use household measures:

> 1 tablespoon = 1 Tb = 15 ml
>
> 1 teaspoon = 1 tsp = 5 ml

So, for example:

Amoxicillin tablets come in 2 sizes:

If you need to take: 'amoxicillin 500 mg 1 tablet 2 times a day', but you only have 250 mg tablets, you need to take 2 tablets each time.

 250 mg and 500 mg

250 mg + 250 mg = 500 mg

Dosing by weight

In this book we have given dosages for adult women. But for some medicines, especially ones that can be dangerous, it is better to figure out the dosage according to a person's weight (if you have a scale). For example, if you need to take gentamicin, and the dosage says 5 mg/kg/day, this means that each day you would give 5 milligrams (mg) of the medicine for each kilogram (kg) the person weighs. So a 50 kg woman would receive 250 mg of gentamicin during 24 hours. This amount should be divided up depending on how many times it is given each day. Gentamicin is given 3 times a day so you would give 80 mg in the morning, 80 mg in the afternoon, and 80 mg in the evening.

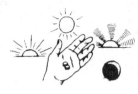

WHEN TO TAKE MEDICINES

It is important to take medicines at the right time. Some medicines should be taken only once a day, but others must be taken more often. You do not need a clock. If the directions say 'I pill every 8 hours', or '3 pills a day', take one at sunrise, one in the afternoon, and one at night. If they say 'I pill every 6 hours', or '4 pills a day', take one in the morning, one at midday, one in the late afternoon, and one at night. If the directions say 'I every 4 hours', take 6 pills a day, allowing about the same time between pills.

IMPORTANT

* *If possible, take medicines while standing or sitting up. Also, try to drink a glass of liquid each time you take a medicine.*
* *If you vomit and can see the medicine in the vomit, you will need to take the medicine again.*
* *If you vomit within 3 hours after taking a birth-control pill, take another one to make sure you will not get pregnant.*

If you are writing a note for someone who does not read well, draw them a note like this:

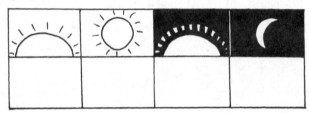

In the blanks at the bottom, draw the amount of medicine to take and carefully explain what it means. For example:

This means they should take I tablet 4 times a day: I at sunrise, I at midday, I in the late afternoon, and I at night.

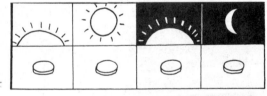

This means ½ tablet 4 times a day.

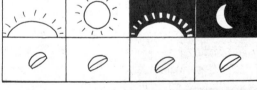

This means I capsule 3 times a day.

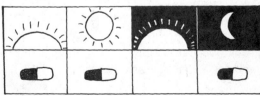

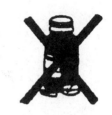

WHO SHOULD NOT TAKE A CERTAIN MEDICINE

Some medicines can be dangerous for certain people, or during certain times of their lives. You should be especially careful if:

- you are **pregnant or breastfeeding**. Many of the medicines that you take during pregnancy and breastfeeding will be passed on to your baby. **Before you take any medicine, find out if it will harm your baby.** Medicines in this book that are harmful during pregnancy and breastfeeding are marked with a warning.

  But if you are sick, it is important that you get treated. Do take medicines to treat serious illnesses and anemia. It is possible to find medicines that will not harm your baby.

 CAUTION = read carefully if you are pregnant

 CAUTION = read carefully if you are breastfeeding

 = do not take if pregnant

 = do not take if breastfeeding

➤ *In the Green Pages, medicines that may be harmful during pregnancy and breastfeeding will be marked with the above signs.*

- you have **long-term *liver* or *kidney* disease**. Your liver and kidneys clear the medicine from your body. If they are not working well, the medicine may build up and become poisonous.

- you have a **stomach *ulcer*** or a stomach that upsets easily (*heartburn*). Medicines such as aspirin and ibuprofen can cause bleeding in the stomach and a painful or burning feeling. If you must take a medicine that bothers your stomach, take it with food.

- you are **allergic** to the medicine. If you have ever had any of these signs after taking a medicine, you are probably allergic to that medicine:

  - a skin rash (raised, red and itchy, usually with swelling)

  - swelling

  - trouble breathing or swallowing

Being allergic means your body fights against the medicine rather than using it to fight disease. Allergic reactions happen more often with antibiotics from the penicillin and sulfa families. Avoid taking other medicines from the same 'family' of medicines as the one you are allergic to. You may also be allergic to them. See page 480 for more information about antibiotics and their families.

IMPORTANT *If you have an allergic reaction to a medicine, never take the medicine again. The next time it may cause a more serious reaction or even death.*

 541

treating allergic reactions and allergic shock

IMPORTANT *If you have taken a medicine and then get a severe skin rash, swelling of the mouth or difficulty breathing or swallowing, get medical help immediately.*

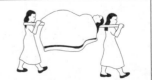

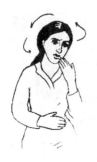

Side effects

Medicines fight disease but can also cause other effects to happen in the body. Some are harmless but annoying. Others are harmful. For example, metronidazole makes your mouth taste bad, which is annoying but harmless. Some very strong antibiotics, such as gentamicin and kanamycin, can cause permanent harm to your kidneys and hearing if too much is taken.

Before you take a medicine, find out what the possible side effects are. When using the medicines in this book you can look at the "Green Pages" to learn about possible side effects.

IMPORTANT: *If you have unusual signs such as dizziness, ringing in the ears, or fast breathing, and these are not listed as side effects for the drug you are taking, see a health worker trained in giving medicines. These signs can mean that you are taking too much medicine.*

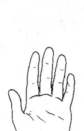

Precautions (warnings)

Some medicines have specific warnings you should learn about. But you should check with a health worker before taking the medicine if:

- you are taking other medicines. Medicines that are safe when taken alone can be harmful when taken with another medicine, or they can be made weaker.
- giving medicine to a child. Children have smaller bodies and may need to take less medicine. Check with a pharmacist or health worker for the right dose for a child.
- you are **older**. Older people sometimes need smaller doses because medicine will stay in their bodies longer.
- you are **very small, thin or poorly nourished**. You may need a smaller dose of some medicines, such as medicines for *tuberculosis*, *high blood pressure*, and *seizures* and other problems.

Information you should know

Food and medicine

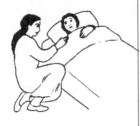

With most medicine, you can continue eating the foods you normally eat. Some medicines work better if you take them when your stomach is empty—when it has been more than 2 hours since you last ate.

Medicines that upset the stomach should be taken with food or just after eating.

If you have *nausea* or vomiting, take the medicine with a dry food that calms the stomach—like rice, bread, or a biscuit.

Taking too much medicine

Some people think that taking more medicine will heal the body faster. This is not true and can be dangerous! If you take too much medicine at one time or too often, or if you take some medicines for too long, the medicine may harm you.

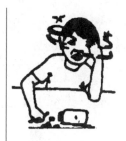

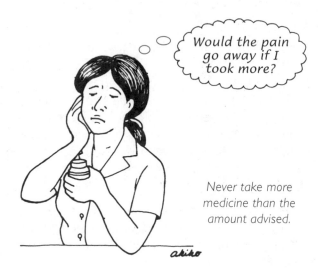

Would the pain go away if I took more?

Never take more medicine than the amount advised.

Some common signs of taking too much of a medicine are:
- nausea
- vomiting
- pain in the stomach
- headache
- *dizziness*
- ringing in the ears
- fast breathing

But these can also be side effects for some medicines. If you have one or more of these signs and they are not common side effects of the medicine you are taking, then you should talk to a health worker trained in giving medicines.

Poisoning. Taking too much of a medicine (for example, half a bottle or more) can poison a person, especially children. You should do the following:

- try to make the person throw up. She may be able to get the extra medicine out of her body before it harms her more.
- give activated charcoal (see page 492). Activated charcoal can absorb some kinds of drugs and keep them from acting as poison.
- Get medical help immediately.

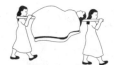

TRANSPORT!

Kinds of Medicines

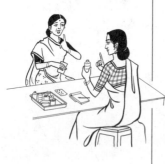

Different medicines are used to treat different problems. Some cure the problem itself and others relieve only the signs of the problem. Sometimes you cannot take the best medicine for your problem because:

- it is not available where you live.
- it is not safe if you are pregnant or breastfeeding.
- you are allergic to it.
- it no longer works where you live, because of drug resistance (see box below).

When this happens, you can substitute one medicine for another, but only if you are sure it will work. The treatments we recommend in this book often give you choices if for some reason you cannot use the best medicine. If you are unsure of what medicines to take, talk to a health worker.

ANTIBIOTICS

Antibiotics are important medicines that are used to fight infections caused by *bacteria*. They do not fight *viruses* or cure the common cold. But not all kinds of antibiotics will fight all kinds of infections. Antibiotics that share the same chemical make-up are said to be from the same family. It is important to know about the families of antibiotics for 2 reasons:

1) antibiotics from the same family can often treat the same problems. This means you can use a different medicine from the same family.

2) if you are allergic to an antibiotic of one family, you will also be allergic to the other members of the same family of antibiotics. This means you will have to take a medicine from another family instead.

The major families of antibiotics used in this book are:

Penicillins: amoxicillin, ampicillin, benzathine penicillin, benzyl penicillin, dicloxacillin, procaine penicillin, and others.

Medicines of the penicillin family are very effective for a variety of infections. They have very few side effects and are safe to take if pregnant or breastfeeding. They are widely available, cheap, and come in oral and injectable forms, but they cause more problems with allergic reactions than many other medicines. They have been overused and some diseases are now resistant to penicillins.

Macrolides: azithromycin, erythromycin, and others

Erythromycin is an older, commonly used and widely available antibiotic that works for many of the same infections as penicillin and doxycycline. It is often a good substitute for doxycycline when a woman is pregnant or breastfeeding, or if there is penicillin allergy.

Tetracyclines: doxycycline, tetracycline

Tetracycline and doxycycline both treat many different infections and are cheap and widely available. Neither drug should be taken by pregnant or breastfeeding women or by children under 8 years of age.

Sulfas (sulfonamides): sulfamethoxazole (part of co-trimoxazole), sulfisoxazole

These medicines fight many different kinds of infections and they are cheap and widely available. But they are less effective now because some infections are resistant to them. They cause more problems with allergic reactions than other medicines. They can be taken during pregnancy, but it is better to take a different medicine just before you give birth and during the first few weeks of the baby's life. Stop using sulfonamides immediately if you develop signs of allergy (see page 483).

Aminoglycosides: gentamicin, streptomycin, and others

These are effective and strong medicines, but most of them can cause serious side effects and can only be given by injection. They should only be used when infection is severe and no safer drug is available.

Cephalosporins: cefixime, ceftriaxone, cephalexin, and others

These are a large family of new and powerful drugs that treat many women's infections that have become resistant to the older antibiotics. They are often safer and have fewer side effects than the older antibiotics but can be quite expensive and hard to find. They are safe to use during pregnancy and breastfeeding.

Quinolones: ciprofloxacin, norfloxacin, and others

Ciprofloxacin and norfloxacin are new and powerful antibiotics. They are expensive and may be hard to find. They cannot be taken while pregnant and breastfeeding or by children less than 16 years old.

Use antibiotics only when necessary

Many antibiotics, especially penicillin, are used too often. Use antibiotics only when necessary because:

- while they kill some germs, antibiotics allow others—ones that are normally in the body and usually harmless—to grow out of control. This can cause problems like diarrhea and vaginal *yeast infections*.

- some antibiotics can cause serious side effects and allergic reactions.

- using antibiotics when they are not needed or for diseases they cannot cure has made some harmful germs stronger and *resistant* to the medicine. This means the medicine can no longer cure the disease.

For example: In the past it was easy to cure gonorrhea, a sexually transmitted disease, with penicillin. But penicillin has been used incorrectly and too often for many other, less serious problems.

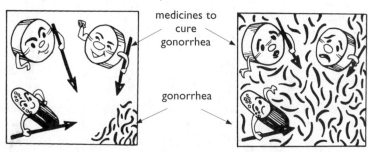

medicines to cure gonorrhea

gonorrhea

Now there are new kinds of gonorrhea that resist penicillin and other antibiotics. These new kinds are harder and more expensive to cure.

MEDICINES FOR PAIN

Pain is a sign of a problem, such as an injury or infection. So it is very important to treat the problem that is causing the pain, and not just the pain. But during the treatment, the pain can be eased with pain medicines. With some illnesses that cannot be cured, like AIDS and cancer, pain can be disabling and last a long time.

When treating pain:
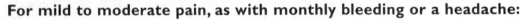
- try to find and treat the cause of the pain.
- try the weakest pain medicines first and use stronger ones only if needed.
- treatment for ongoing pain should be given regularly. Don't wait until the pain returns before the next dose.
- think about other ways to relieve pain: relaxation exercises, acupressure, or putting heat or cold where the pain is (see pages 423 and 542).

For mild to moderate pain, as with monthly bleeding or a headache:

Paracetamol is widely available and cheap. It is the safest pain medicine for pregnant and breastfeeding women, and it also works to reduce *fever*. Do not take it with alcohol or to treat a hangover, or if you have liver or kidney problems.

Aspirin is also widely available, cheap, and works well to lower fever and to treat pain and inflammation in muscles and joints, and for pain with monthly bleeding. Breastfeeding women can use aspirin one week after the baby is born, but pregnant women should use paracetamol instead. It is safe when taken in the correct amounts, but it can irritate the stomach, so it should not be taken by people with stomach ulcers. Aspirin keeps blood from clotting normally, so it should not be taken if the person is bleeding or before any *surgery*.

Ibuprofen is widely available but more expensive than aspirin or paracetamol. Like aspirin, it is very effective in lower doses for pain with monthly bleeding, and for muscle and joint pain and inflammation. Ibuprofen is a good medicine for the lasting pain of arthritis. It can also cause irritation of the stomach and bleeding problems, so it should not be taken before surgery or by people with stomach ulcers. Breastfeeding women can use ibuprofen but pregnant women should not use it during the last 3 months of pregnancy.

For moderate to severe pain:

Ibuprofen in larger doses can be effective (up to 800 mg 3 to 4 times daily).

Codeine is a drug of the opiate family which is useful for pain after surgery or an injury. Taking codeine for too long can cause *addiction*.

For severe or ongoing pain:

Codeine in higher doses can be used for severe pain.

Morphine is a very strong medicine of the opiate family that is good for pain during the last stages of cancer or *AIDS*. Morphine is usually difficult to get unless you are in a hospital, but it may be available with a doctor's prescription. It is highly addictive.

MEDICINES FOR HEAVY BLEEDING FROM THE VAGINA AFTER BIRTH OR ABORTION

Medicines that contain ergometrine or oxytocin cause contractions of the womb and its blood vessels. They are important medicines to control heavy bleeding after childbirth.

Ergometrine is used to prevent or control severe bleeding **after the placenta has come out**. Do not inject ergometrine into the vein (IV). It should be injected into a large muscle. Never give this medicine before the baby is born or the placenta has come out! Do not give this medicine to a woman with high blood pressure.

Oxytocin is used to help stop severe bleeding of the mother **after the baby is born**. It is very rare for oxytocin to be needed before the baby is born. For this pupose, it should only be given in the vein by a doctor or trained birth attendant. Using oxytocin to speed up labor or give strength to the mother in labor can be dangerous to both mother and child.

MEDICINES FOR ALLERGIC REACTIONS

A person can be allergic to medicines, foods, or things that are breathed in or touched. Reactions may be mild—with itching, hives or rash, or sneezing—or they can be moderate or severe. Some reactions can worsen and bring on allergic shock. Severe reactions and allergic shock can be life-threatening and must be treated.

541

how to treat
allergic reaction
and allergic shock

In this book, we talk about how some medicines may cause allergic reactions. Any medicine that causes an allergic reaction should be stopped and never given again—even if the reaction was mild.

Depending on how strong the reaction is, allergic reactions are treated with 1, 2, or 3 kinds of medicines:

1. **Antihistamines**, like diphenhydramine, hydroxizine, or promethazine. None of these medicines are good for pregnant or breastfeeding women, but promethazine is the least dangerous of them. Otherwise diphenhydramine is usually the cheapest and most widely available.

2. **Steroids**, like dexamethasone or hydrocortisone. Dexamethasone is a better choice for pregnant or breastfeeding women.

3. **Epinephrine** or **adrenaline**. These medicines are safe for pregnant or breastfeeding women.

Medicines that Can Save a Woman's Life

Starting a community emergency medicine kit is one way you can help save the lives of women where you live. The medicines in this chart will help you start treatment until other medical help is available. Make sure these medicines are in your kit or at the nearest health post. If you need to buy them, try meeting with leaders in your community. Explain how these medicines can help, and see if you can find ways together to buy them.

What to include in a medicine kit:

Problem	Medicine
pelvic infection (PID)	tablets: doxycycline, tetracycline, norfloxacin, metronidazole
kidney infection	ampicillin, gentamicin, co-trimoxazole
bleeding after birth, abortion, or miscarriage	oxytocin or ergometrine
infection after birth, abortion, or miscarriage	ampicillin or penicillin, gentamicin, chloramphenicol
toxemia during or after birth	diazepam or magnesium sulfate
emergency pregnancy prevention (after rape, broken condom, or other emergency)	*Lo-Femenal* (low dose) or *Ovral*, *Neogynon* (high dose) birth control pills. See the "Green Pages" for other common brand names.
allergic reaction to antibiotic	epinephrine, diphenhydramine, hydrocortisone or dexamethasone

HOW TO USE THE GREEN PAGES

This section gives information about the medicines mentioned in this book. For general information about medicines, be sure to read the chapter called "Use of Medicines in Women's Health" beginning on page 468. For specific information about each medicine, you can look it up in these Green Pages. Medicines are listed by their generic (scientific) names, the same names used in the chapters. The medicines are arranged in the order of the alphabet:

a b c d e f g h i j k l m n o p q r s t u v w x y z

For example, if you are looking up **h**ydroxyzine, it comes after **d**oxycycline but before **m**etronidazole.

You can also find a medicine in the Green Pages by using:

- the **problem index** on page 486. This index lists the health problems discussed in this book and medicines used to treat them. The index gives the page number where information about the health problem can be found. Be sure to read about the problem before treating it with medicine. Remember: good health does not depend only on medicines! The most important 'medicine' for good health is good health information.

- the **medicine index** on page 487. This index lists the generic names of medicines and some common brand (commercial) names. If there is a medicine you want to use, you can look it up here to find the number of the page where you can learn more about that medicine.

Both the problem and medicine indexes are arranged in the order of the alphabet.

Information about specific medicines

Information about specific medicines begins on page 489.

The information about each medicine appears in a box like this:

The generic name is shown in heavy letters:

Some brand names are shown in slanted letters:

These pictures appear with the word *CAUTION* when pregnant or breastfeeding women need to take special care. If the medicine should not be used by a woman who is pregnant or breastfeeding, the picture is crossed out.

General information about the medicine is found here:

The rest of the chart gives other important information about using the medicine safely.

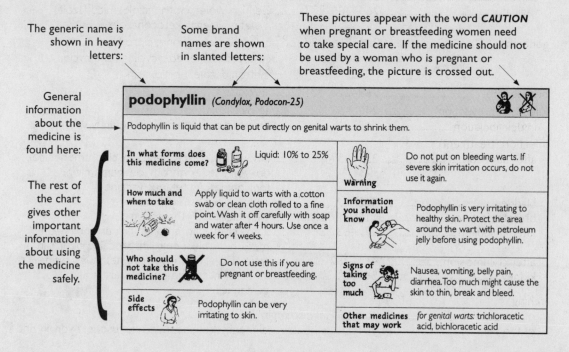

podophyllin *(Condylox, Podocon-25)*

Podophyllin is liquid that can be put directly on genital warts to shrink them.

In what forms does this medicine come?	Liquid: 10% to 25%
How much and when to take	Apply liquid to warts with a cotton swab or clean cloth rolled to a fine point. Wash it off carefully with soap and water after 4 hours. Use once a week for 4 weeks.
Who should not take this medicine?	Do not use this if you are pregnant or breastfeeding.
Side effects	Podophyllin can be very irritating to skin.
Warning	Do not put on bleeding warts. If severe skin irritation occurs, do not use it again.
Information you should know	Podophyllin is very irritating to healthy skin. Protect the area around the wart with petroleum jelly before using podophyllin.
Signs of taking too much	Nausea, vomiting, belly pain, diarrhea. Too much might cause the skin to thin, break and bleed.
Other medicines that may work	*for genital warts:* trichloracetic acid, bichloracetic acid

Problem Index

   This is a list of the health problems discussed in this book that are sometimes treated with medicines. The problems are listed in order of the alphabet in the column on the left. The column in the middle has the numbers of the pages in the book where you can read about each problem. You should read these pages before taking any medicine. The list on the right has medicines that can be used to treat each problem on the left. To learn more about a medicine, look it up in the medicine tables that start on page 490.

Problem	See pages	See medicines
arthritis	133	aspirin, ibuprofen
bleeding from the vagina		
after abortion	251–253	ergometrine
after childbirth	92–93	ergometrine, oxytocin
around menopause	129	medroxyprogesterone
chancroid	268–269, 278	ceftriaxone, ciprofloxacin, erythromycin, co-trimoxazole
chlamydia	264–266, 277	co-trimoxazole, doxycycline, erythromycin, tetracycline
cough	303	codeine
diarrhea	298–299	co-trimoxazole, metronidazole, norfloxacin
emergency birth control	224–225	low-dose birth control pills (groups 2 and 3)
fever	297	aspirin, paracetamol, ibuprofen
after abortion	255–256	amoxicillin, doxycycline, metronidazole
after childbirth	97	amoxicillin, metronidazole, procaine penicillin, chloramphenicol.
during labor	86	ampicillin, procaine penicillin
fits during pregnancy	87	diazepam, magnesium sulfate
fungal infection		
mouth (thrush)	305	Gentian Violet, ketoconazole, nystatin
skin	300	Gentian Violet, ketoconazole, nystatin
vagina	264–266, 277	Gentian Violet, clotrimazole, miconazole, nystatin, vinegar, ketoconazole
gonorrhea	264–266, 277	cefixime, ceftriaxone, ciprofloxacin, co-trimoxazole, doxycycline,kanamycin, metronidazole, norfloxacin
herpes sores	269–270, 301	acyclovir
infection (prevention)	249, 465	amoxicillin, doxycycline,
in deinfibulation	465	amoxicillin, erythromycin, tetanus vaccine
infection (treatment)		
after abortion	255–257	amoxicillin, benzyl penicillin, chloramphenicol, doxycycline, erythromycin, gentamicin, metronidazole, tetanus vaccine
bladder	368	amoxicillin, co-trimoxazole
breast infection	116–117	dicloxacillin, erythromycin
after childbirth	97, 465	amoxicillin, chloramphenicol, erythromycin, metronidazole, penicillin, procaine penicillin
after circumcision	461–462	dicloxacillin, erythromycin, tetanus vaccine
kidney	368	amoxicillin, co-trimoxazole, ampicillin, gentamicin
itching		
of the genitals	*(see vaginal discharge)*	
of the skin	301	diphenhydramine, hydrocortisone, hydroxyzine

List of Medicines

This list of medicines has two different kinds of names—brand (commercial) names and generic (scientific) names. You can look up the the name of a medicine you want to use here to find the page number in the Green Pages where you can learn more about it. Brand names are shown *in slanted letters like this*. Brand names have the generic name of the medicine next to it.

acetaminophen *or* paracetamol *(APAP, Panadol, Tempra, Tylenol, others)*

Acetaminophen and paracetamol are 2 names for the same drug that is used to ease pain and lower fever. It is one of the safest pain killers. It does not cause stomach irritation and can be used instead of aspirin by people with stomach ulcers. It can also be used by pregnant women. *See paracetamol, page 511.*

acyclovir *(Zovirax)* CAUTION

Acyclovir is a medicine that kills viruses and is used to fight herpes, which can cause painful blisters on the genitals, and anus, and in the mouth. Acyclovir will not stop herpes from coming back, but it makes it less painful and keeps it from spreading.

In what forms does this medicine come?	Tablets: 200, 400 or 800 mg Ointment: 5%	Information you should know	The tablets are much more effective than the ointment. Take with lots of water.
How much and when to take	*For genital herpes infection:* Take 200 mg by mouth 5 times a day for 7 to 10 days. *For cold sores:* Apply ointment on sores 6 times a day for 7 days.	Side effects	May sometimes cause headache, dizziness, nausea, vomiting.
Who should not take this medicine? 	Someone with kidney damage.	Signs of taking too much 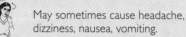	Headache, loss of memory, nausea, cannot pass urine.

adrenaline *or* epinephrine *(Adrenalin)*

Adrenaline and epinephrine are two names for the same drug. It is used for severe allergic reactions or allergic shock, for example, allergic reaction to penicillin. It is also used for severe asthma attacks. *See epinephrine, page 500.*

amoxicillin *(Amoxifar, Amoxil, Himox, Megamox, Sumoxil)*

Amoxicillin is an antibiotic of the penicillin family used to treat womb infections, urine system infections, pneumonia, and other infections. It is now used instead of ampicillin in many places.

In what forms does this medicine come?	Tablets: 250 and 500 mg Liquid: 125 or 250 mg per 5 ml	Who should not take this medicine?	Do not use if allergic to medicines of the penicillin family.
How much and when to take	*For chlamydia, PID, or breast infection:* 500 mg by mouth 3 times a day for 10 days *(for drug combinations to treat vaginal discharge, see page 277; for PID, see page 278).* *For kidney infection:* Take 500 mg by mouth 3 times a day for 14 days. *For infection of the womb after childbirth:* Take 1 gram 3 times a day for 10 days *(also use other drugs, see page 97).* *To prevent infection after abortion:* Take 500 mg by mouth 3 times a day for 5 days. *For bladder infection or infection after abortion:* 3 grams by mouth one time only *(see pages 255 to 257 for drug combinations to treat infection after an abortion).*	Side effects	May cause diarrhea, rash, nausea or vomiting. May cause yeast infection in women or diaper rash in children.
		Information you should know	If you do not start to get better in 3 days, look for medical help; you may need a different medicine. Take with food.
		Other medicines that may work	*for bladder or kidney infection:* ampicillin, co-trimoxazole, gentamicin, norfloxacin *for breast infection:* cephalexin, dicloxacillin, erythromycin *to prevent infection after abortion:* doxycycline

amoxicillin with clavulanate potassium *(Augmentin)*

Amoxicillin with clavulanate potassium *(Augmentin)* is an antibiotic of the penicillin family used to treat gonorrhea and other infections. In some places, however, gonorrhea is now resistent to this drug. It is much more effective for some infections than amoxicillin alone but is expensive and often hard to find outside of rich countries. Unfortunately, clavulanate potassium cannot be purchased by itself and combined with regular amoxicillin.

In what forms does this medicine come? 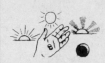	Tablets: 125, 200, 250, 400, 500 and 875 mg Liquid: 125, 200, 250, and 400 mg per 5 ml	**Who should not take this medicine?**	Do not use if allergic to medicines of the penicillin family.
How much and when to take	**For gonorrhea:** Take 3 grams of amoxicillin with clavulanate potassium *(Augmentin)* plus 1 gram of probenecid, 1 time only.	**Other medicines that may work**	*for gonorrhea: see drug combinations, pages 266 and 277.*

ampicillin *(Amcil, Ampicin, Omnipen, Penbritin, Polycillin)*

Ampicillin is an antibiotic of the penicillin family used to treat many kinds of infections.

In what forms does this medicine come?	Tablets and Capsules: 250 or 500 mg Liquid: 125 or 250 mg per 5 ml Powder for mixing injections: 500 mg	**Who should not take this medicine?** 	Do not use ampicillin if you are allergic to medicines of the penicillin family.
		Side effects	May cause stomach upset and diarrhea. May cause rash.
How much and when to take	**For breast infection or PID:** Take 250 to 500 mg by mouth 4 times a day for 7 days *(see page 278 for drug combinations to treat PID).*	**Warning**	If you do not start to get better in 3 days, look for medical help; you may need another medicine.
	For bladder infection: Take 3 grams all at once unless you are pregnant. If you are pregnant, take 250 mg by mouth 4 times a day for 7 days. **For kidney infection:** Take 500 mg by mouth 4 times a day for 14 days. If vomiting, inject 500 mg into muscle 4 times a day and change to tablets when the vomiting stops. **For fever during pregnancy:** Take 500 mg 4 times a day until you can get medical attention.	**Information you should know**	Take this medicine before eating.
		Other medicines that may work	*for bladder or kidney infection:* amoxicillin, co-trimoxazole, norfloxacin *for breast infection:* amoxicillin, cephalexin, dicloxacillin, erythromycin

aspirin *(acetylsalicylic acid, ASA, others)*

CAUTION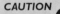

Aspirin works against pain, swelling, and fever.

In what forms does this medicine come?	Tablets: 300, 500 mg and other sizes.	**Side effects** May cause stomach upset, stomach pain, or bleeding problems.
How much and when to take	*For pain, swelling or fever:* 300 to 600 mg by mouth no more than 6 times a day as needed.	**Information you should know** Aspirin treats some sicknesses like arthritis and heart problems, but is usually used to ease pain and fever. It is important to find the cause of the pain or fever and cure that. If pain lasts more than 10 days or fever more than 3 days, get medical help.
Who should not take this medicine? 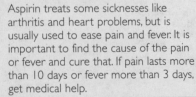	Women should not take aspirin during the last 3 months of pregnancy. People with stomach ulcers or bleeding problems should not take aspirin. Do not use before surgery. Do not use if breastfeeding in the first week of the baby's life. Do not give to children for fever, colds or chicken pox.	**Signs of taking too much** Ringing in the ears, headache, dizziness, confusion, fast breathing.
		Other medicines that may work *for pain or fever:* paracetamol *for pain, fever, or swelling:* ibuprofen *for severe pain:* codeine

azithromycin *(Zithromax)*

CAUTION

Azithromycin is an antibiotic of the macrolide family used to treat many STDs. It is expensive and often hard to find, but it works well against STDs when many other antibiotics do not.

In what forms does this medicine come?	Capsules: 250 mg	**Information you should know**  Take at least 1 hour before eating or at least 2 hours after eating.
How much and when to take	*For women at risk for STDs:* Take 1 gram by mouth 1 time only.	Azithromycin is an excellent treatment for most STDs that cause discharge or genital sores. It is good for treating STDs where there is resistance to other medicines.
Who should not take this medicine?	People with allergies to erythromycin and other antibiotics of the macrolide family.	
Side effects	Diarrhea, nausea, vomiting, abdominal pain.	**Other medicines that may work** *for vaginal discharge with an STD:* see page 277. *for genital ulcers:* see page 278.

AZT *(azidothymidine, Retrovir, zidovudine)*

AZT is a medicine used to treat AIDS and to help prevent passing the HIV virus to a baby during pregnancy and birth. It is a difficult drug to use, and should be given in a hospital or under the care of a qualified health worker. Also, it is very expensive and often hard to find in poor countries.

benzathine penicillin *(Bicillin L-A, Penadur L-A, Permapen)*

Benzathine penicillin is a long-acting antibiotic of the penicillin family used to treat syphilis, genital ulcers, and other infections, including some sore throats. It is always given as an injection into muscle.

In what forms does this medicine come? 	Powder for mixing for injection: 1.2 or 2.4 million Units in a 5 ml vial.	**Who should not take this medicine?** 	People who are allergic to medicines of the penicillin family.
How much and when to take	*For genital ulcers, early syphilis or syphilis prevention after sexual assault or exposure:* Inject 2.4 million Units into muscle one time only. *For late syphilis:* Inject 2.4 million Units into muscle every week for 3 weeks.	**Warning**	Have epinephrine on hand whenever you inject penicillin. Watch for allergic reactions and allergic shock which could start within 30 minutes.
		Other medicines that may work	*for syphilis:* doxycycline, tetracycline, erythromycin *also treat for chancroid, see page 278*

benzylpenicillin *(Celinex, Hi-Do-Pen, penicillin G potassium or sodium)*

Benzylpenicillin is an antibiotic of the penicillin family used to treat many serious infections, including infection after an abortion.

In what forms does this medicine come?	Powder for mixing for injection: 1 or 5 million Units	**Warning**	Watch for allergic reactions and signs of shock.
How much and when to take	*For serious infection after an abortion:* Inject 5 million Units into muscle 1 time only (*also give other medicines, see page 257*).	**Other medicines that may work**	*for serious infection after an abortion:* ampicillin, cephalexin, ciprofloxacin, norfloxacin (see pages 256 and 257 for medicine combinations).
Who should not take this medicine?	People who are allergic to medicines of the penicillin family.		

cefixime *(Suprax)*   **CAUTION**

Cefixime is an antibiotic of the cephalosporin family that is used to treat many infections including gonorrhea, pelvic inflammatory disease, and others.

In what forms does this medicine come?	Tablets: 200 or 400 mg Liquid: 100 mg in 5 ml	**Side effects** 	Nausea, diarrhea, headache.
How much and when to take	*For gonorrhea or PID:* Take 400 mg by mouth one time only (*see page 277 for drug combinations to treat vaginal discharge from STDs; see page 278 for PID*).	**Warning**	Watch for allergic reaction. People who have liver problems should be watched carefully when taking cefixime.
Who should not take this medicine?	Do not use if you are allergic to antibiotics of the cephalosporin family.	**Other medicines that may work**	*for gonorrhea:* ceftriaxone, ciprofloxacin, co-trimoxazole kanamicin, norfloxacin *for PID:* ceftriaxone, norfloxacin

ceftriaxone *(Nitrocephin, Rocephin)*

 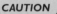

Ceftriaxone is a very strong antibiotic of the cephalosporin family that is injected into muscle. It is used for many infections including gonorrhea, pelvic inflammatory disease (PID), kidney infections, and serious infections after abortion, childbirth, or miscarriage.

In what forms does this medicine come?

In vials for injection: 250, 500 mg and 1 gram, 2 grams and 10 grams

How much and when to take

For severe infections after abortion or childbirth: Inject 1 gram into muscle once a day for 10 days.

For gonorrhea, chancroid, or PID: Inject 250 mg into muscle one time only *(see pages 277 and 278 for drug combinations to treat STDs).*

Who should not take this medicine?

Do not use if you are allergic to antibiotics of the cephalosporin family.

Warning

Watch for allergic reaction.

Always be prepared to treat for allergic reaction and shock when injecting antibiotics.

Other medicines that may work
for severe infections: amoxicillin with clavulanate potassium *(Augmentin),* *for gonorrhea, chancroid, or PID:* kanamicin

cephalexin *(Ceporex, Keflex, Keftab)*

Cephalexin is an antibiotic of the cephalosporin family used to treat breast and bladder infections, bronchitis and some skin infections.

In what forms does this medicine come?
Tablets: 250 or 500 mg
Liquid: 125 or 250 mg per 5 ml

How much and when to take

For breast or bladder infection: 250 mg by mouth 4 times a day for 7 days.

Who should not take this medicine?

Do not take cephalexin if you are allergic to antibiotics of the cephalosporin family.

Side effects

Nausea, vomiting, and diarrhea. In rare cases, the beginning of bloody diarrhea with fever.

Warning
Watch for allergic reaction.

Information you should know

If you start having bloody diarrhea with fever, stop taking cephalexin and treat with metronidazole *(see page 507).*

Other medicines that may work
for breast or skin infection: erythromycin, dicloxacillin, amoxicillin

for bladder infection: amoxicillin, co-trimoxazole, erythromycin, norfloxacin

activated charcoal *(Activated Carbon, Liquid Antidote)*

Activated charcoal is a specially prepared charcoal used to treat some poisonings by drugs like aspirin, acetaminophen, phenobarbitol, or other medicines or chemicals, or poisonous mushrooms. After giving activated charcoal, get medical help immediately.

In what forms does this medicine come?	Liquid: 25 g per 120 ml Powder: 15 g	
How much and when to take	Take 30 to 100 g by mouth all at one time.	
Who should not take this medicine?	Do not take if you have swallowed lighter fluid, fuel, kerosene or petroleum products.	

Side effects	Black stools, vomiting, diarrhea.
Warning	Get medical help immediately. People who take too much of a drug can get very sick and may need much more help than activated charcoal.

chloramphenicol *(Chloromycetin, Kemicetine, Mychel, Pharex)*

Chloramphenicol is a very strong antibiotic used for serious infections after childbirth, miscarriage, or abortion. It should only be used when less dangerous drugs do not work or are not safe to take. As an ointment, it is also used for baby eye care if tetracycline or erythromycin ointments are not available.

In what forms does this medicine come?	Capsules: 250 mg Liquid: 150 mg per 5 ml Powder for mixing for injection: 1 g Ointment: 1% Liquid for eye care: 0.5%

How much and when to take

For infection after childbirth: Take 1 g by mouth one time only and then 500 mg by mouth 4 times a day for 7 days *(also use other medicines, see page 97).*

For serious infection after abortion: Inject 1 g into vein (IV) 4 times a day *(also use other medicines, see page 257).*

For baby eye care: put a little in each eye at birth.

Who should not take this medicine?	Women who are pregnant or breastfeeding.
Side effects	Upset stomach, vision problems.

Warning	Use other antibiotics if possible. Risk of permanent harm to the blood or even death in some people.
Information you should know	For serious infections, choramphenicol should be taken with 10 million Units of benzyl penicillin.
Signs of taking too much	Bleeding or bruising easily, vision problems.
Other medicines that may work	*for serious infection:* after birth, see page 97. after abortion, see page 257. *for baby eye care:* tetracycline or erythromycin ointments are better.

ciprofloxacin *(Ciloxan, Cipro, Ciprobay)*

Ciprofloxacin is a strong antibiotic of the quinolone family that is used to treat skin and kidney infections, and some STDs like gonorrhea, chancroid and PID.

In what forms does this medicine come?
Tablets: 250, 500 or 750 mg

How much and when to take
For gonorrhea, PID, or chancroid: 500 mg by mouth one time only *(see pages 277 and 278 for drug combinations to treat STDs).*

For kidney infection: Take 500 mg by mouth 2 times a day for 10 days.

Who should not take this medicine?
Do not use if you are pregnant, breastfeeding or younger than 16 years old.

Side effects
Nausea, diarrhea, vomiting, headache.

Warning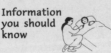
This medicine reacts with caffeine (in coffee, chocolate, cola drinks, etc.), making the caffeine even stronger. Do not take with dairy products.

Information you should know
Drink lots of water. You can eat while taking ciprofloxacin, just avoid dairy products.

Other medicines that may work
for gonorrhea: ceftriaxone, kanamicin, norfloxacin
for chancroid: erythromycin, co-trimoxazole
for PID: norfloxacin, doxycycline, metronidazole
for kidney infection: amoxicillin, co-trimoxazole

clotrimazole *(Canesten, Fungistin, Gyne-lotrimin, Mycelex-G)*

Clotrimazole is used to treat yeast infections of the vagina, mouth and throat.

In what forms does this medicine come?
Inserts: 100 or 500 mg
Cream: 1%
Lozenge: 10 mg

How much and when to take
For vaginal yeast infections:
Inserts: Put one 500 mg insert in the vagina at bedtime one time only; or, put two 100 mg inserts in the vagina at bedtime every night for 3 nights.
Cream: Put 5 g in the vagina each night at bedtime for 7 to 14 days.

For mouth and throat infections: Take a 10 mg lozenge by mouth 5 times a day for 14 days.

Who should not take this medicine?
Do not use if you have had allergic reactions to this drug.

Side effects
Mild burning or itching. Nausea or vomiting if taken by mouth.

Warning
If clotrimazole burns the vagina, stop using it. Avoid having sex for 3-4 days so you do not pass the infection to your partner.

Information you should know
The single, larger dose works better for pregnant women.

Other medicines that may work
for yeast infections: nystatin, miconazole, Gentian Violet or vinegar.
for AIDS patients: ketaconazole.

codeine

 CAUTION

Codeine is a pain killer of the opiate family that also calms coughs and helps you relax and sleep. Only use codeine to calm very bad coughs after you have treated the cause for the cough. Only use codeine for pain when milder pain medicines do not work.

In what forms does this medicine come? 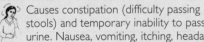	Liquid: 15 mg per ml Tablets: 15, 30, or 60 mg Cough syrup: Different strengths	**Signs of taking too much**	Sleepiness, stupor, coma.
How much and when to take	**For coughs:** 7 to 15 mg 4 times a day, only as needed. **For severe pain:** 30 to 60 mg 4 to 6 times a day, as needed.	**Treatment for taking too much**	Naloxone *(Narcan)* can be given as an injection to someone who has taken too much codeine. Seek medical help.
Side effects	Causes constipation (difficulty passing stools) and temporary inability to pass urine. Nausea, vomiting, itching, headaches.	**Other medicines that may work**	*for pain:* acetaminophen, aspirin, ibuprofen. *for severe pain:* morphine *for cough:* drink plenty of water, use home-made cough syrup *(see page 303).*
Information you should know	Codeine is habit forming (addictive). If you use it for more than a few days, you will need more and more of it for the medicine to work.		

co-trimoxazole = trimethoprim + sulfamethoxazole

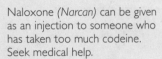 CAUTION

(AzoGantanol, Bactrim, Coptin, Gantanol, Pologrim, Septra, Sulfatrim, TMP/SMX, Trimpex, others)

Co-trimoxazole is a combination of 2 antibiotics (one from the sulfa family) that is used to treat bladder and kidney infections, vaginal discharge caused by gonorrhea, and chancroid. It also helps prevent diarrhea and pneumonia for people with AIDS.

In what forms does this medicine come?	Tablets: 120 mg (20 mg trimethoprim + 100 mg sulfamethoxazole) 480 mg (80 mg trimethoprim + 400 mg sulfamethoxazole), and 960 mg (160 mg trimethoprim + 800 mg sulfamethoxazole) Liquid: 240 mg (40 mg trimethoprim + 200 mg sulfamethoxazole) per 5 ml	**Who should not take this medicine?**	Women in the last 3 months of pregnancy should not use this medicine. If you are allergic to sulfa antibiotics, do not take this drug.
How much and when to take	**For bladder infection:** Take four 480 tablets by mouth one time only. **For kidney infection:** Take two 480 tablets by mouth 2 times a day for 10 days.	**Side effects**	Stop taking it if it causes allergic reactions like itching or skin rashes. Also may cause nausea and vomiting.
		Warning	Take with lots of water.
		Signs of taking too much	Nausea, vomiting, diarrhea, confusion, sweating.

For vaginal discharges caused by STDs: Take ten 480 tablets once a day for 3 days *(see page 266 for drug combinations to treat STDs).*

For prevention of pneumonia and diarrhea for people with AIDS: Take one 480 tablet every day or two 480 tablets two times a week.

For bloody diarrhea, or pneumonia for people with AIDS: Take two 480 tablets by mouth 2 times a day for 10 days.

For PID or chancroid: Take five 480 tablets by mouth 2 times a day for 3 days; or, if this makes you nauseous, take two 480 tablets by mouth 2 times a day for 7 days *(see page 278 for drug combinations to treat PID*

Other medicines that may work	*for bladder and kidney infection:* amoxicillin, nitrofurantoin, norfloxacin *for gonorrhea:* ceftriaxone, kanamicin, norfloxacin

for chancroid: ciprofloxacin, ceftriaxone, erythromycin, kanamycin
for PID: see drug combinations, page 278.
for diarrhea for people with AIDS: norfloxacin, metronidazole

dexamethasone *(Decadron, Decilone, Inflam, Maxidex)*

Dexamethasone is a steroid medicine used to treat allergic shock *(see page 541)*.

In what forms does this medicine come?	Tablets: 0.25, 0.5, 0.75, 1, 1.5, 2, or 4 mg Liquid: 0.5 mg per 5 ml, or 1 mg per 1 ml For injection: 4, 8, 10, 16, or 20 mg per ml	**Side effects** 	If the person has diabetes, it could make it worse for a few hours. Also, it might raise blood pressure.
How much and when to take	*For allergic shock:* Inject 20 mg into muscle. If signs return, take 20 mg by mouth and repeat once if needed.	**Other medicines that may work**	*for allergic shock:* hydrocortisone

diazepam *(Anxionil, Calmpose, Valium)*   *CAUTION*

Diazepam is a tranquilizer used to treat and prevent convulsions and seizures. It also relieves anxiety and helps promote sleep.

In what forms does this medicine come?	Tablets: 5 or 10 mg For injections: 5 mg per 1 ml or 10 mg per 2 ml	**Side effects**	Frequent or large doses of diazepam during pregnancy can cause birth defects.
How much and when to take	*For convulsions:* Use 20 mg of injectable diazepam in the anus using a syringe **without a needle** *(see page 87)*. Repeat if needed using 15 mg after every convulsion. Use crushed up tablets in water if you do not have injectable diazepam. *To prevent seizures during alcohol withdrawl:* Take 10 to 20 mg by mouth. Repeat after 1 hour if needed. If signs continue, give every 4 to 5 hours while seeking medical help. *For anxiety or sleeplessness:* Take 2.5 to 5 mg by mouth.	**Warning**	Diazepam is an addictive (habit-forming) drug. Avoid taking with other drugs that will make you sleepy, especially alcohol.
		Information you should know	Diazepam does not treat pain. It is very habit-forming.
		Signs of taking too much	Sleepiness, loss of balance, confusion.
Who should not take this medicine?	Pregnant or breast-feeding women should only use diazepam in an emergency.	**Other medicines that may work**	*for convulsions:* magnesium sulfate *for sleep:* diphenhydramine *for anxiety:* hydroxyzine

dicloxacillin

Dicloxacillin is an antibiotic of the penicillin family used to treat breast and skin infections.

In what forms does this medicine come?	Capsules: 125, 250 or 500 mg Liquid: 62.5 mg per 5 ml	**Side effects**	Nausea, vomiting, diarrhea.
How much and when to take	*For breast or skin infections:* Take 250 mg 4 times a day for 10 days.	**Warning**	Watch for allergic reations or shock.
Who should not take this medicine?	Do not take this drug if you are allergic to penicillin.	**Other medicines that may work**	*for breast or skin infections:* amoxicillin, cephalexin, erythromycin

diphenhydramine hydrochloride (Bectivo, Benadryl)

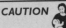 **CAUTION**

Diphenhydramine is an antihistamine that dries up mucus in the nose and also makes you sleepy. It is useful for treating chronic itching and sleep problems for people with AIDS. It is also a treatment for allergic reactions and allergic shock.

In what forms does this medicine come?	Tablets or capsules: 25 or 50 mg Syrup: 12.5 mg per 5 ml Ampules for injection: 10, 30 or 50 mg in 1 ml

Warning
Do not use if you need to be alert. Makes the effects of tranquilizers and alcohol dangerously stronger.

How much and when to take
For allergies, mild to moderate allergic reaction, or itching: Take 25 mg by mouth 3 or 4 times a day as needed. *For sleep:* Take 25 to 50 mg at bedtime. *For allergic shock:* Inject 50 mg into muscle, repeat in 8 hours or sooner if needed (see page 541).

Information you should know
Only inject diphenhydramine for severe allergic reactions or shock.

Who should not take this medicine?
Pregnant and breastfeeding women should not use this drug as a long-term treatment for allergies. People with asthma should not take it.

Other medicines that may work
for allergies: hydroxyzine, promethazine

for sleep: diazepam

Side effects
Sleepiness, dry mouth. Sometimes causes nausea and vomiting. In rare cases can have the opposite effect and excite rather than calm you.

doxycycline (Biocolyn, Doryx, Monodox, Vibramycin, Vibra-Tabs)

Doxycycline is an antibiotic of the tetracycline family used to treat many different infections including STDs, pelvic infections, infections after abortions, and others. It is used instead of tetracycline.

In what forms does this medicine come? Tablets: 50 and 100 mg

Side effects
Diarrhea or upset stomach. Some people get a rash after staying a long time in the sun.

How much and when to take
For vaginal discharge from an STD: Take 100 mg by mouth 2 times a day for 7 days (also take other drugs, see page 266). *For syphilis:* 100 mg by mouth 2 times a day for 15 days.
For late syphilis: 100 mg by mouth 2 times a day for 28 days.
For PID or infection after female circumcision: Take 100 mg by mouth 2 times a day for 10 days (also take other drugs for PID, see page 278).
For risk of STDs before an abortion or to prevent infection after an abortion: Take 100 mg 2 times a day for 5 days.
For infections after an abortion: Take 100 mg by mouth 2 times a day for 10 days (also take other drugs, see pages 255 to 257).

Warning
Do not take if pregnant or breastfeeding. Do not use doxycycline that is old or has passed the expiration date. Do not take with dairy products or antacids.

Information you should know
Do not take just before laying down. Sit up while taking pills and drink lots of water to prevent the irritation that swallowing this medicine can cause.

Who should not take this medicine?
Pregnant and breastfeeding women and children under 8. Doxycycline can damage a baby's or child's teeth and bones.

Other medicines that may work
for syphilis: benzathine penicillin
for gonorrhea: co-trimoxazole
for chlamydia: erythromycin
to prevent infection after abortion: amoxicillin
for infection after abortion: see pages 255 to 257
for infection after circumcision: erythromycin

epinephrine *or* adrenaline *(Adrenalin)*

Epinephrine and adrenaline are two names for the same drug. It is used for allergic reactions or allergic shock, for example, allergic shock caused by penicillin. It is also used for severe asthma attacks.

In what forms does this medicine come?	Ampules for injection: 1 mg in 1 ml	**Warning**	Be careful never to give more than the recommended amount. Avoid injecting this into the buttocks, instead use the back of the upper arm.
How much and when to take	*For asthma, moderate allergic reaction or allergic shock:* Inject ½ mg (½ ml) just under the skin (not into muscle) of the upper arm. If needed, a second dose can be given after 20-30 minutes, and a third dose after another 20-30 minutes *(also give other drugs, see page 541).*	**Information you should know**	Take the person's pulse before injecting. Do not give more than 3 doses. If the pulse goes up by more than 30 beats per minute after the first injection, do not give another dose.
Side effects	Fear, restlessness, nervousness, tension, headaches, dizzyness, increased heart rate.	**Signs of taking too much**	High blood pressure, fast heart beat, stroke.

ergometrine maleate, methylergonovine maleate
(Anurhage, Ergonovine, Ergotrate, Methergine)

Ergometrine causes contractions of the womb and its blood vessels and is used to control heavy bleeding after childbirth or an abortion. Ergometrine and methylergonovine are the same drug. After giving this medicine, get help.

In what forms does this medicine come?	Tablets: .2 mg For injection: .2, .25 and .5 mg in 1 ml vial.	**Warning**	Do not use these drugs to start labor or make labor stronger. Never give this medicine before the baby and the placenta have come out.
How much and when to take	*For heavy bleeding after childbirth:* After the placenta has come out, inject .5 mg into muscle, *or* give 1 tablet (.2 mg) by mouth 4 to 6 times a day. *For heavy bleeding due to complications after an abortion:* Give an injection of .2 mg into muscle, then give a .2 mg pill or a .1 mg injection every 4 hours for 24 hours.	**Information you should know**	Do not use this drug to cause an abortion because it could kill the woman before making her abort. *(For abortion, see Chapter 15).*
Side effects	Nausea, vomiting, dizziness, sweating.	**Other medicines that may work**	oxytocin

erythromycin *(E.E.S., E-Mycin, Ery-max, Ethril, Ilosone, Ilotycin)*

Erythromycin is an antibiotic of the macrolide family used to treat many infections, including some STDs, respiratory and skin infections. It can be safely used during pregancy and is widely available.

In what forms does this medicine come?
Tablets or capsules: 250 mg
Ointment: 1%
Powder for solution: 125 mg per 5 ml

Who should not take this medicine?
Do not use if you are alergic to antibiotics of the macrolide family.

Side effects
May upset stomach or cause nausea, vomiting, diarrhea.

How much and when to take

For bladder infections or chlamydia: 500 mg by mouth 4 times a day for 7 days *(see page 277 for drug combinations to treat vaginal discharge from STDs).*

For breast infection, PID or infection from female circumcision: 500 mg by mouth 4 times a day for 10 days *(see page 278 for drug combinations to treat PID).*

For chancroid or skin infections: 500 mg by mouth 3 times a day for 7 days *(also use other drugs, see page 269).*

If you are treating genital sores but are allergic to penicillin: 500 mg by mouth 3 times a day.

For early syphilis: 500 mg by mouth 4 times a day for 15 days.

For genital sores caused by chlamydia: 500 mg by mouth 4 times a day for 21 days.

For newborn eye care: Use 1% ointment one time only.

Information you should know
Erythromycin works best when taken 1 hour before or 2 hours after a meal. If this upsets your stomach too much, take with a little food. Do not break up tablets. Many tablets are coated to prevent strong stomach juices from breaking down the drug before it can begin to work.

Other medicines that may work
for breast infection: amoxicillin, cephalexin, dicloxacillin
for bladder infection: ampicillin, co-trimoxazole
for infection after circumcision: doxycycline
for STDs: see pages 277 and 278 for drug combinations to treat STDs
for baby eye-care: tetracycline ointment

estrogen *(ethinyl estradiol, mestranol)*

Chemical forms of estrogen are used in birth control pills and injections. They are similar to the hormone estrogen made in a woman's body. Estrogen can also be used to treat abnormal bleeding or problems of menopause *(see Chapter 8)*. For more information, see the section on birth control pills, injections, and emergency family planning *(see Chapter 13 and pages 517 to 520).*

ethambutol *(Interbutol, Myambutol, Mycrol, Odetol, Triambutol)*

Ethambutol is used to treat tuberculosis (TB) especially where other TB medicines are no longer strong enough. It is used in combination with other drugs. *See Chapter 25.*

In what forms does this medicine come?
Tablets: 100 or 400 mg

Side effects
Ethambutol often causes vision changes in one or both eyes. It might make the area of what you can see smaller, or cause patchy dark spots or "holes" in your vision. This usually goes away when you stop taking the drug.

How much and when to take
The doses for tuberculosis medicines differ from region to region. See a health worker. *(Take ethambutol in combination with other drugs, see page 389).*

Information you should know
It is very important that you take the entire course of treatment for tuberculosis, even if it lasts for a year. If not, you might infect other people.

Who should not take this medicine?
People with serious vision problems, including cataracts, should not take this drug. Neither should people with severe kidney problems.

gentamicin *(Bactiderm, Garamycin, Servigenta)*

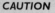 **CAUTION**

Gentamicin is a very strong antibiotic of the aminoglycoside family that is used to treat gonorrhea, kidney and other serious infections, and for pelvic inflammatory disease in combination with other drugs. You should use this drug only when the woman is vomiting and cannot keep other medicines down or no other antibiotic is available.

In what forms does this medicine come?	In vials for injection: 10 or 40 mg per ml	**Warning**	Use a different medicine if hearing problems or ringing in the ears start. Give with plenty of fluids.

How much and when to take
For severe infection after an abortion: Give this medicine according to a woman's weight: inject into muscle 5 mg for every kg of weight, split into 3 doses (morning, afternoon and night) for 5 to 7 days; *or you can use the following average dose:* Inject 80 mg into muscle, then give 60 mg injections 3 times a day for 5 to 7 days *(also use other drugs, see page 257).*

Information you should know Because of the serious side effects and the difficulty of calculating the dosage, this drug should only be used when safer antibiotics are not available.

Signs of taking too much Ringing in the ears or worsening of hearing. Kidney problems.

Who should not take this medicine? Pregnant women or people with kidney problems should use this drug very carefully. Do not use this drug if you are allergic to other antibiotics of the aminoglycoside family.

Side effects This drug can damage the kidneys or cause deafness.

Other medicines that may work
for severe infection: cefixime, ceftriaxone, kanamycin
for kidney infection: amoxicillin, ampicillin, norfloxacin

Gentian Violet *(Crystal Violet, methylrosanilinium chloride)*

Gentian Violet is a disinfectant used to help fight infections of the skin, mouth, and vagina.

In what forms does this medicine come?
Liquid: 0.5%, 1%, 2%
Tincture: 0.5%
Crystals: 1 teaspoon in ½ liter of water makes a 2% liquid.

 Warning Do not have sex while you are using Gentian Violet for a vaginal infection to avoid passing the infection to your partner. Stop using Gentian Violet if it starts to irritate you.

How much and when to take
For vaginal yeast infections: soak clean cotton with 1% liquid and place high in the vagina overnight for 3 nights. Be sure to remove the cotton every morning.
For yeast infections in the mouth (thrush): Rinse the mouth with 1% liquid for 1 minute 2 times a day, but do not swallow.
For skin infections: First wash with soap and water, and dry. Then paint on skin, mouth, or vulva 3 times a day for 5 days.

Information you should know After putting this in an infant's mouth, turn the baby face down so it does not swallow too much. Gentian Violet will stain your skin and clothes purple.

Side effects Long term use causes irritation. Use on a sore or on broken skin may stain that skin purple when it heals.

Other medicines that may work
for skin infections: antibiotic ointments, iodine
for thrush in the mouth: lemon *(not for babies),* nystatin
for vaginal yeast infections: nystatin, miconozole, clotrimazole

hepatitis B vaccine *(Engerix-B, Recombivax HB)*

This vaccine provides immunity to Hepatitis B.

In what forms does this medicine come?	Liquid for injection: 2.5, 5, 10, or 25 mg per ml	**Side effects** Sometimes fever, headache, weakness, tiredness.

How much and when to take

 Always give this vaccine by injection in the upper arm or thigh in 3 doses. Try to give the 2nd dose 1-2 months after the 1st, and the 3rd dose 4-12 months after the 2nd.

Doses for these 2 brands of the vaccine are different:

	Engerix-B	Recombivax HB
Adults:	20 mg	10 mg
Children		
0 to 11 years	10 mg	2.5 mg
11 to 19 years	20 mg	5 mg

Information you should know

This vaccine needs to be stored at 2-8 degrees Centigrade or it loses its strength.
This vaccine should be injected in the upper arm or thigh.

Other medicines that may work

Hepatitis B immune globulin

---

hydrocortisone or cortisol
(Eczacort, Hycotil, Solu-Cortef, others)

CAUTION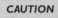

Hydrocortisone is an anti-swelling and anti-itch skin cream used to treat rashes. It is also useful for treating hemorrhoids (piles). In its injection form and as tablets it is an important drug for treating allergic shock.

In what forms does this medicine come?

Cream or ointment: 1%
Tablets: 5, 10, and 20 mg
Liquid for injection and
Powder for mixing for
injection: various strengths

Warning

Do not use cream with a bandage covering. Pregnant and breastfeeding women should use tablets with caution, but can safely use cream.

How much and when to take

For rash, itching or piles: Apply cream directly on skin 3 or 4 times a day.

For allergic shock: Inject 500 mg into muscle, repeat in 4 hours if needed *(also give other drugs, see page 541)*. If signs return later, take 500 to 1000 mg by mouth and repeat once if needed.

Signs of taking too much

High blood pressure, passing more urine than usual.

Side effects

Cream may cause thinning and scarring of skin if used for more than 10 days.

Other medicines that may work

for allergic shock: dexamethasone

for allergies or itching: diphenhydramine

hydroxyzine *(Atarax, Iterax, Marax, My-Pam, Vistaril)*

CAUTION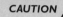

Hydroxyzine is an antihistamine used for allergic reactions, to control itching, and sometimes to treat nausea, vomiting, and anxiety.

In what forms does this medicine come?	Tablets: 25, 50 or 100 mg For injection: 25 or 50 mg	

How much and when to take

For itching: Take 25 to 50 mg by mouth 3 or 4 times a day.

To relieve anxiety: Take 25 to 50 mg by mouth 4 times a day.

For moderate allergic reactions or allergic shock: Inject into muscle: 25 mg for children, 50 mg for adults (*also use other medicines, see page 541*).

Who should not take this medicine?

Do not use during first 3 months of pregnancy. In the rest of pregnancy or if breastfeeding, use only if there is no other choice. Do not use this drug if you must stay alert.

Side effects

Causes dry mouth, sleepiness, and may cause loss of appetite.

Signs of taking too much

Sleepiness

Other medicines that may work

for itching, allergy or allergic shock: diphenhydramine, promethazine

for anxiety: diazepam

---

ibuprofen *(Actiprofen, Advil, Genpril, Motrin, Nuprin, Rufen, others)*

CAUTION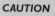

Ibuprofen works against pain, swelling, and fever. It is very useful to relieve discomfort during monthly bleeding and pain from arthritis and AIDS.

In what forms does this medicine come?

Tablets: 200 mg and larger.
Liquid: 100 mg per 5 ml

How much and when to take

Take 200 to 400 mg 4 to 6 times a day. Do not take more than 2400 mg daily.

Who should not take this medicine?

People with stomach ulcers. Pregnant women during the last 3 months.

Side effects

May cause stomach irritation or pain.

Warning

Avoid taking within a week of surgery.

Information you should know

Works best if taken with food, especially dairy products, at mealtimes.

Other medicines that may work

for pain, swelling and fever: aspirin

for pain and fever: acetaminophen

for severe pain: codeine, morphine

isoniazid *(Bisonid, INH, Isoniazdum, isonicotinic acid hydrazide, Odinah, Zidrid)*

Isoniazid is used to treat tuberculosis (TB) in combination with other medicines. *See Chapter 25.*

In what forms does this medicine come?	Tablet: 100 or 300 mg Syrup: 50 mg per 5ml	**Side effects**	May cause pain or numbness in arms and legs. Sometimes isoniazid may cause severe hepatitis with signs like tiredness, loss of appetite, nausea, vomiting, dark urine or yellowing of eyes. If this happens, stop taking this medicine immediately.
How much and when to take	The doses for tuberculosis medicines differ from region to region. See a health worker. *(Take isoniazid in combination with other drugs, see page 389).*	**Information you should know**	Never take more than 300 mg a day. It is important to take the full course of treatment for tuberculosis so you do not infect other people.
Who should not take this medicine?	Anyone who has hepatitis, liver disease, or has taken isoniazid before and had liver problems, should not take this drug.	**Signs of taking too much**	Nausea, vomiting, dizziness, slurred speech, blurred vision. If you take too much, take 1 g of pyridoxine (vitamin B6).

kanamycin *(Kantrex)*

Kanamycin is a very strong antibiotic of the aminoglycoside family that is used to treat gonorrhea and other serious infections. Kanamycin should only be used when other, safer antibiotics are not available.

In what forms does this medicine come?	In vials for injection: 75, 500, or 1000 mg Powder for mixing for injections: 1 g in 2 ml Tablets: 500 mg	**Warning**	Use a different medicine if hearing problems or ringing in the ears start. Give with plenty of fluids.
How much and when to take	*For severe infection:* Give this medicine according to a woman's weight: inject into muscle 15 mg for every kg of weight, divided into 2 doses (morning and night), for 5 to 7 days; *or you can use the following dose:* Inject 500 mg into muscle 2 times a day for 5 to 7 days. *For gonorrhea:* Inject 2 g into muscle 1 time only.	**Information you should know**	Because of the serious side effects and the difficulty of calculating the dosage, this drug should only be used when safer antibiotics are not available.
Who should not take this medicine?	Pregnant women or people with kidney problems should not use this drug. Do not use this drug if you are allergic to other antibiotics of the aminoglycoside family.	**Signs of taking too much**	Ringing in the ears or worsening of hearing. Kidney problems.
Side effects	This drug can damage the kidneys or cause deafness.	**Other medicines that may work**	*for serious infection or for gonorrhea:* cefixime, ceftriaxone, norfloxacin

ketoconazole *(Nizoral)*

Ketoconazole is a strong anti-fungus medicine that is used to treat thrush and other yeast infections. Use only if you have AIDS and other remedies do not work. It is expensive and sometimes hard to find.

In what forms does this medicine come?
Tablets: 200 mg
Also comes as skin cream and shampoo: 2%

Warning
Use with caution if you are pregnant or breastfeeding. Do not put cream or shampoo in vagina. Take with food. If taken by mouth, it may give you hot flashes if you also drink alcohol.

How much and when to take
For fungal infection: Take 200 mg by mouth once a day for 10 days.

For yeast infection inside the mouth (thrush): Take 200 mg by mouth 2 times a day for 14 days.

Information you should know
This medicine works best if taken with orange juice or another citrus fruit.

Side effects
May cause nausea, vomiting.

Other medicines that may work
for yeast infections without STDs: nystatin, clotrimazole.

magnesium sulfate

Magnesium sulfate is the best medicine to prevent convulsions in pregnant women with toxemia.

In what forms does this medicine come?
Injections of 10%, 12.5%, 25%, or 50% solution.

Information you should know
Injecting a large amount needs a big needle and may be uncomfortable. You might want to split the dose in half and give 2 smaller shots, one in each hip.

How much and when to take
For convulsions: Inject 10 g into muscle.

Who should not take this medicine?
Women with kidney problems should not be given this drug.

Signs of taking too much
Sweating, low blood pressure, weakness, problems breathing.

Warning
Only use this drug if a woman's blood pressure is over 160/110. After giving, continue to check her blood pressure. Too much of this medicine can slow down or stop her breathing!

Other medicines that may work
For convulsions: diazepam

medroxyprogesterone acetate
(Amen, Curretab, Cycrin, Depo-Provera, Megestron, Provera)

Medroxyprogesterone acetate is a chemical form of progesterone, a hormone produced naturally in a woman's body. It can be used to treat irregular bleeding caused by changing hormones, especially around the time of menopause. For more information, see Chapter 8 "Older Women." For family planning, see Chapter 13.

In what forms does this medicine come?
Tablets: 2.5, 5, or 10 mg

Who should not take this medicine?
Women with hepatitis, or cancer of the breast or cervix should not take this medicine.

How much and when to take
For heavy bleeding: Take 10 mg once a day for 10 days. If bleeding continues, take for 10 more days.

Warning
If bleeding continues after 20 days of treatment, see a health worker. It could be a serious problem.

methyl ergonovine *(Methergine)*

Methyl ergonovine causes contractions of the womb and its blood vessels and is used to control heavy bleeding after childbirth. It is the same drug as ergometrine and ergonovine. *See ergometrine, page 500.*

---

metronidazole *(Flagyl, Methoprotostat, Metro, Metroxyn, Satric)*   CAUTION

Metronidazole is used for vaginal infections caused by yeast and trichomonas. It is also effective against some bacteria and amoebic dysentery *(also see **Where There is No Doctor**).*

In what forms does this medicine come?	Tablets: 200, 250, 400, or 500 mg Inserts: 500 mg For injection into vein: 500 mg in 100 ml	**Who should not take this medicine?**	People with liver problems like jaundice (yellow eyes).

How much and when to take	*For PID or infection after childbirth:* Take 500 mg by mouth 2 times a day for 10 days *(take in combination with other drugs; for PID, see pages 273 and 278; for infection after childbirth, see page 97).* *For mild vaginal infections:* Put one 500 mg insert in the vagina 2 times a day for 10 days. *For trichomonas, yeast, or bacterial vaginosis:* Take 2 grams by mouth 1 time only, but not if you are pregnant. *If you are pregnant:* Take 400 mg by mouth 2 times a day for 7 days *(to treat abnormal discharge with or without an STD, see drug combinations on pages 266 and 277).* *For serious infection after abortion:* Give 500 mg by mouth 4 times a day *or* inject 1 g into a vein 2 times a day *(see treatment combinations recommended on pages 256 and 257).* *For bloody diarrhea with or without fever:* 500 mg 3 times a day for 7 days.

Side effects	Metallic taste in mouth, dark urine, upset stomach or nausea, headache.
Warning	Stop taking it if you feel numb. If you are in the first 3 months of pregnancy, try not to use this medicine. If you must, do not take the one large dose during pregnancy. But if you are breastfeeding, the 1 large dose is the safest way to take it.
Information you should know	Your sexual partner should also be treated. Do not drink alcohol, not even 1 beer, while you are taking metronidazole. It will make you feel very nauseous.
Other medicines that may work	*for yeast and trichomonas:* tinidazole *for diarrhea for people with AIDS:* co-trimoxazole, norfloxacin

---

miconazole *(Daktarin, Fungtopic, Micatin, Monistat)*   CAUTION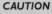

Miconazole is an anti-fungus medicine used to treat vaginal yeast and other fungus infections.

In what forms does this medicine come?	Cream: 2% Inserts: 100 mg and 200 mg	**Side effects**	Irritation

How much and when to take	*For yeast infections:* Cream: put 5 g in the vagina every night for 7 days. 100 mg inserts: put 1 in the vagina every night for 7 days. 200 mg inserts: put 1 in the vagina every night for 3 days.

Warning	If miconazole irritates you, stop using it. Avoid having sex for 3-4 days so you do not pass it to your partner. Keep it out of your eyes.
Who should not take this medicine?	Women in the first 3 months of pregnancy.
Other medicines that may work	*for yeast infections:* nystatin, clotrimazole, Gentian Violet or ketaconazole

mifepristone *(RU 486)*

Mifepristone, used together with misoprostol or other drugs, can be used for abortion. This drug is available now only through special programs in some countries, and is given in clinics and hospitals where the woman can be watched and treated for complications.

In what forms does this medicine come?	Tablets: 200 mg	

How much and when to take

For medical abortion: 600 mg is given 1 time before the woman is 2 months pregnant. After 48 hours, another medicine such as misoprostol (400 mcg) is placed high in the vagina.

Who should not take this medicine?

Women who are more than 9 weeks from their last monthly bleeding.

Information you should know

After cramping and heavy bleeding, the abortion is usually completed within 48 hours after the second medicine is given.

If this medicine fails, an abortion by manual vacuum aspiration (MVA) or dilation and cuterage (D and C) may be necessary. *(See Chapter 15, "Abortion.")*

Other medicines that may work

misoprostol

---

misoprostol *(Cytotec)*

Misoprostol is used for stomach ulcers. It can be used for abortion because it makes the womb contract, bleed, and expel the pregnancy.

In what forms does this medicine come?

Tablets: 100 or 200 mcg

How much and when to take

For medical abortion: Place 400 mcg high in the vagina. If bleeding has not started in 12 hours, repeat. If bleeding still has not started, wait 2 weeks and try again.

Who should not take this medicine?

Women after the third month of pregnancy must not use this medicine. It could cause the womb to split open.

Side effects

May cause nausea, vomiting, diarrhea and headache. If breastfeeding, will cause diarrhea in infants.

Warning

Do not use more than 400 mcg at once or take it more often than every 12 hours because it can make the womb split open.

Information you should know

An abortion caused by misoprostol may take several hours to several days to finish. Most of the time, complete abortion does not occur. See a health worker after bleeding has begun to have the womb emptied completely.

Signs of taking too much

Severe pain in the belly and very heavy bleeding. Get medical help immediately.

nitrofurantoin *(Furadantin, Macrobid, Macrodantin)*

 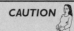

Nitrofurantoin is an antibiotic used to treat kidney and bladder infections.

In what forms does this medicine come?	Tablets: 25, 50 or 100 mg	Side effects	Nausea or vomiting, headaches, passing gas.
How much and when to take	For bladder infections: 50 mg 4 times a day for 7 days. For kidney infections: 100 mg 4 times a day for 7 days.	Signs of taking too much	Vomiting, chest pains.
Who should not take this medicine?	People with kidneys that did not work well before they got an infection. Women in their last month of pregnancy.	Other medicines that may work	for bladder or kidney infections: ampicillin, amoxicillin, co-trimoxazole, erythromycin, norfloxacin

norfloxacin *(Lexinor, Noroxin, Uritracin)*

Norfloxacin is an antibiotic of the quinolone family used to treat gonorrhea, bladder and kidney infections, and serious cases of diarrhea.

In what forms does this medicine come?	Tablets: 400 mg	Side effects	May cause lightheadedness and increase the effect of caffeine.
How much and when to take	For bladder infections: Take 1 tablet 2 times a day for 3 days, either 1 hour before eating or 2 hours after eating. For kidney infections: Take 1 tablet 2 times a day either 1 hour before eating or 2 hours after eating for 10 days. For PID, gonorrhea, or vaginal discharge with STDs: Take 800 mg one time only (see pages 277 and 278 for combinations of medicines needed to treat STDs). For diarrhea for people with AIDS: Take 400 mg 2 times a day for 5 days.	Warning	Take with lots of water. Do not take this drug while using antacids or vitamins that contain iron or zinc. If norfloxacin gives you an allergic reaction, stop using it.
Who should not take this medicine?	Women who are pregnant, breastfeeding, or under 16 years old should not take norfloxacin. People with allergies to quinolone antibiotics should not take norfloxacin.	Other medicines that work	for bladder or kidney infections: ampicillin, amoxicillin, nitrofurantoin, co-trimoxazole, erythromycin for gonorrhea: ciprofloxacin, ceftriaxone, cefixime, kanamycin for diarrhea for people with AIDS: metronidazole, co-trimoxazole

nystatin *(Dermodex, Mycostatin, Nilstat, Nystat)*

Nystatin is an anti-fungus medicine used to treat yeast infections in the mouth (thrush), the vagina, or the skin.

In what forms does this medicine come?
Inserts: 100,000 U
Lozenges for the mouth: 100,000 U
Cream: 100,000 U per gram
Liquid: 100,000 U per ml

How much and when to take
For mouth or throat infections: Three or four times a day, put 1 ml of liquid in mouth, swish around both sides of mouth for 1 minute and swallow. **Do this for 5 days.**

For skin infections: Keep area dry and apply ointment 3 times a day.

For vaginal infections: Put cream inside the vagina twice daily for 10-14 days; or put 100,000 U insert inside the vagina at bedtime for 10-14 days.

For vaginal discharge not caused by STDs: Put 100,000 U insert in the vagina at bedtime for 7 nights.

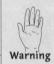
Warning
If nystatin causes you irritation, stop using it. Avoid having sex for 3-4 days so you do not pass the infection to your partner.

Information you should know
Nystatin works only against candida yeast infections, while miconazole works against other fungal infections as well. Clotrimazole may be less costly and easier to use.

Other medicines that may work
for yeast infections: miconazole, ketoconazole, clotrimazole, vinegar or Gentian Violet

oxytocin *(Oxtimon, Pitocin, Syntocinon, Uteracon)*

Oxytocin is used to cause contractions of the womb and its blood vessels to control heavy bleeding after childbirth or if the placenta takes more than 1 hour to come out.

In what forms does this medicine come?
For injection:
10 Units in 1 ml

How much and when to take
Inject 10 Units into muscle after the baby is born. Repeat every 10 minutes if needed.

Side effects
Oxytocin can cause the womb to contract so strongly that it will not relax after and may even tear the womb. Also, oxytocin can cause high blood pressure.

Warning
Do not use this drug to cause an abortion, because it could kill the woman before making her abort. *(See Chapter 15, "Abortion.")*

Using oxytocin to speed up labor or give strength to the mother in labor can be dangerous to both mother and child. Do not give it before the baby is out.

Other medicines that may work
for heavy bleeding after childbirth: ergometrine

paracetamol, acetaminophen *(APAP, Panadol, Tempra, Tylenol, others)*

Paracetamol and acetaminophen are 2 names for the same drug that is used to ease pain and lower fever. It is one of the safest pain killers. It does not cause stomach irritation and so it can be used instead of aspirin or ibuprofen by people with stomach ulcers. It can also be used by pregnant women, and is safe at lower doses for children.

In what forms does this medicine come?	Tablets: 100, 325 and 500 mg Liquid: 120 or 160 mg per 5 ml Inserts: 300 mg Drops: 80 mg per 0.8 ml	**Information you should know**	Acetominophen does not cure the sickness, it only eases the pain or the fever. It is important to find the cause of the pain or fever and cure that.
How much and when to take	500 to 1000 mg by mouth 4 to 6 times a day.		
Who should not take this medicine?	Do not take acetaminophen if you have liver or kidney damage.	**Signs of taking too much**	Nausea Vomiting Pain in the stomach
 Warning	If your fever or pain lasts for more than 3 days, get medical help. Acetaminophen can cause liver damage if you take too much or if taken with or after drinking alcohol.	**Other medicines that may work**	*for pain, fever, or swelling:* aspirin, ibuprofen (do not take either if you are pregnant) *for severe pain:* codeine

penicillin *(Betapen VK, PenVee K, phenoxymethyl penicillin)*

Penicillin is an antibiotic used to treat mouth, tooth, skin, womb and many other infections.

In what forms does this medicine come?	Tablets: 250, 500 mg Liquid: 125 or 250 mg per 5 ml	**Side effects**	Rash
How much and when to take	*For womb infection after childbirth:* 250 mg (which is the same as 400,000 U) by mouth 4 times a day for 7 days *(also take other medicines for womb infection, see page 97).* *For skin infection:* 250 mg by mouth 4 times a day for 10 days.	 **Warning**	Watch for allergic reactions and allergic shock (see *page 541*).
Who should not take this medicine?	Do not take if you are allergic to any antibiotics of the penicillin family.	**Other medicines that may work**	*for skin infection:* ampicillin, amoxicillin, erythromycin *for infection after childbirth:* procaine penicillin, amoxicillin, metronidazole

podophyllin *(Condylox, Podocon-25)*

Podophyllin is a liquid that can be put directly on genital warts to shrink them.

In what forms does this medicine come?	Liquid: 10% to 25%	**Warning**	Do not put on bleeding warts. If severe skin irritation occurs, do not use it again.
How much and when to take	Apply liquid to warts with a cotton swab or clean cloth rolled to a fine point. Wash it off carefully with soap and water after 4 hours. Use once a week for 4 weeks.	**Information you should know** 	Podophyllin is very irritating to healthy skin. Protect the area around the wart with petroleum gel before using podophyllin.
Who should not take this medicine?	Do not use this if you are pregnant or breastfeeding.	**Signs of taking too much**	Nausea, vomiting, belly pain, diarrhea. Too much might cause the skin to thin, break, and bleed.
Side effects	Podophyllin can be very irritating to skin.	**Other medicines that may work**	*for genital warts:* trichloracetic acid, bichloracetic acid

probenecid *(Benemid, Probalan)*

CAUTION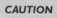

Used with some antibiotics of the penicillin family, probenecid increases the amount of penicillin in the blood and makes it last longer, increasing the effectiveness of treatment.

In what forms does this medicine come?	Tablets: 500 mg	**Side effects**	It sometimes causes headache, nausea, or vomiting.
How much and when to take	Take 500 mg to 1 gram by mouth each time you use an antibiotic from the penicillin family.	**Warning**	Use with caution during pregnancy and breastfeeding, and if you have a stomach ulcer.
Who should not take this medicine?	Do not give probenecid to children under 2 years old.	**Signs of taking too much**	Vomiting

procaine penicillin *(Benzylpenicillin Procaine, Bicillin C-R, Crysticillin, Duracillin AS, Penadur, Pfizepen AS, Wycillin)*

Procaine penicillin is an antibiotic used to treat womb and other infections.

In what forms does this medicine come?	For injection: vials of 300,000, 400,00 or 600,000 Units Powder for mixing for injection: I gram = I million Units	**Warning**	Use with caution if you have asthma. Do not use with tetracycline. Never inject this into the vein.
How much and when to take	**For womb infection after childbirth:** Inject 800,000 Units into muscle 2 times a day for 7 days *(also take other medicines, see page 97).* **For fever during pregnancy:** Inject 1.2 million Units every 12 hours while you take the woman for medical treatment.	**Information you should know**	When taken with probenecid, the amount of penicillin in the blood increases and lasts longer, making the treatment more effective.
Who should not take this medicine?	Do not use this drug if you are allergic to antibiotics of the penicillin family.	**Other medicines that may work**	*for fever during pregnancy:* ampicillin *for womb infection after childbirth:* amoxicillin, metronidazole, penicillin

progesterone, progestin

Progestin is a chemical found in birth control pills and injections that is similar to the hormone progesterone produced in women's bodies. It is also used to treat irregular bleeding caused by changing levels of hormones. For information about birth control pills, injections, and emergency pills, **see Chapter 13** and **pages 517 to 520.**

promethazine *(Mepergan, Phenergan, Thaprozine)*   CAUTION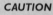

Promethazine is an antihistamine that dries up mucus and makes you drowsy. It is used for allergic reactions, to sleep at night, and to help stop uncontrollable vomiting.

In what forms does this medicine come?	Tablets: 10, 12.5 or 25 mg Syrup: 5 mg per 5 ml Injection: ampules of 25 mg in 1 ml Rectal inserts: 12.5, 25, or 50 mg	**Who should not take this medicine?**	Pregnant and breastfeeding women should not use this drug for long-term treatment. Do not take this if you need to stay alert.
How much and when to take	**For moderate allergic reaction:** Give 25 mg by mouth or injection into muscle. Repeat in 8 hours or sooner if needed. **For allergic shock:** Inject 50 mg into muscle. Repeat in 8 hours or sooner if needed. *(See page 541 for information on treating allergic reactions and shock.)* **For vomiting:** Inject 25 to 50 mg every 6 hours as needed. **For sleep:** Take 25 to 50 mg at bedtime.	**Side effects**	Often causes dry mouth and blurry vision. In rare cases, may cause twitching movements of body, face or eyes.
		Warning	Pregnant and breastfeeding women should take with caution. Do not drive or use heavy machines if you are taking this medicine.
		Signs of taking too much	Unconsciousness, seizures.
		Other medicines that may work	*for allergy or allergic reaction:* diphenhydramine, hydroxyzine

pyrazinamide *(Isopas, Pyzamed, PZA, Zinamide, Zinastat)*

Pyrazinamide is used to treat tuberculosis (TB) *(see Chapter 25).*

In what forms does this medicine come?	Tablets: 500 mg

How much and when to take	The doses for tuberculosis medicines differ from region to region. See a health worker. *(Take pyrazinamide in combination with other drugs, see page 389).*

Who should not take this medicine?	People with liver damage or hepatitis should not take this medicine.

Side effects	Yellow skin or eyes, fever, loss of appetite, tiredness, liver tenderness, gout or arthritis. If you have any of these problems, get medical help.

Warning 	Pregnant and breastfeeding women should avoid this drug since its effects on the baby are not known. It is very important that you take the entire course of treatment for tuberculosis. If not, you might infect other people.

rifampicin *(Resimin, rifampin, Rifastat)*

CAUTION

Rifampicin is an antibiotic used to treat tuberculosis (TB) *(see Chapter 25)* and other kinds of infections, including leprosy (Hansen's Disease).

In what forms does this medicine come?	Tablets: 150 or 300 mg Liquid: 50 mg per 5 ml Ampules for injection: 600 mg

How much and when to take	Doses for tuberculosis medicines differ from region to region. See a health worker. *(Take rifampicin in combination with other drugs, see page 389).*

Who should not take this medicine?	People with liver damage or liver disease should not take this medicine.

Side effects	• Nausea, vomiting, loss of appetite, diarrhea, cramps • Hot face, itching, rash • Headaches, fever, chills, bone pain • Yellow skin or eyes

Except for yellow skin or eyes, these side effects usually happen 2 to 3 hours after taking this medicine and can sometimes be avoided by taking the medicine with food.

Information you should know	May turn your urine, stool, tears, sweat, or spit a red-orange color. It is very important that you take the entire course of treatment for tuberculosis so you do not infect others.

streptomycin

Streptomycin is an antibiotic of the aminoglycoside family used to treat tuberculosis (TB). It is given only by injection into muscle. It is used for TB in combination with other medicines. *See Chapter 25.*

In what forms does this medicine come?	Liquid for injection: 400 mg per ml

How much and when to take	The doses for tuberculosis medicines differ from region to region. See a health worker. *(Take streptomycin in combination with other drugs, see page 389).*

Who should not take this medicine?	Pregnant women should not use streptomycin because it can cause deafness in the baby. People with allergies to antibiotics of the aminoglycoside family like gentamicin should not take this drug. People with kidney problems should use with caution.

Side effects	May damage hearing or balance, and can cause a rash.

Information you should know	Wear gloves if you touch this medicine often because it can cause a serious rash. It is very important that you take the entire course of treatment for tuberculosis. If not, you might infect other people.

sulfisoxazole *(Gantrisin)*

Sulfisoxazole is an antibiotic of the sulfonamide family used to treat bladder infections.

In what forms does this medicine come?
Tablets: 500 mg
Liquid: 500 mg per 5 ml

How much and when to take
For bladder infections: Take 1,000 mg by mouth 4 times a day for 10 days.

Side effects
Nausea, vomiting, diarrhea, rashes, headaches.

Who should not take this medicine?
Pregnant women should not take this drug in the last 3 months. Do not give sulfisoxazole to anyone who has allergies to sulfa antibiotics or kidney problems.

Information you should know
Drink at least 2 liters of water every day when you are taking sulfisoxazole.

Other medicines that may work
for bladder infection: amoxicillin, ampicillin, co-trimoxazole

tetanus toxoid *(Tetavax)*

Tetanus toxoid is an immunization given to prevent a tetanus infection. It can be given during or after pregnancy, or after an abortion. If a woman gets 2 injections (or better still, 3 injections) when pregnant, it will also prevent this deadly infection in her newborn baby.

In what forms does this medicine come?
Liquid for injection: 4, 5, or 10 U per .5 ml

How much and when to take
To be safe from tetanus for your entire life, you must get 5 immunization injections, and then one injection every 10 years.
For each immunization: Give 1 injection of .5 ml into the muscle of the upper arm.

Side effects
Pain, redness, warmth, slight swelling.

Information you should know
Tetanus immunizations should be given to everyone, starting in childhood. Tetanus immunization is often given to children as part of a combined immunization called DPT, and the three DPT immunizations are equal to the first 2 tetanus toxoid immunizations.

The schedule below gives the *minimum* time in between injections for adults.

First .... As soon as possible
Second .... 4 weeks after the first
Third .... 6 months after the second
Fourth........................... 1 year after the third
Fifth .... 1 year after the fourth

tetracycline *(Achromycin, Sumycin, Terramycin, Theracine, Unimycin)*

Tetracycline is an antibiotic of the tetracycline family. It is used to treat many infections including chlamydia, syphilis, pelvic inflammatory disease, kidney and bladder infections, respiratory infections, diarrhea, and other infections. Doxycycline works for all the same infections, costs less and is easier to take *(see page 499)*.

In what forms does this medicine come?	Capsules: 100, 250, or 500 mg Ointment: 1%

Warning	Do not take within 1 hour of eating dairy products or antacids. Do not take if past expiration date.

How much and when to take 	**For chlamydia:** 500 mg 4 times a day for 7 days *(also take other medicines, see page 277)*. **For syphilis:** 500 mg 4 times a day for 15 days *(also take other medicines, see page 278)*. **For PID:** 500 mg 4 times a day for 10 days *(take other drugs, see page 278)*. **For baby eye care:** a bit of ointment in each eye at birth, one time only.

Information you should know 	Tetracycline does no good in fighting common colds or preventing STD infections.
Side effects 	If you spend a lot of time in the sun it can cause skin rashes. It may cause diarrhea or upset stomach.

Who should not take this medicine? 	Do not use tetracycline if you are pregnant or breastfeeding. Do not give to children under 9 years old except for baby eye care. Do not take if allergic to antibiotics of the tetracycline family.

Other medicines that may work	for *chlamydia:* amoxicillin, erythromycin for *syphilis:* benzathine penicillin for *PID:* amoxicillin for *baby eye care:* erythromycin ointment

thiacetazone

CAUTION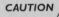

This drug is combined with isoniazid to fight tuberculosis (TB). *People who have the HIV virus must not take this drug! See Chapter 25.*

In what forms does this medicine come?	Tablets: 50 mg with 100 mg of isoniazid

How much and when to take 	The doses for tuberculosis medicines differ from region to region. See a health worker. *(Take thiacetazone in combination with other drugs, see page 389)*.

Who should not take this medicine? 	People who have the HIV virus must not take this drug because it can cause severe, even deadly allergic reactions, and can make their skin peel off. People with liver or kidney problems should also not use this drug.
Side effects 	Rashes, vomiting, dizziness, loss of appetite. Sometimes causes uncontrollable laughing.

trichloroacetic acid, bichloroacetic acid

Either trichloroacetic acid or bichloroacetic acid can be used to treat genital warts.

In what forms does this medicine come?	Liquids in strengths between 10% and 35%

Warning	Use very carefully. It can burn normal skin badly enough to cause a scar.

How much and when to take 	Put only on wart once a week for 1 to 3 weeks as needed.

Information you should know	First protect the area around the wart with petroleum gel. Then put on trichloroacetic acid. It will hurt for 15 to 30 minutes. If it spills onto normal skin, wash it off with soap and water. You can also put baby powder (talc) or baking soda on spills.

Side effects	Trichloroacetic acid will hurt or destroy normal skin if spilled.

Other medicines that may work	for genital warts: podophyllin

ORAL CONTRACEPTIVES (BIRTH CONTROL PILLS)

Most birth control pills contain 2 hormones similar to those produced in a woman's body to control her monthly bleeding. These hormones are called estrogen and progesterone (progestin). The pills come under many different brand names with different strengths and combinations for the 2 hormones. A few of the brand names are listed in the groups below.

Usually, brands that contain a smaller amount of both hormones are the safest and work best for most women. These "low dose" pills are found in Groups 1, 2, and 3.

Group 1 - Triphasic pills

These contain low amounts of both estrogen and progestin in a mix that changes throughout the month. Since the amounts change, it is important to take the pills in order.

Brand names: Logynon   Tricyclen   Trinovum   Triphasil
              Synophase   Trinordiol   Triquilar

Group 2 - Low dose pills

These contain low amounts of estrogen (35 mcg of the estrogen "ethinyl estradiol" or 50 mcg of the estrogen "mestranol") and progestin in a mix that stays the same throughout the month.

Brand names:
Brevicon 1 + 35   Norinyl 1 + 35, 1 + 50   50   Neocon
Noriday 1 + 50   Ortho-Novum 1/35, 1/   Ovysmen 1/35   Norimin
                                                               Perle

---

Group 3 - Low dose pills

These pills are high in progestin and low in estrogen (30 or 35 mcg of the estrogen "ethinyl estradiol").

Brand names: Lo-Ovral   Microvlar
Lo-Femenal   Microgynon 30   Nordette

To assure effectiveness and minimize spotting (small amounts of bleeding at other times than your normal monthly bleeding), take the pill at the same time each day, especially with pills that have low amounts of hormones. If spotting continues after 3 or 4 months, try one of the brands in Group 3. If there is still spotting after 3 months, try a brand from Group 4 (see the next page).

As a rule, women who take birth control pills have less heavy monthly bleeding. This may be a good thing, especially for women who are anemic. But if a woman misses her monthly bleeding for months or is disturbed by the very light monthly bleeding, she can change to a brand with more estrogen from Group 4.

For a woman who has very heavy monthly bleeding or whose breasts become painful before her monthly bleeding begins, a brand low in estrogen but high in progestin may be better. These pills are found in Group 3.

The higher progestin pills in Group 3 may sometimes cause or increase pimples or hair growth on your arms or upper lip. If this bothers you, you may want to change to a pill that is lower in progestin.

Women who continue to have spotting or miss their monthly bleeding when using a brand from Group 3, or who became pregnant before while using another type of pill, can change to a pill that has a little more estrogen. These "high dose" pills are found in Group 4.

Group 4 - High dose pills

These pills are higher in estrogen (50 mcg of the estrogen "ethinyl estradiol") and most are also higher in progestin.

Brand names:

Eugynon	Norlestrin
Femenal	Ovcon 50
Minovlar	Ovral
Neogynon	Primovlar
Nordiol	

If spotting continues even when taking pills from Group 4, the brands Ovulen and Demulen will often stop it. But these are very strong in estrogen and so are rarely recommended. They are sometimes useful for women with severe acne.

Women who are disturbed by morning sickness or other side effects after 2 or 3 months of taking birth control pills, and women who have a higher risk for blood clots, should try a Triphasic birth control pill, low in both estrogen and progestin, from Group 1.

Women who are breastfeeding, or who should not use regular pills because of headaches or mild high blood pressure, may want to use a pill with only progestin. These pills in Group 5 are also called "mini-pills."

Group 5 - Progestin only pills

These pills, also known as "mini-pills," contain only progestin.

Brand names:
Femulen
Mocrolut
Micronor
Mocronovum
Nor-Q D
Ovrette

These pills should be taken at the same time every day, even during the monthly bleeding. Menstrual bleeding is often irregular. There is also an increased chance of pregnancy if even a single pill is forgotten.

EMERGENCY FAMILY PLANNING (EMERGENCY PILLS)

Emergency pills are special doses of certain birth control pills for a woman who has had unprotected sex and wants to avoid pregnancy. Using birth control pills this way is safe, even for many women who should not use pills all the time.

Dose:

The sooner you take the pills after unprotected sex, the more likely you will not get pregnant. For emergency family planning, carefully follow these instructions:

> Take 2 "high dose" birth control pills from GROUP 4 within 3 days of unprotected sex, followed by 2 more GROUP 4 pills 12 hours later.
>
> **or**
>
> Take 4 "low dose" birth control pills from GROUP 2 or GROUP 3 within 3 days of unprotected sex, followed by 4 more GROUP 2 or GROUP 3 pills 12 hours later.
>
> **or**
>
> Take 20 progestin only pills or "mini-pills" from GROUP 5 within 2 days of unprotected sex, followed by 20 more GROUP 5 pills 12 hours later.

New birth control pills have been developed just for emergency family planning and may be available where you live. Some brand names include: **PC4**, **Postinor-2**, and **Tetragynon**. With **Postinor-2**, for example, which contains only progestin, you take 1 pill within 2 days of unprotected sex, followed by 1 more pill 12 hours later.

Side effects:

More than half of all women who use emergency pills will have nausea and even vomiting. If vomiting occurs within 3 hours after taking the pills, another dose must be taken. If vomiting is a problem for you, you can take 25 mg of promethazine by mouth 2 times a day (see *Green Pages page 513*). Or, instead of taking the emergency pills by mouth you can place them high in the vagina. This method works just as well to prevent pregnancy. It does not reduce the side effects of nausea or vomiting, but it does prevent you from vomiting the pills.

Progestin only pills cause less nausea and vomiting, but must be taken within 2 days of unprotected sex.

INJECTABLE CONTRACEPTIVES

With this type of family planning, an injection of hormones is given to a woman every 1, 2 or 3 months, depending on the brand. It is very effective.

Two brand names, **Depo Provera** (DMPA) and **Noristerat** (Net-En) are progestin only injections. Like the mini-pill and implants, these injections may be a good choice for women who cannot take the regular pill because of medical risks or side effects. The dose for **Depo Provera** (DMPA) is 150 mg once every 3 months, and the dose for **Noristerat** (Net-En) is 200 mg once every 2 months.

Sometimes these injections cause sore breasts or nausea, or make women feel tired. This usually goes away after two months. Some women have headaches or feel nervous, depressed or dizzy. Any side effects may last until the injection wears off. While some women can get pregnant 3 or 4 months after their last injection, other women have to wait up to 18 months to get pregnant again.

Do not use injectable contraceptives if you think you might be pregnant, if you have vaginal bleeding and do not know why, if you have liver problems, breast cancer, or blood clots in the legs, lungs, or eyes.

Two other brand names, *Cyclofem* and *Mesigyna*, are injections of both progestin and estrogen. These injections do not cause the problems with irregular bleeding that progestin only injections cause, but women who cannot take regular birth control pills because of medical risks or side effects should not use them. The dose for *Cyclofem* is 25 mg DMPA with 5 mg estradiol cypionate once every month, and the dose for *Mesigyna* is 50 mg Net-En with 5 mg estradiol valerate once every month.

With all injectable contraceptives, monthly bleeding may be irregular and often becomes very light or stops after the first year. This is not serious, but it worries some women. Older women may mistake this for menopause, stop getting injections and then become pregnant. If very heavy bleeding occurs, seek medical advice.

CONTRACEPTIVE IMPLANT (NORPLANT)

Implants are a very convenient and effective form of birth control. Because they contain only progestin, they can be used by women who should not use regular pills because of headaches or mild high blood pressure.

Six small rubber tubes are put under the skin in a woman's upper arm by a specially trained health worker. They prevent pregnancy for about 5 years, but can be removed sooner if the woman wants to become pregnant. The tubes should be inserted 5-7 days after the woman starts her monthly bleeding.

SPERMICIDES

Spermicides are foams, jellies, and tablets which are placed in the vagina to kill sperm and prevent pregnancy. Some spermicides contain nonoxynol-9, which may also prevent some STDs, but not all brands have this. Remember, no spermicide can prevent the passing of the HIV virus which can give you AIDS. Use a condom.

Contraceptive foam (Delfen, Emko, Koromex)

Contraceptive foam is put in the vagina with a special applicator. The foam will kill sperm for 1 to 2 hours. You must put in another applicator full of foam every time you have sex. Foam prevents pregnancy better than inserts, jellies, or creams, and is very effective when used together with a condom.

Contraceptive inserts (Encare, Koromex, Neo Sampoon)

This is a tablet containing spermicide that a woman puts deep in her vagina near her cervix. The insert should be put in 10 to 15 minutes before having sex, and works for up to one hour. It is a fairly effective method of birth control alone, and very effective if used with a condom. Use one insert each time you have sex.

Contraceptive jellies and creams (Conceptrol, Koromex, Ortho Gynol)

Jellies and creams work best with a diaphragm. They do not cover the vagina as well as foam or inserts. They are put in the vagina with an applicator and kill sperm for at least 1 hour. Used with a diaphragm, they work for 6 to 8 hours. For even better protection against pregnancy and to prevent STDs or HIV infection, also use a condom.

Health Care Skills

In many parts of this book we refer to certain skills that can help a person give the best care to someone who is ill. These skills include preventing infection, giving an exam and getting information about a person's body, giving life-saving fluids, and giving injections.

This section gives more complete information about these skills. You may think of these as 'doctor's' or 'nurse's' skills, but they are all skills that anyone can learn with time and practice. Some skills, like giving an *exam* or an *injection*, are best learned by having a skilled person show you how. Once learned, all of these skills can make a careful person better able to help others safely.

Preventing Infection

Infections cause many kinds of sickness. People who are already sick or hurt are often more at risk for getting an infection, and getting one can make them much sicker. So it is important to do everything you can to keep infections from developing. It is also important to protect yourself from getting an infection from those you care for.

Infections are caused by germs, such as bacteria and viruses, that are too small to see. Every person carries bacteria on her skin, and in her mouth, *intestines*, and *genitals* all the time. These germs do not usually cause problems, but they can cause infections if passed to sick people. Germs also live on the equipment and tools used when caring for a sick person and can easily be passed to others you help.

You can *prevent* infection by following the guidelines in this chapter. For other ways to prevent infection, see page 149.

IMPORTANT *You must follow these guidelines every time you help someone, whether you use your hands, tools, or special equipment. If you do not, you may get a dangerous infection, or pass an infection to the people you are helping.*

WASHING YOUR HANDS

Wash your hands before and after caring for another person. It the most important way to kill germs living on your skin. You need to wash your hands even more thoroughly and for a longer time:

Let your hands dry in the air instead of using a towel. Do not touch anything until your hands are dry.

- before and after helping someone give birth.
- before and after touching a wound or broken skin.
- before and after giving an injection, or cutting or piercing a body part.
  - after touching blood, *urine*, *stool*, *mucus*, or fluid from the *vagina*.
  - after removing gloves.

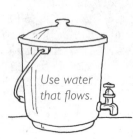

Use water that flows.

Use soap to remove dirt and germs. Count to 30 as you scrub your hands all over with the soapy lather. Use a brush or soft stick to clean under your nails. Then rinse. Use water that flows. Do not reuse water if your hands must be very clean.

Try making a Tippy Tap. It will save water and will make it easy to keep a supply of clean water for washing hands.

Use a large, clean plastic bottle with a handle.

1. Pinch the handle together here with a pair of hot pliers or a hot knife.

2. Make a small hole in the handle, just above where you sealed it.

3. To hang the tippy tap, make 2 more holes in the other side of the bottle and pass a string through them. Now you can hang it on a peg or tree branch.

4. Fill the bottle with clean water and replace the lid.

5. When you tip the bottle forward, the water will flow out, so you can wash your hands. Do not make the hole too large or it will waste water.

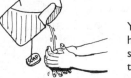

You can also hang a bar of soap from the string.

HOW TO DISINFECT EQUIPMENT AND TOOLS

Cleaning tools and equipment to get rid of nearly all the germs is called *high-level disinfection*.

Tools must **first** be washed and **then** disinfected if they are used to:

- cut, pierce, or tattoo skin.
- give an injection.
- cut the cord during childbirth.
- examine the vagina, especially during or after childbirth, a *miscarriage*, or an *abortion*.
- when giving fluids in the *rectum*.

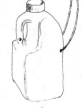

High-level disinfection: 3 steps

Steps 1 and 2 should be done right after using your tools. Try not to let blood and mucus dry on them. Step 3 should be done right before you use the tools again. All the steps can be done together if you can store your tools so they will stay disinfected (see the next page).

1. **Soaking**: Soak your tools for 10 minutes. If possible, use a 0.5% solution of bleach *(chlorine)*. Soaking your tools in bleach solution first will help protect you from infection when cleaning the tools. If you do not have bleach, soak your tools in water.

How to make a disinfecting solution of 0.5% bleach:

If your bleach says:	*Use:*
2% available chlorine	1 part bleach to 3 parts water
5% available chlorine	1 part bleach to 9 parts water
10% available chlorine	1 part bleach to 19 parts water
15% available chlorine	1 part bleach to 29 parts water

For example:

If your bleach says 5% available chlorine, use this much bleach: and this much water:

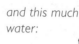

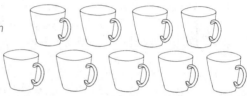

Mix just enough solution for one day. **Do not use it again the next day**. It will not be strong enough to kill germs anymore.

---

2. **Washing**: Wash all tools with soapy water and a brush until each one looks very clean, and rinse them with clean water. Be careful not to cut yourself on sharp edges or points. If possible, use heavy gloves, or any gloves you may have.

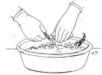

3. **Disinfecting**: Steam or boil the tools for 20 minutes (as long as it takes to cook rice).

To steam them, you need a pot with a lid. The water does not need to cover the tools, but use enough water to keep steam coming out the sides of the lid for 20 minutes.

To boil them, you do not need to fill the whole pot with water. But you should make sure water covers everything in the pot the entire time. If possible, put a lid on the pot.

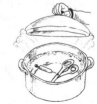

For both steaming and boiling, start to count the 20 minutes after the water is fully boiling. Do not add anything new to the pot once you begin to count.

IMPORTANT *Never use a tool on more than one person without washing and disinfecting all the parts between each use.*

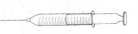

Storing your tools

If you store your tools properly you can do Steps 1, 2, and 3 at one time, and the tools will be ready to use whenever you need them. To store tools:

- After boiling, pour off the water and let the tools dry by themselves. Do not dry them with a cloth. Put a lid or a thin, clean cloth over the pot to prevent flies and dust from getting in. Be sure to let the tools dry completely. Metal objects will rust if they are not dry.

- Do not let the tools touch your hands or anything else.

- Store the tools in a covered pot that has been disinfected. You can use the pot that was used for boiling with a lid, or the steamer that was used for steaming, or a glass jar and lid that have been boiled. If possible, put everything in a clean plastic bag to protect from dust.

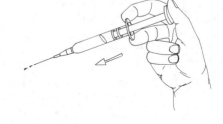

Make sure the pot and lid where you store the tools have also been disinfected.

Disinfecting needles and syringes, gloves, and bandages

Needles and syringes. If a needle and *syringe* can be used more than once (reusable), squirt bleach or soapy water through the syringe 3 times right after using it. Then take everything apart and follow Step 2 and then Step 3 on page 523. Carefully store the syringe until the next use. Be sure not to touch the needle or the plunger.

If you are not able to store things in a clean and dry place, boil or steam them again before use.

If a needle and syringe can be used one time only (disposable), carefully put them in a covered container that cannot be pierced by the needle, and bury the container deeply. If you cannot dispose of the needle safely, squirt bleach solution through it 3 times.

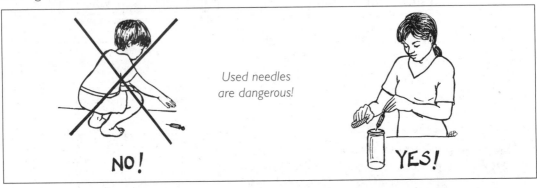

Used needles are dangerous!

NO!   YES!

Gloves

Gloves protect both you and the people you help against the spread of infection. If you do not have gloves, use clean plastic bags to cover your hands.

Sometimes it is OK to use gloves that are clean but not disinfected—as long as you are not reusing them. But you should **always use high-level disinfected gloves when:**

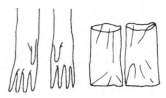

If you do not have gloves, you can use clean plastic bags to cover your hands.

- putting your hand inside the vagina during an emergency exam before or after childbirth or abortion.
- touching broken skin.

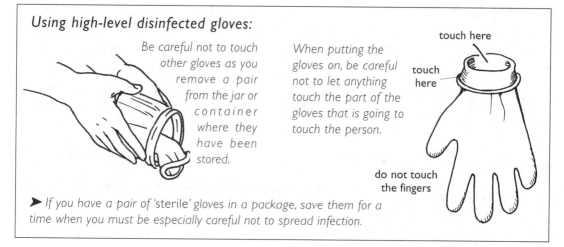

Using high-level disinfected gloves:

Be careful not to touch other gloves as you remove a pair from the jar or container where they have been stored.

When putting the gloves on, be careful not to let anything touch the part of the gloves that is going to touch the person.

touch here

touch here

do not touch the fingers

➤ *If you have a pair of 'sterile' gloves in a package, save them for a time when you must be especially careful not to spread infection.*

If you use gloves more than one time, they should be cleaned, disinfected, and stored following the instructions on pages 523 and 524. Always check washed gloves for holes, and throw away any that are torn.

If possible, it is best to steam gloves rather than boil them because they can stay in the pot they were steamed in until they are dry. If you are unable to steam gloves and must boil them, try to dry them in the sun. You will probably have to touch them to do this, so they will no longer be disinfected, but they will be clean. Keep them in a clean, dry place.

Cloth dressings

If you do not have sterile *gauze*, use cloth dressings. Follow the instructions for disinfection and storage on page 523 and 524. Dry the dressings in the sun, but be sure to keep them off the ground, and to protect them from dust, flies, and other insects.

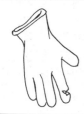

Any items that have touched blood or body fluids (urine, stool, semen, fluid from the bag of waters, pus) should be burned, or disposed of carefully so that children or animals will not find them. This includes supplies that are no longer useful but are contaminated, such as syringes, torn gloves or gloves that can only be used once, gauze, or cotton.

How to Take Temperature, Pulse, Respiration, and Blood Pressure

When a person is sick or has a health problem, her basic physical signs may change. The next few pages tell how to measure these signs to know if a person has a problem.

TEMPERATURE

If you need to know a person's temperature and do not have a thermometer, touch the back of your hand to the person's skin, and compare it with your own skin. If her skin feels much warmer, she probably has a fever. To learn what to do for a fever, see page 297.

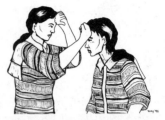

If you have a thermometer, you can take a person's temperature in the mouth, armpit, or rectum. A person's temperature is normally cooler in the armpit, warmer in the mouth, and warmest in the rectum. There are 2 kinds of thermometer scales. Either can be used to measure a person's temperature. Here is how they compare:

Centigrade (C)

Fahrenheit (F)

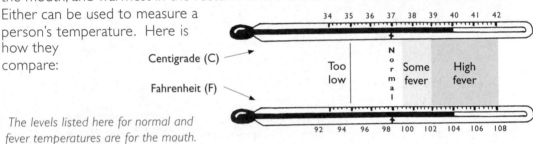

The levels listed here for normal and fever temperatures are for the mouth.

How to take the temperature
(using a thermometer marked in degrees centigrade—°C)

1. Clean the thermometer well with soap and cold water, or alcohol. Hold it at the end without the silver (or red) and shake it hard, with a snap of the wrist, until it reads less than 36 degrees.

2. Put the thermometer . . .

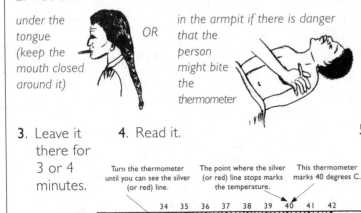

under the tongue (keep the mouth closed around it)   OR   *in the armpit if there is danger that the person might bite the thermometer*   OR   *carefully, in the rectum (wet or apply petroleum gel first).*

3. Leave it there for 3 or 4 minutes.

4. Read it.

Turn the thermometer until you can see the silver (or red) line.   The point where the silver (or red) line stops marks the temperature.   This thermometer marks 40 degrees C.

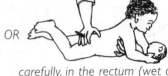

Normal   Fever   High fever

5. Wash the thermometer well with soap and cold water. Then, if you can, soak it for 20 minutes in a bleach solution (see page 523) and rinse with clean water.

PULSE (HEARTBEAT)

The pulse tells how fast the heart is beating and how hard it is working. After hard work or exercise, the heart of a healthy person beats fast, but slows back to normal in a few minutes. The heart usually increases 20 beats a minute for each degree (C) rise in fever.

A normal pulse in an adult is between 60 and 90 beats per minute. A fast pulse can be a sign of:

- blood loss or fluid loss, or *shock* (see page 254).
- fever and infection.
- problems with the lungs and breathing system, or with the heart.
- *thyroid* problems.

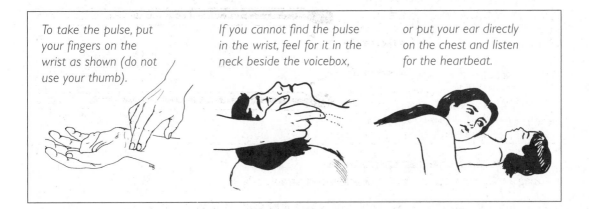

To take the pulse, put your fingers on the wrist as shown (do not use your thumb).

If you cannot find the pulse in the wrist, feel for it in the neck beside the voicebox,

or put your ear directly on the chest and listen for the heartbeat.

RESPIRATION (BREATHING RATE)

The breathing rate tells you about health of the lungs and breathing system. It can also give information about a person's general health. To take the breathing rate, watch the chest rise and fall when a person is at rest. Normal breathing in an adult is 12 to 20 total breaths per minute (a complete breath equals one breath in and one breath out).

Breathing usually speeds up (along with the pulse) when there is infection, fever, blood loss or *dehydration*, shock, lung problems, or other emergencies.

Very slow pulse and breathing in a very sick person can mean she is near death.

Fast, shallow breathing can be a sign of infection of the breathing system. A breathing rate of more than 30 breaths per minute may be a sign of *pneumonia* (see page 304).

BLOOD PRESSURE

Blood pressure is a measure of how hard the blood presses on the inside of the blood vessels.

It is useful to know a woman's blood pressure at these times:

- during pregnancy, childbirth, miscarriage, or abortion.
- if she is using or planning to use birth control pills.
- in emergencies, such as shock, severe abdominal pain, or a difficult childbirth.

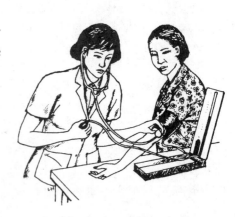

What the numbers mean

A blood pressure measurement (BP) has two numbers:

$$BP \frac{120}{80} \quad \text{or} \quad BP\ 120/80$$

120 is the top (systolic) reading

80 is the bottom (diastolic) reading

Normal blood pressure for an adult is usually around 120/80, but anything from 90/60 to 140/85 can be considered normal.

The bottom number usually gives more information about a person's health. For example, if a person's blood pressure is 140/90, there is not much need for concern. But if it is 225/110, a person has seriously **high blood pressure** and should lose weight (if she is fat) or get treatment. A bottom number of over 100 usually means the blood pressure is high enough to require attention (diet and perhaps medicine).

If a person regularly has **low blood pressure**, there is no need to worry. In fact, blood pressure on the low side of normal—90/60 to 110/70—means a person is likely to live long and is less likely to suffer from heart trouble or stroke.

A **sudden drop in blood pressure** is a danger sign, especially if it falls below 90/60. Watch for any sudden drop in the blood pressure of persons who are losing blood or at risk of shock. If you get an abnormal blood pressure reading and you do not think the person is in shock, wait a few minutes and take the blood pressure again.

You will often need to watch a person's blood pressure over time (for example, during a woman's pregnancy) to see how it changes. It will help to keep a record:

Sept 13	100/60
Oct 12	110/62
Nov 15	90/58
Dec 10	112/60
Jan 12	110/70

This woman's blood pressure goes up and down a little from month to month. This is normal.

How to take blood pressure

There are several types of blood pressure equipment. Some have a tall gauge that looks like a thermometer. Others have a round dial.

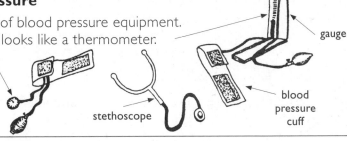

gauge

Blood pressure equipment usually comes with a *stethoscope*.

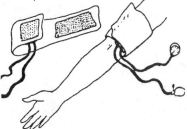

stethoscope

blood pressure cuff

To take a person's blood pressure, first tell her what you are going to do. Then follow these steps:

1. Fasten the cuff around the bare upper arm.

2. Close the valve on the rubber bulb by turning the screw to the right. The valve will get shorter.

3. Feel for a pulse just below the elbow, on the inside of the arm, and put the stethoscope over the pulse. Sometimes you may not feel the pulse. If you cannot, put the stethoscope over the center of the skin crease inside the elbow.

4. Pump the cuff up by squeezing the bulb.

5. As you pump, the needle will move.

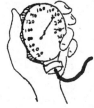

When it reaches 200, stop pumping.

6. Then release the valve a little so that the air leaks out slowly.

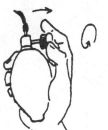

7. The needle will begin to go back down. (If the valve is closed, it will stay at 200.)

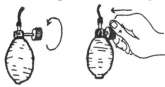

As the air leaks out, you will start to hear the person's pulse through your stethoscope. Notice where the needle or the silver bar is when you start to hear the pulse (this will be the top number) and when the pulse disappears or gets very soft (this will be the bottom number).

If you...   do not hear anything when the needle is here...

...or here

but start to hear a pulse about here →

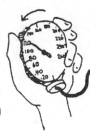

and then lose it again when the needle is about here

then the blood pressure is: 100/70.

How to Examine the Abdomen

If a woman has pain in the lower *abdomen*, first read the chapter on "Pain in the Lower Abdomen" and ask the woman the questions on page 357.

Then examine her abdomen:

1. Ask her to undress so that you can see her abdomen from just below her breasts down to the hair between her legs.

2. Ask her to lie flat on her back on a firm bed, a table, or a clean floor, with her knees bent and her feet close to her buttocks. Ask her to relax her abdominal muscles as much as she can. This may be difficult for someone who is in pain.

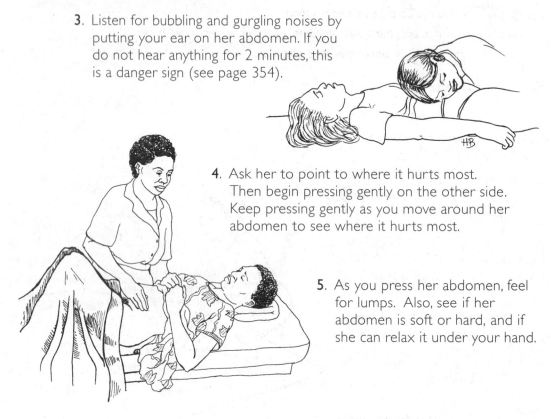

3. Listen for bubbling and gurgling noises by putting your ear on her abdomen. If you do not hear anything for 2 minutes, this is a danger sign (see page 354).

4. Ask her to point to where it hurts most. Then begin pressing gently on the other side. Keep pressing gently as you move around her abdomen to see where it hurts most.

5. As you press her abdomen, feel for lumps. Also, see if her abdomen is soft or hard, and if she can relax it under your hand.

6. To make sure she does not have another problem like *appendicitis*, an infection in her gut, or a *pelvic infection (PID)*, slowly but firmly press on her abdomen on the left side, just above where the leg joins the body (the groin). Press until it hurts a little. Then quickly remove the hand. If a very sharp pain (rebound pain) happens when the hand is removed, she may have a serious infection. Take her immediately to a health center or hospital to see if she needs surgery. If she does not have rebound pain, continue to examine her by looking at the outside of her genitals for sores, *discharge*, bleeding, or other signs of *sexually transmitted diseases (STDs)*. For signs and treatment of STDs, see page 261. If you know how, do a pelvic exam (see the next page).

How to Examine a Woman's Genitals (the *Pelvic* Exam)

Knowing how to examine a woman's genitals can save lives. It is necessary for giving some *family planning* methods and for finding out about many serious women's health problems, such as *pregnancy in the tubes, cancer* of the *cervix* and of the *womb (uterus),* many STDs, and complications from abortion. It is not difficult to learn, and with practice, most women or health workers can:

- examine the outer genitals.
- feel the *reproductive parts* inside the abdomen.

But only do a pelvic exam if it is really necessary. Any time you put something inside a woman's vagina you increase her risk of infection.

IMPORTANT *Do not do a pelvic examination:*
- *when a woman is pregnant and bleeding, or if her waters have broken.*
- *after a normal birth or uncomplicated abortion.*

Before you start:

1. Ask the woman to pass urine.
2. Wash your hands well with clean water and soap.
3. Ask her to loosen her clothing. Use a sheet or her clothing to cover her.
4. Have her lie on her back, with her heels close to her bottom and her knees up. Explain what you are about to do.
5. Put a clean glove on the hand you will put inside the vagina.

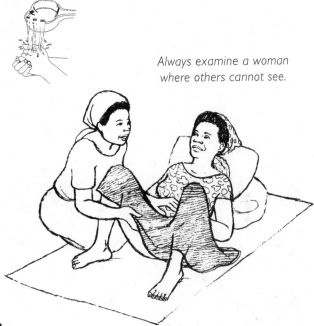

Always examine a woman where others cannot see.

Look at the outside genitals:

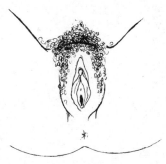

Using the gloved hand to gently touch the woman, look for lumps, swelling, unusual discharge, sores, tears, and scars around the genitals and in between the skin folds of the *vulva.* Some diseases have signs that appear on the outside of the genitals (see the chapter on STDs).

How to do a speculum exam

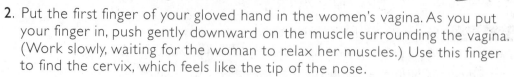

A speculum is useful for looking at the cervix and vagina. If you have one, follow the steps below and then continue with the exam on the next page. If you do not have a speculum, you can get much of the same information by following the steps on the next page.

1. Be sure the speculum has been disinfected before you use it (see page 523). Wet the speculum with clean water before using it.

2. Put the first finger of your gloved hand in the women's vagina. As you put your finger in, push gently downward on the muscle surrounding the vagina. (Work slowly, waiting for the woman to relax her muscles.) Use this finger to find the cervix, which feels like the tip of the nose.

3. With the other hand, hold the speculum blades together between the pointing finger and the middle finger. Turn the blades sideways and slip them into the vagina. (Be careful not to press on the urine hole or *clitoris*, because these areas are very sensitive.) When the speculum is half way in, turn it so the handle is down. Remove your gloved finger.

4. Gently open the blades a little and look for the cervix. Move the speculum slowly and gently until you can see the cervix between the blades. Tighten the screw on the speculum so it will stay in place.

5. Check the cervix, which should look pink and round and smooth. Notice if the opening is open or closed, and whether there is any discharge or bleeding. If you are examining the woman because she is bleeding from the vagina after birth, abortion, or miscarriage, look for flesh coming from the opening of the cervix. If you think she may have an infection, check for green or yellow discharge, or bleeding from the cervix. If the woman has been leaking urine or stool, gently turn the speculum to look at the walls of the vagina. Bring the blades closer together to do this.

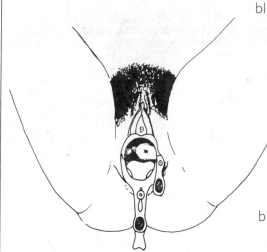

6. To remove the speculum, gently pull it toward you until the blades are clear of the cervix. Then bring the blades together and gently pull back. Be sure to disinfect your speculum again.

How to feel the reproductive parts inside the abdomen

1. Put the pointing finger of your gloved hand in the woman's vagina. As you put your finger in, push gently downward on the muscle surrounding the vagina. When the woman's body relaxes, put the middle finger in too. Turn the palm of your hand up.

2. Feel the opening of her womb (cervix) to see if it is firm and round. Then put one finger on either side of the cervix and move the cervix gently. It should move easily, without causing pain. If it does cause pain, she may have an infection of the womb, tubes, or ovaries. If her cervix feels soft, she may be pregnant.

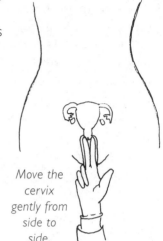

Move the cervix gently from side to side.

3. Feel the womb by gently pushing on her lower abdomen with your outside hand. This moves the inside parts (womb, *tubes*, and *ovaries*) closer to your inside hand. The womb may be tipped forward or backward. If you do not feel it in front of the cervix, gently lift the cervix and feel around it for the body of the womb. If you feel it under the cervix, it is pointed to the back.

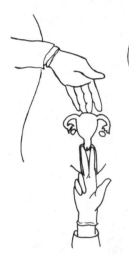

4. When you find the womb, feel for its size and shape. Do this by moving your inside fingers to the sides of the cervix, and then 'walk' your outside fingers around the womb. It should feel firm, smooth, and smaller than a lemon.

If the womb:

- feels soft and large, she is probably pregnant.

- feels lumpy and hard, she may have a *fibroid* or other growth (see page 380).

- hurts when you touch it, she probably has an infection inside.

- does not move freely, she could have scars from an old infection *(pelvic inflammatory disease – PID,* see page 272).

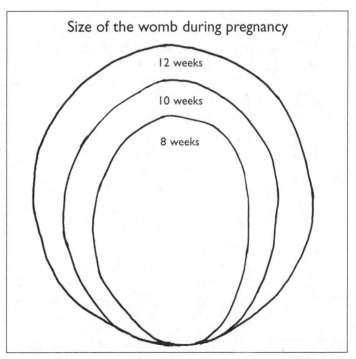

Size of the womb during pregnancy

12 weeks

10 weeks

8 weeks

5. Feel her tubes and ovaries. If these are normal, they will be hard to feel. But if you feel any lumps that are bigger than an almond (this size) or that cause severe pain, she could have an infection or other emergency. If she has a painful lump, and her monthly bleeding is late, she could be pregnant in the tube. She needs medical help right away.

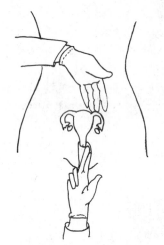

6. Move your finger and feel along the inside of the vagina. If she has a problem with leaking urine or stool, check for a tear (see page 370). Make sure there are no unusual lumps or sores.

7. Have the woman cough, or push down as if she were passing stool. Watch to see if something bulges out of the vagina. If it does, she could have a fallen womb or fallen *bladder* (see page 131).

8. When you are finished, clean and disinfect your glove (see page 523). Wash your hands well with soap and water.

Caring for Burns

Burns are a common injury for women and children (see page 394). All burns should first be cooled for 15 minutes with ice, cold water, or cloths soaked in cold water. After cooling, treatment depends on how serious the burn is. It is very important to keep burns as clean as possible. Protect them from dirt, dust, flies, and other insects. For better healing, never put grease, fat, animal skins, coffee, herbs, or stool on a burn. It is important for persons who have been burned to eat body-building foods (*protein*). There is no type of food that needs to be avoided.

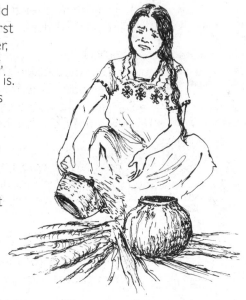

There are 3 basic kinds of burns:

1. Minor burns (1st degree)

These burns do not form blisters, but the skin will get darker or red. After cooling, no other treatment is needed. Use aspirin or paracetamol for pain.

IMPORTANT: *Wash your hands carefully before caring for burns to prevent infection.*

2. Burns that cause blisters (2nd degree)

After cooling, do not break the blisters. Do not make a hole in the blister or take out the liquid inside—not even with a needle and syringe that has been disinfected. If the blister does break, use scissors that have been disinfected to gently remove all the dead skin. Then use mild soap and boiled, cooled water on sterile cotton or gauze, or disinfected cloth, to gently clean the burn. You can also use *hydrogen peroxide*. Remove any remaining burned skin on and around the burn until you see the fresh pink skin underneath. Cover this fresh skin with a piece of sterile gauze or disinfected cloth. If the cloth sticks to the burn when you want to remove it, wet it with water that has been boiled and cooled.

To prevent infection in the burn area, apply a sterile gauze or disinfected cloth that has been soaked in a salt water solution for 15 minutes, 3 times a day. Each time you change the cloth, remove the dead skin and flesh carefully with very clean tweezers, until you see fresh pink skin.

To make a salt solution:

Use 1 teaspoon of salt for 1 liter or quart of water. Boil both the cloth and water before use and cool before putting on the burn.

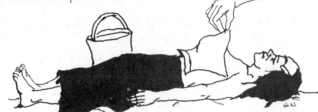

If the burn does become infected, it will be even more painful, more swollen, and the skin spreading out away from the burn will become hard and red. Use an *antibiotic*, such as penicillin or ampicillin, 250 mg, 4 times each day for 7 days. But if the infection has not gone away after 5 days, change to dicloxicillin or erythromycin, 250 mg, 4 times a day for 7 to 10 days. Give the person plenty of liquids.

3. Deep Burns (3rd Degree)

These are burns that destroy the skin and expose blackened and charred flesh. **These burns are always serious.** Take the person for medical help at once. In the meantime, wrap the burned part with a disinfected damp cloth or towel. Make sure the water used to dampen the cloth has been boiled and cooled. Give the person plenty of fluids.

If it is impossible to get medical help, treat the burn as you would a 2nd degree burn. To protect the burn from dust and insects, cover it with a loose, sterile cotton cloth or sheet. Change the cloth at least 4 times a day, or 2 times a day if the cloth stays dry.

Give 'rehydration drink' (see page 536) as often as possible, until the person passes urine frequently. If the person is *unconscious* or cannot swallow, give the rehydration drink in the rectum (see page 537 for how to do this).

Any person who has been badly burned can easily go into shock, caused by the loss of body fluids from the oozing burn.

Comfort and reassure the burned person, and treat her or him for shock if necessary. Give any strong pain medicine you have. Bathing open wounds in slightly salty cold water also helps ease pain.

How to Give Fluids to Treat Shock

If a women loses a lot of blood—for example, during childbirth, after a complicated miscarriage or abortion, or if she is badly burned—she may go into shock (see page 254).

When this happens a woman needs fluids fast in order to save her life. If she is awake and can drink fluids, let her do so. Also, if you know how, you can start an *intravenous* drip (IV). In an emergency, an *enema* can be used instead (see the next page). But enemas should be used for emergencies only. Using too many enemas can be harmful.

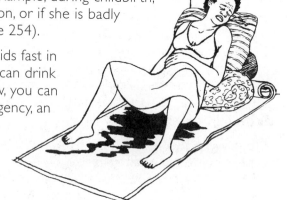

How to make rehydration drink

2 ways to make rehydration drink

If you can, add half a cup of fruit juice, coconut water, or mashed ripe banana to either drink. These contain potassium, a mineral which helps a sick person accept more food and drink.

1. With sugar and salt. (You can use raw sugar or molasses instead of sugar.)

In 1 liter of clean WATER put half of a level teaspoon of SALT and 8 level teaspoons of SUGAR.

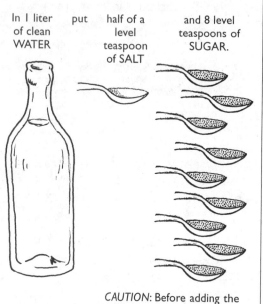

CAUTION: Before adding the sugar, taste the drink and be sure it is less salty than tears.

2. With powdered cereal and salt. (Powdered rice is best. But you can use finely ground maize, wheat flour, sorghum, or cooked and mashed potatoes.)

In 1 liter of clean WATER put half of a level teaspoon of SALT and 8 heaping teaspoons of powdered CEREAL.

Boil for 5 to 7 minutes to form a liquid gruel or watery porridge. Cool the drink quickly and begin to give it to the sick person.

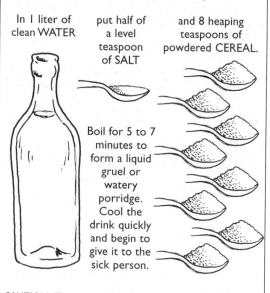

CAUTION: Taste the drink each time before you give it to make sure that it has not spoiled. Cereal drinks can spoil within a few hours in hot weather.

Rehydration drink will also help treat and prevent dehydration, especially in cases of severe watery *diarrhea*.

How to give rectal fluids

You will need:
- a clean enema bag, or a can or tin with tubing.
- a cloth to place under the person.
- 600 ml (a little more than ½ a liter bottle) of warm (not hot) drinking water. If you have them, sugar and salt rehydration drink or a bag of IV solution can be used instead.

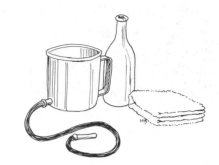

What to do:

1. Tell the woman what you are doing and why.

2. Wash your hands.

3. Ask her to lie on her left side if she can. If possible, her body should be a little higher than her head.

4. If you have them, put on clean gloves.

5. Let the water come down to the end of the tube to get the air out. Then pinch the tubing to stop the flow.

6. Wet the end of the tube with water, and slide it into the anus. Ask her to take slow, deep breaths to help her relax.

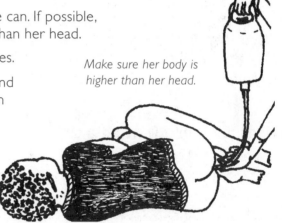

Make sure her body is higher than her head.

Do not put the tube in more than this much.

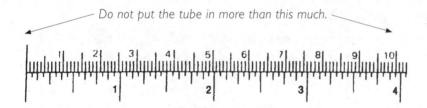

7. Hold the bag or can just high enough for the water to run in very slowly (about the level of the woman's hips). It should take about 20 minutes. If the water runs out of her body, the bag may be too high. Lower the bag so the water runs in more slowly.

8. Gently remove the tube. Tell her to try and keep the water inside, and that the urge to pass stool will go away soon. If the woman is unconscious, you can hold her *buttocks* together.

9. Clean and dry the woman. Then remove your gloves and wash your hands.

10. Transport the woman for medical help right away. If the woman is still in shock, you can give another enema one hour later. If she is not in shock, try to give sips of rehydration drink as you transport her.

How to Give an Injection

Injections are not needed often. Many medicines sometimes given by injection are safer when given by mouth. But it can be necessary to give an injection:

- when the medicine does not come in a form that can be given by mouth.
- when the person cannot swallow or keep medicine down without *vomiting*.
- in some emergencies, such as bleeding or infections after childbirth or abortion.

It is important to give injections properly. They can be dangerous when given in the wrong place, in the wrong way, or without properly cleaning the syringe, hands, and injection site. Carefully follow all of the instructions on 'How to inject,' page 540.

Preventing infection

Needles and syringes that are not cleaned and disinfected properly can pass a disease like *HIV/AIDS* or liver disease (*hepatitis*) to another person. They can also cause a serious infection at the injection site or in the blood.

- **Never** use the same needle and syringe to inject more than one person without cleaning and disinfecting the needle and syringe first. Follow the steps on page 524.
- After the needle has boiled, do not touch it with anything that has not been disinfected.
- If needles are for one-time use only, see page 524 for how to dispose of them safely.

Wʜᴇʀᴇ ᴛᴏ ɢɪᴠᴇ ᴀɴ ɪɴᴊᴇᴄᴛɪᴏɴ

There are 2 basic kinds of injections:

- injections that go into a muscle (intramuscular or IM)
- injections that go into the fatty layer under the skin (subcutaneous).

Where you choose to inject depends on how much medicine you need to inject, the size of the person receiving the injection, and what kind of medicine you are using. For information about how to give both kinds of injections, see page 540.

Most of the medicines in this book that need to be injected should go into the muscle. IM injections can be given in a large muscle in the buttock, upper arm, or thigh. It is best to use the buttock or thigh instead of the arm if:

- the amount to inject is more than 2 ml (2 cc). (But you should never inject more than 3 ml (3 cc) in a single dose. Use 2 injections instead.)
- the medicine is likely to cause pain when injected.
- the person being given the injection is very small or poorly nourished.

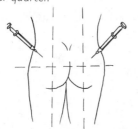

In the buttock, always inject in the upper, outer quarter.

In the upper arm, keep the arm relaxed against the body. Measure 2 finger widths down from the bone at the edge of the shoulder.

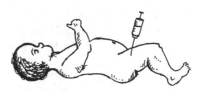

In the thigh, inject into the upper outer part. (This is the best way to inject babies.)

HOW TO PREPARE A SYRINGE FOR INJECTION

Before preparing a syringe, **wash your hands with soap and water**. If the syringe is reuseable, start with step 1. If you have a disposable syringe, open the package carefully and start with step 2.

1. Follow the instructions for disinfecting syringes on page 524.

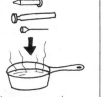

2. Put the needle and syringe together, touching only the base of the needle and the end of the plunger.

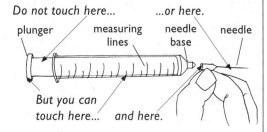

Do not touch here... *...or here.*

plunger   measuring   needle   needle
lines   base

But you can touch here...   and here.

3. Some medicines come ready to use. If you have this kind of medicine, follow steps 4, 5, and 10. If the medicine needs to be mixed with distilled water, follow steps 4 through 10.

4. Clean the glass container (ampule) of medicine or distilled water. Then break off the top.

5. Fill the syringe. Be careful that the needle does not touch the outside of the ampule.

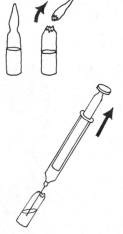

6. Rub the rubber top of the medicine bottle with a clean cloth or cotton that is wet with alcohol or boiled water.

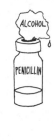

ALCOHOL
PENICILLIN

7. Inject the distilled water into the bottle with the powdered medicine.

8. Shake until the medicine mixes completely with the water.

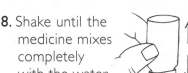

9. Fill the syringe again.

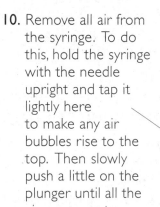

10. Remove all air from the syringe. To do this, hold the syringe with the needle upright and tap it lightly here to make any air bubbles rise to the top. Then slowly push a little on the plunger until all the air comes out through the needle.

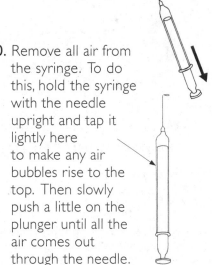

Be very careful not to touch the needle with anything—not even the cloth or cotton that is wet with alcohol. If the needle touches anything, boil it again.

HOW TO INJECT INTO THE MUSCLE (INTRAMUSCULAR, OR **IM**)

The pictures below show how to inject into the buttock. Steps 2 through 6 are the same for injections into the arm or thigh.

1. The person should sit or lie down. Pointing the toes together will relax the muscle to be injected.

2. Clean the skin with alcohol, or soap and water (it will hurt less if you let the alcohol dry before injecting).

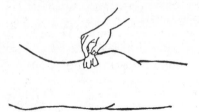

3. Put the needle straight in, all the way. If it is done with one quick movement, it hurts less.

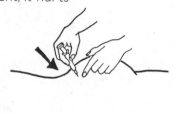

4. Before injecting the medicine, gently pull back on the plunger a little bit (do not pull until the plunger falls out). If blood enters the syringe, take the needle out and put it back in somewhere else close by in the area you have cleaned.

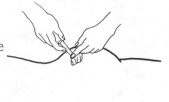

5. Pull back on the plunger again. If no blood enters, inject the medicine slowly.

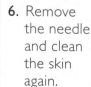

6. Remove the needle and clean the skin again.

TO GIVE AN INJECTION UNDER THE SKIN (SUBCUTANEOUS INJECTION)

- Grab the fatty part on the underside of the arm. Hold the skin like this:
- Put the needle under the skin at this angle. Make sure the needle does not go into the muscle.

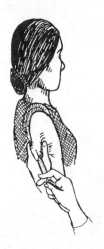

Be prepared to treat allergic reaction and allergic shock

Some medicines, especially antibiotics like penicillin and ampicillin, can produce an allergic reaction, usually within 30 minutes after an injection. An allergic reaction can progress to allergic shock, which is an emergency. To prevent allergic reaction and allergic shock, before giving an injection ask the person: "Have you ever had a reaction to this medicine—like hives, itching, swelling, or trouble breathing?" If the answer is yes, do not use that medicine in any form, or any medicine from the same family of medicines. Whenever you inject medicines, watch for signs of allergic reaction and allergic shock and have medicines for treating them nearby.

Mild allergic reaction

Signs:
- itching
- sneezing
- hives or rash

Treatment:
Give 25 mg diphenhydramine by mouth 3 times a day until the signs disappear.

Pregnant or breastfeeding women may find the discomfort of a mild allergic reaction better than the risks of taking an antihistamine.

Moderate to severe allergic reaction

Signs:
- itching
- hives
- swollen mouth and tongue
- difficulty breathing

Treatment:
1. Inject 0.5 mg of epinephrine immediately under the skin. See the drawing on page 540. Give a second injection in 20 minutes if the signs do not get better.

2. Give 25 mg diphenhydramine or promethazine by mouth or by injection into a muscle. Repeat in 8 hours or less if the signs do not get better.

3. Watch the person for at least 4 hours to make sure the reaction does not progress to allergic shock.

Allergic shock

Signs:
- itching or hives
- sudden paleness or cool, moist skin (cold sweats)
- swollen mouth and tongue
- difficulty breathing
- weak, rapid pulse or heartbeat (more than 100 beats per minute)
- loss of consciousness

Treatment:
1. Inject 0.5 mg of epinephrine immediately under the skin. See the drawing on page 540. Give a second injection in 20 minutes if the signs do not get better.

2. Inject 50 mg diphenhydramine or promethazine into muscle. Repeat in 8 hours or less if the signs do not get better.

3. Inject 500 mg hydrocortisone (cortisol) into muscle and repeat in 4 hours if needed. **Or** inject 20 mg dexamethasone into muscle and repeat in 6 hours if needed.

4. Watch the person for 8 to 12 hours to make sure the signs do not come back. Leave her with steroid medicines to take by mouth if her signs return. She should take 500 to 1000 mg of hydrocortisone and repeat after 4 hours if needed. Or she can take 20 mg of dexamethasone and repeat after 6 hours if needed.

Acupressure Massage

Pressing on special 'points' on the body can help relieve some of the common health problems of women. These points come from an ancient Chinese way of healing called acupressure. Local healers may know other kinds of massage.

Use your own sense of how long and how often to press on these points (an average amount of time is 3 to 10 minutes). Many women feel tender at these points. If a point is very tender, be careful not to irritate it. If there is an injury, do not use acupressure in that area.

Sometimes there are several points to help the same problem. You can try all these points. If one seems tender or makes you feel better, focus on that point. If not, use all of the points in any order.

IMPORTANT *Pressing on some of these points can cause problems during pregnancy. If you are pregnant, watch for the warnings mentioned below.*

General pain from monthly bleeding

(For information about monthly bleeding, see page 48.)

1. To help prevent general discomfort during monthly bleeding, such as sore breasts, feeling tired, and a full feeling in the lower abdomen:

press here

2. To lessen pain and cramps during monthly bleeding, firmly hold and massage the tender place on your hand you will find between your thumb and first finger. Pressing hard on this spot can ease many kinds of pain.

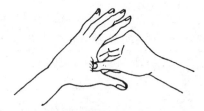

You can also press on these points on the inside of the foot and leg.

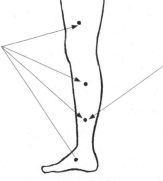

But do not press too hard on this point or it will cause injury. Do not press on this point if a woman is pregnant. This point can cause labor to begin.

The following massage is also useful to relieve pain and *cramps*, as well as signs of pre-menstrual syndrome (PMS). See page 51.

Massage in between the toes, around the ankle bones, and up the ankles on the outside of the feet. Look for areas that are sensitive and massage these places longer. **For a pregnant woman, do not massage the outside of the big toe, the arch or the middle of the bottom of the foot or above the outside of the ankle. It can make labor start.**

Hand, wrist, and ear massage can also help with pain or signs of PMS.

Pregnancy and childbirth
(See the chapter on "Pregnancy and Childbirth," page 67.)

To relieve nausea (morning sickness):

To help with a difficult or painful birth:

To help stop bleeding after birth:

To bring on labor, or to make a weak labor stronger:

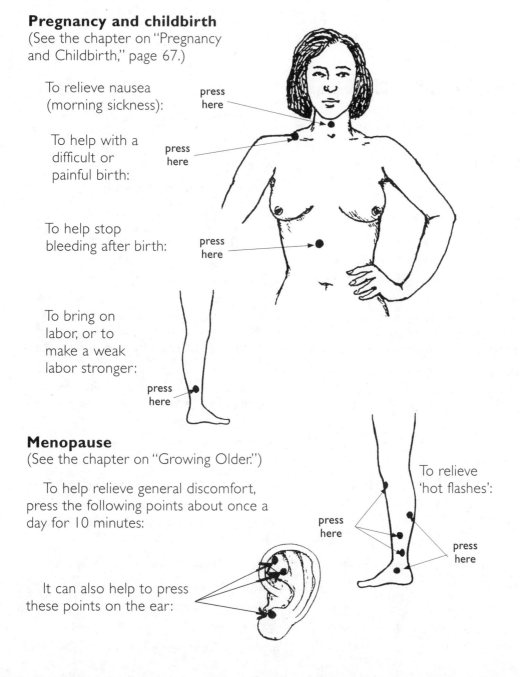

press
here

press
here

press
here

press
here

Menopause
(See the chapter on "Growing Older.")

To help relieve general discomfort, press the following points about once a day for 10 minutes:

It can also help to press these points on the ear:

To relieve 'hot flashes':

press
here

press
here

LIST OF DIFFICULT WORDS

Here is a list of words that may be difficult to understand. Knowing what these words mean can help you use the book better.

Some of the words included here are explained in the chapters, but many are not. The first time they are used in a chapter, the words are written in *slanted letters*. Some of the explanations here in this vocabulary also contain words written in *slanted letters*. This is because an explanation for these words can be found somewhere else in this list.

This vocabulary is listed in the order of the alphabet:

A B C D E F G H I J K L M N O P Q R S T U V W X Y Z

A

abdomen The part of the body that contains the *stomach, liver*, guts and *reproductive organs*. The belly.

abnormal bleeding Bleeding that is different from what is usual, natural, or average. Not normal.

abortion When a woman does something to end a pregnancy.

abscess A raised, red, painful lump on the skin that is filled with *pus* (for example, a boil).

abuse When someone hurts another person's body (physical abuse), humiliates or insults a person (emotional abuse) or makes a person do sexual things against her will (sexual abuse).

access (to health services) When health services are available, and a woman has the freedom, the money, and the time to use them.

acute When something happens suddenly, lasts for a short time, and is usually serious or strong—for example, acute pain or acute *infection*. Compare with *chronic*.

addiction When the body feels a strong need for alcohol or a *drug*.

afterbirth See *placenta*.

AIDS (acquired immune deficiency syndrome) A *sexually transmitted disease* caused by the HIV virus. A person has AIDS (rather than just being infected with HIV) when the *immune system* gets so weak it can no longer fight off common *infections* and illnesses.

allergy, allergic reaction, allergic shock A problem—such as itching, sneezing, hives or rash, and sometimes difficult breathing or shock—that affects certain people when specific things are breathed in, eaten, *injected*, or touched. Allergic shock is a severe form of allergic reaction.

anal sex Having sex in the *anus*.

anemia A disease in which the blood gets weak and thin because it lacks red blood cells. This happens when blood is lost or destroyed faster than the body can replace it.

anesthesia General anesthesia is when you are given medicine to make you sleep during an *operation* so you will not feel pain. Local anesthesia is when you are given an *injection* in one place so that you will not feel pain in that area.

antacid Medicine used to control too much *stomach* acid and to calm stomach upset. See *heartburn*.

antibiotic Medicine used to fight *infection* caused by *bacteria*.

antibodies Substances the body makes to fight *infection*.

anus The opening of the *intestine* where waste *(stool)* leaves the body.

anxiety Feeling nervous or worried.

appendicitis An *infection* of the *appendix*.

appendix A finger-like sac attached to the large *intestine*.

areola The dark, bumpy area around the *nipple*.

artery A thin, tube-like vessel that carries blood from the heart through the body. Arteries have a *pulse*. *Veins*, which return blood to the heart, have no pulse.

arthritis Pain and swelling in the *joints*.

asthma A disease of the lungs, which causes attacks of difficult breathing. There is often a hissing or wheezing sound when a person breathes out.

B

bacteria *Germs* that cause many different *infectious diseases*. Bacteria are too small to see without a *microscope*.

bacterial vaginosis An *infection* of the *vagina* caused by bacteria.

bag of waters The sac (or amniotic sac) inside the *womb* that holds the baby. When the sac breaks and releases fluid, this usually means that *labor* has begun.

balls Part of the man's outer *genitals*. Also called the *testicles*.

barrier methods *Family planning methods* that prevent pregnancy by keeping the *sperm* from reaching the egg.

Bartholin's glands Small *glands* on either side of the vaginal opening that make a liquid to keep the *vagina* wet.

benefit The good that something may bring.

bile A liquid found in the *gallbladder* that helps digest fatty foods.

bilharzia An *infection* caused by a kind of worm that gets into the bloodstream.

biopsy When a piece of *tissue* or fluid is taken from somewhere on or in the body and examined to see if it is healthy or diseased.

birth canal See *vagina*.

birth control See *family planning*.

birth control pills A *hormonal family planning method*.

birth defects Physical or mental problems a child is born with, like a *cleft lip* or *cleft palate*, or an extra finger or toe.

birth spacing Using *family planning methods* to space your children.

blackouts When you are using too much alcohol or other *drugs* and wake up not knowing what happened.

bladder The bag inside the *abdomen* that stores *urine*. As the bladder fills, it stretches and gets bigger.

blood clots Soft, dark red, shiny lumps in the blood that look like liver.

blood pressure The force or pressure of the blood upon the walls of the blood vessels (*arteries* and *veins*). Blood pressure varies with the age and health of the person.

blood transfusion When someone's blood is given to another person, in a *vein* and using a special needle, to replace blood the person may have lost.

blurred eyesight When the eyes cannot see things clearly.

bowels The *intestines*.

brand name The name for a medicine that is given by the company that makes it. Compare with *generic*.

breast exam Checking the breasts for lumps that might be a sign of *cancer*.

breast infection (mastitis) An *infection* inside the breast that can be very painful for the mother, and make it difficult for the baby to suck the *nipple*.

breech When a baby is born feet or buttocks first, instead of head first. This can be dangerous for the baby.

bronchitis An *infection* of the large tubes in the lungs.

buttocks The round, fleshy part of the body a person sits on.

C

caffeine A *drug* found in coffee, tea, and cola drinks that causes the heart to beat faster and makes a person feel more awake.

calcium A *mineral* found in some foods that helps make bones and teeth strong.

cancer A serious disease that causes *cells* to change and grow in an abnormal way, causing growths. Cancer can affect many different parts of the body.

cannula A small tube used to suction out the contents of the *womb*.

cassava (manioc root) A starchy root grown in the tropics.

cataracts An eye problem in which the lens or covering of the eye becomes cloudy, making it more and more difficult to see. The dark, round, center part of the eye (pupil) looks gray or white when a light is shined on it.

cell The smallest unit of living matter in the body.

cervix The opening of the *womb* at the back of the *vagina*.

cesarean section (c-section) When it is dangerous for a baby to be born through the *vagina*, the woman can have an *operation* in which her *abdomen* is cut open and the baby is taken out.

chart A file where information about a person's illnesses and treatments is kept.

chemicals Substances found in all living and nonliving things. Many chemicals used in women's work cause harm to the body.

child spacing Having children at least 2 or 3 years apart so that a woman's body has a chance to get strong again between pregnancies.

chlamydia A *sexually transmitted disease*.

chlorine solution A *chemical* liquid that can be used to kill *germs*. Also known as bleach.

cholera A serious *infectious disease* with severe *vomiting* and bloody *diarrhea*.

chronic Something that lasts for a long time, or that occurs often. Compare with *acute*.

circulation Blood flowing through the *arteries* and *veins* in the body.

circumcision (in a man) When the loose fold of skin at the end of a man's *penis* is cut off.

circumcision (in a woman) When part or all of a girl or woman's outer *genitals* are cut off.

cleft lip An opening or gap on a baby's upper lip, often connecting to the nostril.

cleft palate A split or abnormal opening in the roof of the baby's mouth.

climax When the body reaches its peak of sexual pleasure.

clitoris The part of the *vulva* most sensitive to touch.

clots See *blood clots*.

cold sores See *herpes*.

colostrum The yellow-colored milk that comes from the breasts for the first 2 or 3 days after birth.

community health workers Health workers who work in the community and may or may not have formal training.

complications Problems or things that go wrong.

compost A mixture of plant and animal waste that is allowed to rot for use as a fertilizer. Hay, dead leaves, vegetable waste, animal droppings, and manure all make good compost.

compress A folded cloth or pad that is put on a part of the body. The compress may be soaked in hot or cold liquid.

conception When the egg and *sperm* join to begin making a baby.

condom (rubber) A narrow bag of thin rubber that the man wears on his *penis* during sex. The bag traps the man's *sperm* so that it cannot get into the woman's *womb* and make her pregnant. Condoms also help prevent the spread of *sexually transmitted diseases*.

condom for women See *female condom*.

constipation When a person has a difficult time passing *stool*.

contagious An illness that can be spread easily from one person to another.

contaminated When medical supplies or food contain harmful *germs*.

contraception (birth control) Any method of preventing pregnancy. See *family planning*.

contraceptive gel A slippery gel or cream that is put into the *vagina* before sex to prevent pregnancy.

contractions (pains, labor pains) When the *womb* squeezes and becomes hard. Contractions open the *cervix* and help push the baby out of the *womb*.

convulsion An uncontrolled *fit*. A sudden jerking of part or all of the body.

cord (umbilical cord) The cord that connects the baby at its navel (belly button) to the *placenta*.

counseling When a trained person helps you think about your situation or decisions you need to make. For example, some people are trained especially to help people cope with *HIV/AIDS*.

cramps A painful tightening or *contraction* of a muscle. Many woman have cramps that begin just before *monthly bleeding* or just after it starts.

cretinism When a baby is born mentally slow because its mother did not have enough *iodine* in her diet during pregnancy.

curette A small tool used to scrape out the lining of the *womb* during a *dilation and curettage (D and C)*.

D

D and C See *dilation and curettage*.

date rape When a woman is forced to have sex by a man she is dating or courting.

dehydration When the body loses more liquid than it takes in.

dementia When a person has severe difficulty remembering things and thinking clearly.

dengue fever A serious illness caused by a *virus* that is spread by mosquitoes.

dependence When the mind feels an overpowering need for a *drug*.

depression When a person feels extremely sad or feels nothing at all.

diabetes When a person has too much sugar in her blood.

diaphragm A *family planning method* in which a soft rubber cup, usually filled with *contraceptive* gel or cream, is worn over the *cervix* during sex.

diarrhea Passing 3 or more loose, watery stools in a day.

digestion When food is broken down by the *stomach* and *intestines* to be used by the body or to pass out of the body as waste.

dilation and curettage (D and C) To gradually open the *cervix* and then scrape out the *womb*. Often used for an *abortion* or to find the cause of *abnormal bleeding* from the *vagina*.

disability Physical or mental limitations that affect daily living.

discharge (from the vagina) The wetness or fluid that comes out of the *vagina*.

discrimination When people are ignored or treated badly because of who they are (for example, because they are women or old or poor).

disinfection Cleaning tools and equipment in a certain way to get rid of nearly all the germs. Also called high-level disinfection.

divorce To legally end a marriage.

dizziness Feeling lightheaded or unsteady.

dose The amount of a medicine you should take at one time.

douche Washing out the *vagina*. This can cause harm because it washes out the natural wetness in the vagina.

drugs Substances, like alcohol and cocaine, that can be used in harmful ways to alter the mind, to feel good, or to cope with life.

dysentery *Diarrhea* with *mucus* or blood in it, usually caused by an *infection*.

E

ectopic pregnancy See *pregnancy in the tube*.

ejaculate When a man reaches his peak of sexual pleasure and his *semen* comes out.

embryo An unborn baby is called an embryo between the second and eighth weeks after *conception*.

emphysema A serious lung disease.

enema A solution of water put up the *anus* to make a person pass *stool* or to increase the amount of fluid in the body.

epilepsy A disease in which a person has *convulsions* and *loss of consciousness*.

erection When a man becomes sexually excited and his *penis* gets hard.

esophagus The tube connecting the mouth and the *stomach* that food goes down.

estrogen A female *hormone*.

examination (exam) When a health worker, nurse, or doctor looks at, listens to, or feels parts of the body to find out what is wrong.

exhaustion Extreme tiredness.

F

fainting See *loss of consciousness*.

fallen womb. See *prolapse*.

fallopian tubes The tubes that lead from the *ovaries* to the *womb*. When the *ovary* releases an egg, it travels down these tubes to the *womb*.

family planning When a woman uses methods to prevent pregnancy, so that she can have the number of children she wants, when she wants them.

farsighted Being able to see things that are far away but not things close by. Often happens after age 40.

fats Foods, like oils and butter, that give the body energy.

female condom A thin piece of rubber that fits into the *vagina* and covers the outer folds of the *vulva*. The condom prevents a man's *sperm* from reaching the woman's *womb*.

fertile time The time in a woman's cycle when she can get pregnant. For most women, this time starts about 10 days after the last *monthly bleeding* and lasts for about 6 days.

fertility awareness (Natural Family Planning) A *family planning* method that teaches a woman how to know her fertile time.

fertilization See *conception*.

fertilizer A material used to make the land richer so that more crops can be produced.

fetoscope A tool for listening to and counting the heartbeat of the baby inside the mother's *womb*.

fetus The baby growing inside the *womb*.

fever When the body *temperature* is higher than normal.

fiber Parts of certain plants that when eaten help the body pass stool.

fibroids Growths in the *womb* that can cause abnormal bleeding from the *vagina*, pain, and repeated *miscarriage*.

fistula A hole in the skin between the *vagina* and the urine tube or *rectum* that causes *urine* or *stool* to leak from the *vagina*.

fit See *seizure*.

flashback When a person suddenly remembers something from the past as if it is happening now.

flexibility When the muscles and *joints* can move easily, without stiffness or pain.

folic acid or **folate** A B-*vitamin* that helps make healthy red blood cells. It is especially important that a pregnant woman get enough folic acid in her diet in order to prevent *birth defects* in the baby.

fumes Vapors that can contain harmful *chemicals*.

G

gallbladder A small, muscular sac attached to the *liver*. The gallbladder collects a liquid that helps digest fatty foods.

gallstones Hard material that forms in the *gallbladder* and can cause severe pain.

gang rape when a woman or girl is *raped* by more than one man.

gangrene When skin and *tissue* dies because of a lack of blood to that area.

gauze Soft, loosely woven kind of cloth used for bandages.

gender discrimination See *discrimination*.

gender role The way a community defines what it means to be a woman or man.

generic The name of the main ingredient in a medicine.

genital herpes A *sexually transmitted disease* that produces sores on the *genitals* or on the mouth.

genital warts Growths on the *genitals*, which are caused by a *virus* spread during sex.

genitals The sexual parts both inside and outside a woman's body.

German measles A disease spread by a *virus* that can harm a baby growing in the *womb*.

germs Very small organisms that can grow in the body and cause some infectious diseases.

gland A small sac that produces fluid.

glaucoma A disease of the eye in which too much pressure builds up inside the eyeball and damages vision. Glaucoma can happen slowly (*chronic* glaucoma) or suddenly (*acute* glaucoma).

glaze The liquid coating on a clay pot that hardens when fired and keeps water from seeping through the clay.

goiter A swelling on the lower front of the neck (enlargement of the *thyroid gland*) caused by lack of *iodine* in the diet.

gonorrhea A *sexually transmitted disease*.

groin the very top of the leg where it joins the body in the front, next to the *genitals*.

gut thread A special thread for sewing or stitching tears from childbirth. The gut thread is slowly absorbed (disappears) so that the stitches do not need to be taken out.

H

hallucinations Seeing strange things or hearing voices that others do not see or hear.

health centers Places that provide a middle level of health care, usually in larger towns. Health centers may have trained nurses and doctors.

health posts A place that provides health care like *immunizations*, *prenatal care*, *family planning*, and health *exams*.

heartburn A burning feeling in the throat that is common in later pregnancy.

helper foods Foods that provide *nutrition*—like *protein*, *vitamins*, *minerals*, *fats*, and *sugar*—that are needed in addition to the main food.

hemorrhage Heavy bleeding.

hemorrhoids Small, painful bumps or lumps at the edge of the *anus* or inside it. They are a type of swollen *veins* that may burn, hurt, or itch.

hepatitis A serious disease of the *liver* caused by a *virus*. Some forms of hepatitis can be *sexually transmitted*.

herbicides Chemicals used to kill unwanted plants.

herpes A disease caused by a *virus* that causes sores on the mouth or *genitals*. Herpes can be sexually transmitted.

herpes zoster (shingles) A painful rash caused by the herpes *virus*, with blisters on the face, back, and chest.

high blood pressure When the force or pressure of the blood upon the walls of the *arteries* and *veins* is harder than normal.

HIV/AIDS HIV, or human immune-deficiency *virus*, is the virus that causes *AIDS*. We sometimes use the word 'HIV/AIDS' since *infection* with HIV eventually leads to AIDS.

HIV virus See *HIV/AIDS*.

hives Hard, thick, raised spots on the skin that itch severely. They may come and go all at once or move from one place to another. A sign of *allergic reaction*.

home remedies Traditional ways of healing.

hookworm A *parasitic* worm that infects the *intestines*.

hormonal methods *Family planning methods* that prevent the woman's *ovary* from releasing an egg and keep the lining of the *womb* from supporting a pregnancy.

hormones *Chemicals* the body makes that tell it how and when to grow. *Estrogen* and *progesterone* are the most important hormones for women.

hospital A medical center with doctors, nurses, and special equipment for finding or treating serious illnesses.

hydrogen peroxide A chemical that kills *germs*, often used for cleaning wounds.

hymen A thin piece of skin that partially closes off the *vaginal* opening. In some communities, a woman is no longer considered a *virgin* if her hymen is torn, even though it can be torn by activities other than sex.

hysterectomy An *operation* in which the *womb* is removed. In a 'total hysterectomy', the *tubes* and *ovaries* are also removed.

I

immune system The parts of the body that recognize harmful *germs* and try to fight off *infection*.

immunization See *vaccination*.

implantation When the *fertilized* egg attaches to the *womb* wall at the beginning of pregnancy.

implants A *family planning method* in which small tubes containing *hormones* are put under the skin.

impotence When a man is unable to have sex, usually because his *penis* will not get or stay hard.

incest Sexual relations between family members or relatives.

incision A cut made into the body.

incomplete abortion When part of a pregnancy remains in the *womb* after an *abortion*.

indigestion See *heartburn*.

infant formula Artificial milk for babies used instead of breast milk. Infant formula does not have the same health benefits as breast milk.

infection A sickness caused by *bacteria*, *viruses*, or other organisms. Infections may affect part of the body or all of it.

infectious disease Diseases caused by *germs* or *parasites* that can be spread from one person to another.

infertility When a woman has had sex regularly during her *fertile time* for one year but has been unable to get pregnant. A woman with repeated *miscarriages* is also considered infertile.

infibulation A form of female *circumcision* in which the outside *genitals* are cut away and the opening to the *vagina* is sewn almost closed.

inheritance The possessions, property, or money a person receives after someone dies.

injections When medicine or other liquid is put into the body using a *syringe* and needle.

inner folds The part of a woman's *genitals* that lie just inside the hairy outer folds of the *vulva*. The inner folds are soft flaps of skin without hair that are sensitive to touch.

intestines The guts or tube-like part of the food canal that carries food and finally waste from the *stomach* to the *anus*.

intimacy Sharing your private thoughts and feelings with someone.

intramuscular injection (IM) *Injection* deep into the muscle.

intra-uterine device (IUD, IUCD) A small object that is put into the *womb* to prevent pregnancy.

intravenous (IV) When medicines or fluids are put into a vein.

iodine A *mineral* found in the ground and some foods that prevents *goiter* and mental slowness at birth.

iron A *mineral* found in some foods that helps make the blood healthy.

J

jaundice Yellow color of the skin and eyes. Jaundice can be a sign of *hepatitis* or of newborn jaundice.

joints Places in the body where bones come together.

K

Kaposi's sarcoma Brown or purple patches on the skin or in the mouth caused by a *cancer* of the blood vessels or *lymph nodes*. Occurs most often in persons with *AIDS*.

kidneys Two large *organs* in the lower back that make *urine* by cleaning waste from the blood.

L

labia Large and small folds of skin that are part of the *vulva*.

labor The work a woman's body does in childbirth, when her *womb* squeezes or contracts, causes her *cervix* to open, and pushes her baby down through the *vagina* and out of her body.

latex A material like thin rubber. *Condoms* and gloves are often made of latex.

latrine A hole or pit in the ground for passing *urine* or *stool*. A toilet.

laxatives Medicine used for *constipation* to make *stools* softer and more frequent.

lice Tiny insects that attach on the skin or hair of people and other animals.

ligaments Strong fibers in a person's body that help hold muscles and bones in place.

literacy The ability to read and understand written information.

liver A large *organ* under the lower right ribs that helps clean the blood and get rid of poisons.

loss of consciousness When a sick or injured person seems to be asleep and cannot be awakened. Unconscious.

lubricants A slippery cream or gel used to make dry surfaces wet. Lubricants are often used on *condoms* during sex.

lymph nodes Small lumps under the skin in different parts of the body that trap *germs*. Lymph nodes become swollen and painful when they get *infected*.

M

main food The main food, usually low-cost, that is eaten with almost every meal. This main food usually provides most of the body's daily food needs. For good nutrition, the body also needs *helper* foods.

malaria An *infection* that causes chills and high *fever*, which is spread by mosquitoes. The mosquito sucks up the malaria *parasites* in the blood of an infected person and injects them into the next person it bites.

malnutrition When the body does not have enough of the foods it needs to stay healthy.

massage A way of touching the body to relieve pain, tension, or other signs. Massaging the belly can help the *womb contract* and stop heavy bleeding after birth, *miscarriage* or *abortion*.

mastitis See *breast infection*.

masturbation Touching one's own body to bring personal sexual pleasure.

maternal mortality When a woman dies due to problems from pregnancy and birth.

medical abortion Using certain medicines to end a pregnancy.

membranes A thin layer of skin or *tissue* that either covers *organs* inside the body or lines other parts. An example is the sac that surrounds and protects the baby when it is in the mother's *womb*.

menopause When a woman's *monthly bleeding* stops forever.

menstrual cycle See *monthly cycle*.

menstruation See *monthly bleeding*.

microscope An instrument that makes very tiny objects look larger.

midwife Someone with special training or experience to help a woman give birth.

migraines Severe headaches with *blurred eyesight*.

minerals Substances in foods—like *iron*, *calcium*, and *iodine*—that help the body fight disease and recover after injury or illness.

miscarriage When a woman loses a developing baby before it is old enough to survive outside the *womb*.

monthly bleeding (menstruation, monthly period) When a bloody fluid leaves a woman's *womb* and passes through the *vagina* and out of her body. It happens about every 28 days and lasts for a few days.

monthly cycle The period of time between the beginning of one *monthly bleeding* and the beginning of the next. About 2 weeks after a woman starts her monthly bleeding one of her *ovaries* releases an egg, and about 2 weeks after that she starts another monthly bleeding.

monthly period See *monthly bleeding*.

morning sickness See *nausea*.

mucous method When a woman checks the *mucus* in her *vagina* every day to find out when she is most *fertile*.

mucus A thick, slippery wetness that the body makes to protect the inside of the *vagina*, nose, throat, *stomach*, and *intestines*.

mumps A *contagious* disease caused by a *virus* and common in children. Mumps can be *prevented* by *vaccination*.

N

natural methods (of family planning) Methods of preventing pregnancy that do not require any devices or *chemicals*.

nausea When a person feels sick to her *stomach*, as though she wants to *vomit*. This often happens to women during the first 3 or 4 months of pregnancy. Also called 'morning sickness'.

nipple The center of the dark-colored part on the outside of the breast where milk comes out.

nonoxinol-9 A *chemical* that kills *sperm* and so helps prevent pregnancy. It also provides some protection against *gonorrhea* and *chlamydia*.

nutrition Good nutrition is eating enough food and the right kind of food so the body can grow, be healthy, and fight off disease.

O

operation When a doctor makes a cut in the skin in order to repair damage inside, or to change the way the body functions.

oral sex When a person uses his or her mouth on a partner's *genitals* to give the partner sexual pleasure.

organ A part of the body that is more or less complete in itself and does a specific job. For example, the lungs are organs for breathing.

orgasm See *climax*.

osteoporosis Weak, brittle bones that break easily. Osteoporosis is more common in older women, because they produce less *estrogen* after *menopause*.

outer folds The fatty lips of the *vulva* that protect the outside *genitals* and close up when the legs are together.

ovaries Small sacs about the size of an almond or grape, one on each side of the *womb*. Ovaries produce eggs that join with a man's *sperm* to make a baby.

overdose Taking too much of a *drug* or medicine at one time. This can cause serious injury or death.

ovulation When an egg is released from one of the *ovaries* during the middle of a woman's *monthly cycle*.

oxygen A *chemical* in the air that is necessary for life.

P

Pap test A test in which some skin *cells* are scraped from the *cervix* during a *pelvic exam* and then examined under a *microscope* to see if there are any early warning signs of *cancer*.

paralysis Loss of the ability to move part or all of the body.

parasites Tiny worms and animals that can live in a person (or animal) and cause disease.

peer counselor Someone who is trained to talk with another person who is in a similar situation. For example, one young woman may counsel another young woman, or someone who used to drink too much may counsel another person who is trying to quit.

pelvic area Everything between a woman's hips. This is where a woman's *reproductive* parts are.

pelvic exam An examination of a woman's genitals both inside and outside her body. A pelvic exam sometimes includes a *speculum* exam.

pelvic inflammatory disease (PID) An *infection* of the *reproductive parts* in a woman's lower *abdomen*. Also called pelvic infection.

penis The male sex *organ*, also used to pass *urine*. The penis gets hard during sex and releases a fluid called *semen* that contains *sperm*.

pension fund A fund—often set up by a union, employer, or the government—that pays people when they get older and stop working.

period See *monthly bleeding*.

permanent methods (of family planning) See *sterilization*.

pesticides Poisonous *chemicals* used to kill insects that destroy food crops.

PID See *pelvic inflammatory disease*.

piles (hemorrhoids) Swollen *veins* around the *anus*, which can itch, burn, or bleed.

pimp A man who finds clients for a *sex worker* and who often keeps all or part of her money.

pimple A spot or small *infected* swelling that grows, often on the face, due to extra oil on the skin. Common in adolescent girls and boys. Also called acne.

placenta (afterbirth) A spongy *organ* in a woman's *womb* that gives the baby everything it needs to grow during pregnancy. The baby is connected to the placenta by the *cord*. After the baby is born, the placenta also comes out of the *womb*.

plant medicines Flowers, leaves, roots and other parts of plants that can be used to treat diseases.

pneumonia An *infection* of the small breathing tubes deep in the lungs.

polyps Growths found usually in the *womb*. Polyps are almost never caused by *cancer*.

pregnancy in the tube A pregnancy that grows in one of the *fallopian tubes*, instead of in the *womb*.

prenatal The time between when a woman gets pregnant and when she gives birth.

prenatal care Checkups during pregnancy, when a midwife or specially trained health worker examines a pregnant woman to make sure the pregnancy is going well.

premature When a baby is born too early.

prevent Stopping something before it starts.

pressure sores (bed sores) Sores that form over bony parts of the body when a person lies or sits on that part of the body for too long without moving.

privacy When a person gives information to a health worker, nurse, or doctor and knows it will not be overheard by, or repeated to, others.

progesterone A female *hormone*.

progestin A *hormone* made in a laboratory that is similar to the *progesterone* made naturally in a woman's body. It is found in some hormonal *family planning methods*.

progestin only pill A method of *family planning* that contains one *hormone*—progestin—but no *estrogen*.

prolapsed uterus When the muscles that hold up the *womb* become weak, causing it to fall or drop down into the *vagina*.

prostitute See *sex worker*.

proteins Body-building foods necessary for proper growth and strength.

puberty The time when a girl changes into a woman and her *monthly bleeding* begins, or when a boy changes into a man.

pubic bone The front part of the *pelvic* bones, just beneath the hair on a woman's *genitals*.

pulse The heartbeat, which tells how fast and how hard the heart is working. The pulse can be felt at certain points on the body, like the inside of the wrist or the neck.

purification Killing harmful *germs* in water before drinking it.

pus White or yellow fluid that is filled with *germs*, often found inside an *infected* tear or wound.

R

radiation Rays of energy given off by certain elements. Radiation is harmful because it kills *cells* in the body. But it can also be used to treat *cancer* by killing cancer cells.

radiation treatment When a machine sends rays of energy into a person's body to kill *cancer cells*. The rays cannot be seen or felt.

rape When a man puts his *penis*, finger, or any object into a woman's *vagina, anus*, or mouth without her consent.

rectal exam Checking the *rectum* for growths or other problems. A rectal exam can also give information about the wall or lining of the *vagina*.

rectum The lower part of the *intestine* that is connected to the *anus*.

rehydration drink A drink to treat *dehydration*. The drink can be made with boiled water, salt, sugar, or powdered cereal.

reproductive health Health services like *family planning* services or *prenatal care*, that help *prevent* or treat health concerns connected to a woman's *reproductive parts*.

reproductive parts The parts of a man's and a woman's body that allow them to make a baby.

resistance The ability of something to defend itself against something that would normally harm or kill it. Many *bacteria* become resistant to the effects of certain *antibiotics*.

rhythm method A *family planning method* in which a woman counts the days of her *monthly cycle* to find out when she is most *fertile*. She then avoids having sex during her fertile time.

S

safer sex Avoiding direct contact with a sexual partner's *genitals*, blood, *semen*, or *vaginal* wetness.

saliva A person's spit.

sanitation Public cleanliness to prevent disease, such as providing clean drinking water and keeping public places free of waste.

scabies A *contagious* skin disease caused by a *parasite*.

scar A cut or wound that leaves the skin or *tissue* rough and raised after it has healed.

scrotum The bag between a man's legs that holds his *testicles* or *balls*.

seizures See *convulsion*.

self-esteem How a woman feels about herself, and about her role in her family and community.

semen The liquid containing a man's *sperm*, which is released from his *penis* during *ejaculation*.

sepsis A serious *infection* that has spread into the blood.

sex worker Anyone who exchanges sex for money or other favors, goods or services.

sexual abuse See *abuse*.

sexual assault Unwanted sexual contact.

sexual harassment Unwanted sexual attention from anyone who has power over a woman.

sexual health When a woman has control over her sexual life.

sexual intercourse Sex with the *penis* in the *vagina*.

sexual roles The way a community defines what it means to be a woman or a man.

sexually transmitted diseases (STDs) *Infections* passed from one person to another during sex.

shock A dangerous condition with severe weakness or *loss of consciousness*, cold sweats, and fast, weak *pulse*. It can be caused by *dehydration,* heavy bleeding, injury, burns, or a severe illness.

side effects When medicines or *hormonal methods* cause changes in the body other than those needed to fight disease or *prevent* pregnancy.

speculum A small metal or plastic tool that holds the *vagina* open.

sperm Tiny organisms in a man's *semen* that can swim up a woman's *vagina* and *fertilize* an egg. This is how a pregnancy starts.

spermicide A slippery, *lubricating* cream or gel that helps prevent pregnancy by killing *sperm*, and may help prevent some *STDs*.

squeezing exercise An exercise to help strengthen weak muscles that cause a woman to pass *urine* often or to leak urine.

status The importance a person has in her or his family and community.

STDs See *sexually transmitted diseases*.

sterile When something is completely free from *germs*.

sterilization A permanent way of making a woman or man unable to have children.

steroids A class of medicines used to treat many different health problems. Steroids can have serious *side effects* if used for a long time.

stethoscope An instrument used to listen to sounds inside the body, like the heartbeat.

stomach The sac-like *organ* in the belly where food is *digested*.

stool The waste that passes from the *anus* during a *bowel* movement.

stress Any activities or events that put pressure on a woman, causing tension in her body and mind.

stroke A sudden *loss of consciousness*, feeling, or ability to move caused by bleeding or a *clot* inside the brain.

subcutaneous injection An *injection* into the fatty *tissue* under the skin, not into the muscle.

sugar Sweet foods, like honey or sugar cane, that give energy.

support groups When people with a common problem meet together to help one another.

surgery When a doctor cuts into the body to find out what is wrong or to treat an illness. An *operation*.

syphilis A *sexually transmitted disease*.

syringe An instrument used to inject medicine.

T

tampons Cotton, cloth, or sponges that are put inside the *vagina* to catch *monthly bleeding* before it leaves the body.

temperature The degree of heat of a person's body.

testicles The part of the male *genitals* that is inside the *scrotum* and makes the *sperm*.

testosterone The main *hormone* in a man's body.

tetanus A serious disease caused by a *germ* that lives in the *stools* of people or animals. Tetanus enters the body through a wound.

thrush A fungal *infection* that causes white patches and soreness on the skin inside the mouth, on the tongue, and the tube that connects the mouth with the *stomach*.

thyroid gland A *gland* in the front of the throat that makes *hormones* that affect growth and development. The thyroid needs *iodine* to work properly.

thermometer An instrument used to measure how hot a person's body *temperature* is.

tissue The material making up the muscles, fatty areas, and *organs* of the body.

toxemia A dangerous condition during pregnancy, which can lead to *seizures*.

toxic A harmful substance that can cause disease or death when it enters the body is said to be toxic.

toxicity When a person takes too much medicine and it builds up to a dangerous level in the body.

traditional healers Healers who use methods based on beliefs that have been passed down from generation to generation.

trauma When something horrible happens to a person or to someone the person is close to.

trichomonas A disease of the *genitals* that is usually *sexually transmitted*, but not always.

tubal ligation An *operation* in which the *fallopian tubes* are cut or tied so the egg cannot travel to the *womb* to be *fertilized*.

tubal pregnancy See *pregnancy in the tube*.

tuberculosis A serious *infection* caused by a *germ* that usually affects the *lungs*.

tubes See *fallopian tubes*.

tumor Abnormal growth.

U

ulcer A *chronic* open sore of the skin, the *stomach*, or the *intestines*.

ultrasound A machine that uses sound to take a picture of the inside of the body without cutting it open. It is often used during pregnancy to see the baby inside the *womb*.

unconscious See *loss of consciousness*.

unsafe sex Direct contact with a sexual partner's *genitals*, blood, *semen* or *vaginal* wetness—if there is any chance you or your partner has a *sexually transmitted disease* (STD).

urethra A short tube that carries *urine* from the *bladder* to the hole a person urinates from.

urine Liquid waste that collects in the *bladder* and leaves the body through a hole just above the *vagina*.

uristix Special paper strips that change color when dipped in *urine* that has sugar in it. Uristix can be used to find out if a person has *diabetes*.

uterus See *womb*.

V

vaccinations or **vaccines** Medicines that are *injected* to give protection against specific diseases like *tetanus*.

vagina (birth canal) A tube made of muscle that goes from the opening of the woman's *genitals* to the *cervix*.

varicose veins Abnormally swollen *veins*—often blue, lumpy, and winding—on the legs of older people, pregnant women, and women who have had a lot of children. Pregnant women also sometimes have varicose veins in the *genitals*.

vasectomy A permanent method of preventing pregnancy, in which the tubes that carry *sperm* from the *testicles* to the *penis* are cut.

veins Thin, tube-like vessels that carry blood back to the heart. Also see *artery*.

virgin A person who has not had sex.

virus *Germs* smaller than *bacteria*, which cause some *infectious diseases*.

vitamins Foods that the body needs to work properly, to fight disease, and to get better after a sickness or injury.

vomiting Throwing up the contents of the *stomach* through the mouth.

vulva All the parts of a woman's *genitals* that can be seen on the outside of her body between her legs.

W

withdrawal The period of time in which the body gets used to being without a *drug* or alcohol to which it is physically *addicted*.

womb (uterus) A sac of strong muscle inside a woman's belly. *Monthly bleeding* comes from the womb, and the baby grows inside the womb during pregnancy.

X

x-rays Pictures of parts of the inside of the body, like the bones or the lungs, which are created by rays sent through the body. The body does not need to be cut open.

Y

yeast infection A vaginal *infection* with white, lumpy *discharge*, itching, and burning. These infections are common during pregnancy and when taking *antibiotics*.

WHERE TO GET MORE INFORMATION

Here is a small selection of organizations and printed materials that can provide useful information about women's health care. We have tried to list organizations and materials covering as many of the topics in this book as possible, and to include groups working in all areas of the world. Many of the printed materials are easy to adapt and often include other helpful resource lists.

Organizations

AHRTAG (Appropriate Health Resources and Technologies Action Group)

Farringdon's Point, 29-35 Farringdon Road, London EC1M 3JB, UK.   Tel: (44-71)242-0606; Fax: (44-71)242-0041; Email: ahrtag@gn.apc.org

Information on primary health care in developing countries. Publishes several newsletters and resource guides on health topics.

Alcoholics Anonymous

World Services Incorporated, PO Box 459, Grand Central Station, New York, NY 10163, USA

Information about alcoholism and materials on how to start community support groups for persons with drug or alcohol problems. Contact them for information about groups in your area.

Aprovecho Research Center

80574 Hazelton Rd., Cottage Grove, Oregon 97424, USA

Tel: (1-541)942-8198; Fax: (1-541)942-0302

Information and training in organic gardening, sustainable forestry, and appropriate technology. Publishes an excellent book called Capturing Heat— illustrated, easy to follow instructions for making 5 simple cooking stoves that use less fuel and produce less smoke. Useful for any community.

Arab Resource Collective

PO Box 7380, Nicosia, Cyprus

Tel: (357-2)476-741; Fax: (357-2)476-790; Email: arccyp@spidernet.com.cy

Written and audio-visual materials in general health care, community development, skills training, and promotion of networking among grass-roots organizations in the Middle East.

Disabled People International (DPI)

101-7 Evergreen Place, Winnipeg, Manitoba, R3L 2TS Canada

Tel: (1-204)287-8010; Fax: (1-204)453-1367; Email: dpi@dpi.org; Web: htpp://www.dpi.org

Information on a wide range of issues and concerns for persons with disabilities, including women's health care, human rights, independent living, and social justice. Special focus on grass-roots development. Has local offices in many countries.

English Collective of Prostitutes

PO Box 287, London, NW6 5QU, UK

Information and health education materials for women who exchange sex for money or services. Has international connections with other similar groups.

Gender and Learning Team

Policy Department, Oxfam UK/Ireland, 274 Banbury Road, Oxford, OX2 7DZ, UK

Tel: (44-1865)311311; Fax: (44-1865)313133 Email: ssmith@oxfam.org.uk

Provides advice and support on gender and learning issues, including health, natural resources, capacity building and rights. Networks with groups worldwide to exchange experiences and offer mutual support. Also publishes a newsletter called "Links."

Global Fund for Women

425 Sherman Ave., Suite 300, Palo Alto, California 94306-1823, USA

Tel: (1-415)853-8305; Fax: (1-415)328-0384; Email: gfw@igc.apc.org; Web: http://www.globalfundforwomen.org

Gives small grants to community-based women's groups, especially those working on controversial issues and in difficult conditions. Areas of special interest are human rights, communications technology, and economic independence. Contact them for grant request information.

Health Action Information Network (HAIN)

PO Box 1665, Central Post Office, Quezon City, Philippines

Tel: (632)978-805; Fax: (632)721-8290

General health care information. Networking with many general and women's grass-roots health groups, especially in Pacific Island countries.

Health Action International

Jacob Van Lennepkade 334T, 1053 NJ Amsterdam, The Netherlands

Tel: +31(0)20 683 3684; Fax: +31(0)20 685 5002 Email: hai@hai.antenna.nl

Network of 200 consumer, health, development, and other public interest groups involved in health issues and the rational use of drugs. Has contacts in over 70 countries. Contact Amsterdam office for local groups that can help.

Inter-African Committee on Traditional Health Practices Affecting Women

c/o Economic Commission for Africa,
ATRCW, PO Box 3001, Addis Ababa, Ethiopia
c/o Inter-African Committee,
147, rue de Lausanne, CH-1202 Geneva, Switzerland

Monitors world-wide practices harmful to girls and women, including female circumcision.

International Development Research Center (IRDC)

PO Box 8500, Ottowa, Ontario, K1G 3H9 Canada

Magazines, brochures, films, and other publications on health, agriculture, and development. Materials in English, Spanish, French, and Arabic, some at no cost. Write for a catalogue.

International Labour Organization

4, rue des Morillons, CH 1211, Geneva 22, Switzerland
Tel: (41-22)799-7940; Fax: (41-22)788-3894

An agency of the United Nations that promotes international workplace standards for: equality, justice, human rights, worker safety and health, job protection and safety for pregnant women, and the hours children work.

International Planned Parenthood Federation

International Headquarters, Regent's College; Inner Circle, Regent's Park, London NW14NS, UK
Tel: (44-171)486-0741

IPPF promotes and supports family planning activities worldwide. They also publish information on all aspects of family planning.

International Women's Tribune Center

777 United Nations Plaza, New York, NY 10017, USA
Tel: (1-212)687-8633; Fax: (1-212)661-2704

Works to empower women. Some IWTC publications include: The Tech and Tools Book: A guide to technologies women are using worldwide; Women Organizing; Women and Small Business.

ISIS International

Ricardo Lyon 1735, Casilla 2067, Correo Central Santiago, Chile
or
85-A East Maya Street, Philamlife Homes
Quezon City, Phillipines

Information and communication services. Has contact with many women's groups worldwide. Publications, technical assistance and training in communication skills and management.

Musasa Project

112 Harare Street, Box A172, Avondale, Harare, Zimbabwe. Tel/Fax: (263-4)794983

Provides information and support to abused women. Also provides education programs to women, girls and others on domestic violence and rape.

TALC (Teaching Aids at Low Cost)

PO Box 49, St. Albans, Herts, AL1 4AX, UK
Tel: (44)1727-853869; Fax: (44)1727-846852

Publishes low-cost books, slides and accessories in English, French, Spanish and Portuguese in health care and development for use in poor communities. Free booklist.

Voluntary Health Association of India (VHAI)

40, Institutional Area, South of IIT, New Delhi 110016, India. Tel: (91-11)668071 or 668072; Fax: (91-11)6853708

Publishes Health for the Millions, a journal about low-cost health care. Also has teaching materials in English and local Indian languages.

Women in Law and Development in Africa (WiLDAF)

PO Box 4622, Harare, Zimbabwe
Tel: (263-4)752-105; Fax: (263-4)733-670

Umbrella organization for many people and organizations using law to promote women's rights.

Women's Global Network on Reproductive Rights

Nieuwe Zijds Voorburgwal 32, 1012 RZ Amsterdam, Netherlands. Tel: (31-20)20 96 72

Networking; collecting and sharing information; quarterly newsletter; international campaigns; monitoring research in reproductive health.

Women's Health Project

PO Box 1038, Johannesburg 2000, South Africa
Tel: (011)489-9917; Fax: (011) 89-9922

Provides training, research, resource materials, networking, policy development and promotion, and a newsletter on issues concerning women's health. Materials can be adapted for other communities.

World Alliance for Breastfeeding Action (WABA)

PO Box 1200, 10850 Penang, Malaysia
Tel: (604) 658-4816, Fax: (604) 657-2655

A global network of NGOs and individuals whose common goal is to promote, support and protect breastfeeding. Contact WABA for local groups that can help.

World Neighbors

4127 NW 122 Street, Oklahoma City, OK, 73120, USA
Tel: (405) 752-9700; Fax: (405) 752-9393, email: order@wn.org

Teaching materials designed from program experience for use in the specific country and locality. Topics include health and nutrition, family planning, community development and agriculture. In English and local languages.

Printed Materials

Across Borders: Women with Disabilities Working Together

Diane Driedger, Irene Feika, Eileen Giron Batres (Eds.), Council of Canadians with Disabilities, gynergy books, PO Box 2023, Charlottetown, PEI, C1A 7N7 Canada

Accounts of political activism and personal stories of women with disabilities from around the world.

Adding Health to Years

Gill Garrett, HealthAge International, 67-74 Saffron Hill, London EC1R OBE, UK
Fax: (44-171)404-7203; Email: helpage@gn.apc.org

Self-help health guide for older persons. HealthAge also has a network of over 50 organizations worldwide, working to achieve a lasting improvement in the quality of life for older persons.

AIDS Home Care Handbook

World Health Organization, Global Programme on AIDS, 20 avenue Appia, CH-1211 Geneva 27, Switzerland. Tel: (41-22)791-4651 or 4745; Fax: (41-22)791-4187; Email: UNAIDS@WHO.CH

Good information about caring for someone sick with AIDS at home. Designed for health workers and trainers, but useful for anyone caring for someone with AIDS. Written for Africa, but easy to adapt for any community.

Arab Women: A Profile of Diversity & Change

The Population Council
West Asia and North Africa Regional Office
Cairo, PO Box 115, Egypt
Tel: (20-2) 570-1733; Fax: (20-2) 570-1804
New York Office
One Dag Hammarskjold Plaza
New York, NY 10017 USA
Tel: (212) 339-0500; Fax: (212) 755-6052

This book focuses on women's social and political position in Arab countries. It is a source book for women in the region and a tool for advocacy and change.

Asia and Pacific Women's Resource and Action Series: Health

Published by Asian and Pacific Development Centre, Persiaran Duta, Kuala Lumpur, Malaysia

This book reflects the ideas, perspectives, strategies and action in the 1980s of women from all parts of the Region.

Contact

Christian Medical Commission, Box 66, 150 Route de Ferney, 1211 Geneva 20, Switzerland

Newsletter about appropriate health care, published in French, Spanish, English and Portuguese.

South Pacific Community Nutrition Training Project,

The Director, Extension Services, The University of the South Pacific, PO Box 1168, Suva, Fiji

Publishes a series of books on food and nutrition for Pacific Islanders, but useful everywhere. The books include stories, drawings, summaries, and questions to help educate people on making good choices about food and living healthy lives.

Gender and Women's Health

Resource Centre for Primary Health Care
PO Box 117, Bagbazar, Kathmandu, Nepal
Tel./Fax: (977-1)225675

A manual describing a workshop in Nepal that takes a holistic approach to women's health. Useful for group discussions and workshops on women's health care. Could be adapted for any community and region.

Health Alert

Health Action Information Network, PO Box 1665, Central Post Office, Quezon City, Phillipines

Journal that provides news on health-related issues, as well as economic and political developments that shape the health care situation.

Healthy Women Counselling Guide, and Health Workers Training Guide

Gender and Health Research Group, World Health Organization, CH-1211, Geneva 27, Switzerland

Written together with women and health workers in Kenya, Nigeria, Sierra Leone and South Africa. Includes topics in all areas of women's health and gender relations. Useful for any community.

Healthy Women, Healthy Mothers

A.A. Arkutu, Family Care International, Inc. (FCI), 588 Broadway, Suite 503, New York, NY 10012, USA

A book on pregnancy and birth for health workers and others who work with women at the community level. Easy to read and well illustrated. Written for Africa, but useful for all communities.

Also from FCI: **Strengthening Communication Skills for Women's Health: A Training Guide,** by Jill Tabbutt, and **Getting the Message Out: Designing an Information Campaign on Women's Health,** by Ann M. Starrs and Rahna R. Rizzuto.

Helping Mothers to Breastfeed

F. Savage King, African Medical and Research Foundation, Publishing Department, PO Box 30125, Nairobi, Kenya

Summarizes the most current information on breastfeeding, including a section on breastfeeding and family planning.

Managing Drug Supply: The Selection, Procurement, Distribution and Use of Pharmaceuticals (Second Edition)

Edited by J.D. Quick, et al (Management Sciences for Health). Order from: Kumarian Press, Inc., 14 Oakwood Ave., West Hartford, Connecticut 06119-2127, USA. Tel: (1-860)233-5895; Fax: (1-860)233-6072; Email: kpbooks@aol.com

Information on essential drugs management in developing countries. Illustrated with over 300 figures, tables, 'how-to boxes', sample forms, and address lists, this is an excellent resource for anyone who prescribes and dispenses medicines.

Montreal Health Press

Montreal Health Press, PO Box 1000, Station Place du Parc, Montreal, Quebec, H2W 2N1 Canada Tel: (514) 282-1171

Publishes several excellent guides about menopause, birth control, STDs, and sexual assault.

Our Bodies, Ourselves

Boston Women's Health Book Collective, PO Box 192, West Somerville, MA 02144, USA
Published by: Touchstone, Simon & Schuster Building, Rockefeller Center, 1230 Avenue of the Americas, New York, NY 10020, USA

This classic book provides complete information on women's health issues.

Practical guidelines for preventing infections passed by blood or air in health-care settings

AHRTAG, 29-35 Farringdon Road, London EC1M 3JB, UK

Easy to understand and useful for home, clinic, and hospital settings. Free to persons in developing countries.

Primary Clinical Care Series

Health Services Development Unit, Department of Community Health, University of the Witerwatersrand, Medical School, York Road Parktown, Johannesburg 2193, South Africa

A series of manuals to train primary health care workers in rural and developing areas. Topics include: urinary and genital problems, sexually transmitted diseases, infectious diseases, family planning, and basic medical sciences. Written for Africa, but useful for any community.

Reproductive Health in Refugee Situations

United Nations High Commissioner for Refugees Programme and Technical Support Section UNHCR Headquarters, Case postale 2500, CH-1211 Geneva 2 Depot 2, Switzerland Fax: (41 22) 739 73 71

Manual to assist any interested person in promoting reproductive health services in refugee and other emergency situations.

Safe Motherhood Newsletter

World Health Organization, 1211 Geneva 27, Switzerland

Published 3 times a year in English, Arabic and French. Information on pregnancy, the health of mothers and newborns, and general health concerns of women. Contains good resource section. Write for a free subscription.

Sexual and Domestic Violence: Help, Recovery and Action in Zimbabwe

Jill Taylor and Sheelagh, Published by A. von Glehn and J. Taylor in collaboration with Women and Law in Southern Africa, PO Box UA 171, Union Avenue, Harare, Zimbabwe

Designed for people in developing countries to help raise awareness of and develop skills to fight sexual and domestic violence. Can be adapted for any community.

South African Women's Health Book

Oxford University Press, Southern Africa, Harrington House, 37 Barrack Street, Cape Town 8001, South Africa

Comprehensive information on women's health in South Africa including stories from women in local communities. Includes chapters on gender, culture, healthy living, violence, work, sexuality, and reproductive health.

Training Course in Women's Health

Institute for Development Training, 212 East Rosemary Street, Chapel Hill, NC, 27514, USA Tel: (1-919)967-0563; Fax: (1-919) 929-2353

A series of easy-to-read, adaptable clinical training manuals in women's health services for health workers. Series includes trainings in: The Female Reproductive and Sexual System, Communication and Counseling Skills, Infection Control, Gyn Exams and Common Problems, Urine System and Problems, Family Planning, Breastfeeding, Sterilization, Reproductive Tract Infections, FGM, and Abortion.

Understanding and Reacting: Women Partners in Health

Association Genevoise d'Entraide aux Refugies (A.G.E.R.), route de Bardonnex 27b, CH-1228 Geneva, Switzerland

Illustrated, simply-written first aid manual for women in exile.

Women & Health

Patricia Smyke, Zed Books Ltd, 57 Caledonian Road, London N1 9BU, UK

An overview of women, health and development. One book in the "Women and Development" series. Other books in the series are on: economics, disability, the environment, refugees, literacy, work, and the family.

S

OTHER BOOKS FROM THE HESPERIAN FOUNDATION

Where There Is No Doctor, by David Werner with Carol Thuman and Jane Maxwell, is perhaps the most widely used health care manual in the world. The book provides vital, easily understood information on how to diagnose, treat and prevent common diseases. Special importance is placed on ways to prevent health problems, including cleanliness, a healthy diet and vaccinations. The authors also emphasize the active role villagers must take in their own health care. 512 pages.

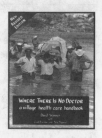

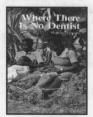

Where There Is No Dentist, by Murray Dickson shows people how to care for their own teeth and gums, and how to prevent tooth and gum problems. Emphasis is placed on sharing this knowledge in the home, community and school. The author also gives detailed and well-illustrated information on using dental equipment, placing fillings, taking out teeth, and suggests ways to teach dental hygiene and nutrition. 208 pages.

Disabled Village Children, by David Werner, contains a wealth of information about most common disabilities of children, including polio, cerebral palsy, juvenile arthritis, blindness and deafness. The author gives suggestions for simplified rehabilitation at the village level and explains how to make a variety of appropriate low-cost aids. Emphasis is placed on how to help disabled children find a role and be accepted in the community. 672 pages.

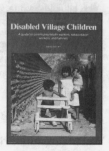

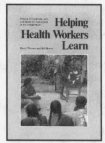

Helping Health Workers Learn, by David Werner and Bill Bower, is an indispensable resource for anyone involved in teaching about health. This heavily illustrated book shows how to make health education fun and effective. Includes activities for mothers and children; pointers for using theater, flannel-boards, and other techniques; and many ideas for producing low-cost teaching aids. Emphasizing a people-centered approach to health care, it presents strategies for effective community involvement through participatory education. 640 pages.

A Book for Midwives, by Susan Klein, is written for midwives, traditional birth attendants, community health workers and anyone concerned about the health of pregnant women and their babies. The book is an invaluable tool for midwives facilitating education and training sessions as well as an essential reference for practice. The author emphasizes helping pregnant women stay healthy; giving good care and dealing with complications during labor, childbirth and after birth; family planning; breastfeeding; and homemade, low cost equipment. 528 pages.

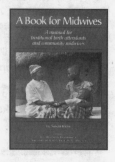

All titles are available from Hesperian in both English and Spanish. For information regarding editions in other languages, for price and ordering information, or for a brochure describing the Foundation's work, please write to us:

The Hesperian Foundation
PO Box 11577
Berkeley, California, 94712-2577, USA
Telephone: (510) 845-4507 Fax: (510) 845-0539
E-mail: hesperianfdn@igc.apc.org